Really Essential Medical Immunology

Arthur Rabson

MB, BCh, FRCPath
Department of Pathology
Tufts University School of Medicine
Boston
USA

Ivan M. Roitt

DSc, HonFRCP, FRCPath, FRS
Department of Immunology & Molecular Pathology
Royal Free & University College Medical School
London
UK

Peter J. Delves

PhD
Department of Immunology & Molecular Pathology
Royal Free & University College Medical School
London
UK

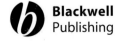
Blackwell
Publishing

© 2005 A. Rabson, I.M. Roitt, P.J. Delves
Published by Blackwell Publishing Ltd
Blackwell Publishing, Inc., 350 Main Street, Malden, Massachusetts 02148-5020, USA
Blackwell Publishing Ltd, 9600 Garsington Road, Oxford OX4 2DQ, UK
Blackwell Publishing Asia Pty Ltd, 550 Swanston Street, Carlton, Victoria 3053, Australia

First published 2000
Reprinted 2001
Second edition 2005

Library of Congress Cataloging-in-Publication Data
Rabson, Arthur.
    Really essential medical immunology / Arthur Rabson, Ivan M. Roitt,
      Peter J. Delves.— 2nd ed.
        p. ;   cm.
    Rev. ed. of: Really essential medical immunology / Ivan Roitt and
Arthur Rabson. 2000.
    Includes bibliographical references and index.
    ISBN 1-4051-2115-7
1. Clinical immunology.
[DNLM: 1. Immunity. QW 540 R116r 2005]   I. Roitt, Ivan M. (Ivan
Maurice)   II. Delves, Peter J.   III. Roitt, Ivan M. (Ivan Maurice). Really
essential medical immunology.   IV. Title.

    RC582.R65 2005
    616.07′9—dc22

                                                                200400393

ISBN 1-4051-2115-7

A catalogue record for this title is available from the British Library

Set in 10/12.5 Palatino by SNP Best-set Typesetter Ltd., Hong Kong
Printed and bound in India by Replika Press Pvt., Ltd

Commissioning Editor: Martin Sugden
Managing Editor: Geraldine Jeffers
Production Editors: Fiona Pattison & Alice Nelson
Production Controller: Kate Charman

For further information on Blackwell Publishing, visit our website:
http://www.blackwellpublishing.com

Contents

Innate immunity

We live in a potentially hostile world filled with a bewildering array of infectious agents against which we have developed a series of defense mechanisms at least their equal in effectiveness and ingenuity. It is these defense mechanisms that can establish a state of immunity against infection (Latin *immunitas*, freedom from) and whose operation provides the basis for the delightful subject called "Immunology."

A number of nonspecific antimicrobial systems (e.g. phagocytosis) have been recognized which are **innate** in the sense that they are not intrinsically affected by prior contact with the infectious agent and are usually present before the onset of the infectious agent. The innate response is not enhanced by previous exposure to the foreign organism and the response time is very rapid usually occurring in minutes or hours. We shall discuss these systems and examine how, in the state of **specific acquired immunity**, their effectiveness can be greatly increased.

EXTERNAL BARRIERS AGAINST INFECTION

The simplest way to avoid infection is to prevent the microorganisms from gaining access to the body. The major line of defense is of course the skin which, when intact, is impermeable to most infectious agents. When there is skin loss, as for example in burns, infection becomes a major problem. Additionally, most bacteria fail to survive for long on the skin because of the direct inhibitory effects of lactic acid and fatty acids in sweat and sebaceous secretions and the low pH which they generate. An exception is *Staphylococcus aureus*, which often infects the relatively vulnerable hair follicles and glands.

Mucus secreted by the membranes lining the inner surfaces of the body acts as a protective barrier to block the adherence of bacteria to epithelial cells. Microbial and other foreign particles trapped within the adhesive mucus are removed by mechanical stratagems such as ciliary movement, coughing and sneezing. Among other mechanical factors that help protect the epithelial surfaces, one should also include the washing action of tears, saliva and urine. Many of the secreted body fluids contain bactericidal components, such as acid in gastric juice, spermine and zinc in semen, lactoperoxidase in milk, and lysozyme in tears, nasal secretions and saliva.

A totally different mechanism is that of microbial antagonism where the normal bacterial flora of the body suppresses the growth of many potentially pathogenic bacteria and fungi. This is due to competition for essential nutrients or by the production of microbicidal substances. For example, pathogen invasion of the vagina is limited by lactic acid produced by commensal organisms which metabolize glycogen secreted by

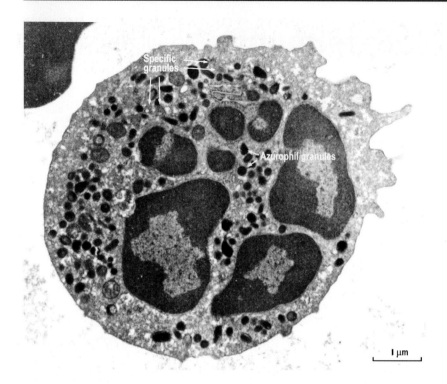

Specific granules

Azurophil granules

1 μm

Figure 1.1 Ultrastructure of neutrophil. The multilobed nucleus and two main types of cytoplasmic granules are well displayed. (Courtesy of Dr D. McLaren.)

the vaginal epithelium. When protective commensals are disturbed by antibiotics, susceptibility to opportunistic infections such as *Candida albicans* and *Clostridium difficile* is increased.

If microorganisms do penetrate the body, two further innate defensive operations come into play, the destructive effect of soluble chemical factors such as bactericidal enzymes and the mechanism of **phagocytosis**—literally "eating" by the cell (Milestone 1.1).

PHAGOCYTIC CELLS KILL MICROORGANISMS

The polymorphonuclear neutrophil

This cell shares a common hematopoietic stem cell precursor with the other formed elements of the blood and is the dominant white cell in the bloodstream. It is a nondividing, short-lived cell with a multilobed nucleus (figures 1.1 & 1.2a,b) and an array of granules which are of two main types (figure 1.1): (i) the **primary azurophil granule**, which develops early and contains myeloperoxidase together with most of the nonoxidative antimicrobial effectors, including defensins, bactericidal/permeability-increasing (BPI) protein and cathepsin G, and (ii) the peroxidase-negative **secondary specific granules**, containing lactoferrin and much of the lysozyme, alkaline phosphatase (figure 1.2c) and membrane-bound cytochrome b_{558}.

The macrophage

These cells derive from bone marrow promonocytes which, after differentiation to blood monocytes (figure 1.2a), finally settle in the tissues as mature macrophages where they constitute the **mononuclear phagocyte system** (figure 1.2d). They are present throughout the connective tissue and around the basement membrane of small blood vessels and are particularly concentrated in the lung (figure 1.2f, alveolar macrophages), liver (Kupffer cells), and lining of spleen sinusoids and lymph node medullary sinuses, where they are strategically placed to filter off foreign material. Other examples are mesangial cells in the kidney glomerulus, brain microglia and osteoclasts in bone. Unlike the polymorphonuclear neutrophils, they are long-lived cells with significant rough-surface endoplasmic reticulum and mitochondria. Whereas the neutrophils provide the major defense against pyogenic (pus-forming) bacteria, as a rough generalization it may be said that macrophages are at their best in combating those bacteria (figure 1.2e), viruses and protozoa that are capable of living within the cells of the host.

Milestone 1.1—Phagocytosis

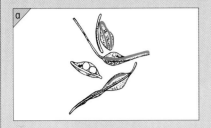
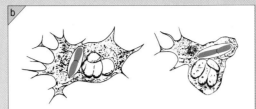
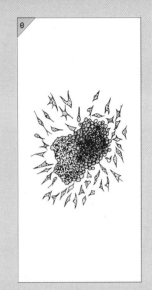
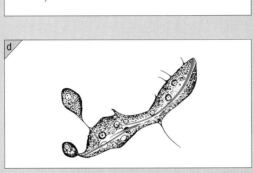

Figure M1.1.1 Reproductions of some of the illustrations in Metchnikoff's book, *Comparative Pathology of Inflammation* (1893). (a) Four leukocytes from the frog, enclosing anthrax bacilli. Some are alive and unstained; others, which have been killed, have taken up the vesuvine dye and have been colored. (b) Drawing of an anthrax bacillus, stained by vesuvine, in a leukocyte of the frog. The two figures represent two phases of movement of the same frog leukocyte which contains stained anthrax bacilli within its phagocytic vacuole. (c and d) A foreign body (colored) in a starfish larva surrounded by phagocytes which have fused to form a multinucleate plasmodium, shown at higher power in (d). (e) This gives a feel for the dynamic attraction of the mobile mesenchymal phagocytes to a foreign intruder within a starfish larva.

The perceptive Russian zoologist, Elie Metchnikoff (1845–1916), recognized that certain specialized cells mediate defense against microbial infections, so fathering the whole concept of cellular immunity. He was intrigued by the motile cells of transparent starfish larvae and made the critical observation that a few hours after the introduction of a rose thorn into these larvae these motile cells surrounded it. A year later, in 1883, he observed that fungal spores can be attacked by the blood cells of *Daphnia*, a tiny metozoan which, also being transparent, can be studied directly under the microscope. He went on to extend his investigations to mammalian leukocytes, showing their ability to engulf microorganisms, a process which he termed **phagocytosis**.

Because he found this process to be even more effective in animals recovering from infection, he came to a somewhat polarized view that phagocytosis provided the main, if not the only, defense against infection. He went on to define the existence of two types of circulating phagocytes: the polymorphonuclear leukocyte, which he termed a "microphage," and the larger "macrophage."

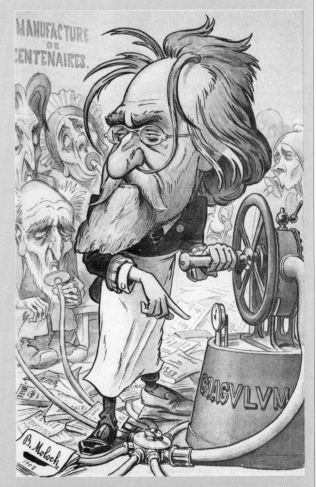

Figure M1.1.2   Caricature of Professor Metchnikoff (from *Chanteclair*, 1908, **4**, p. 7). (Reproduction kindly provided by The Wellcome Institute Library, London.)

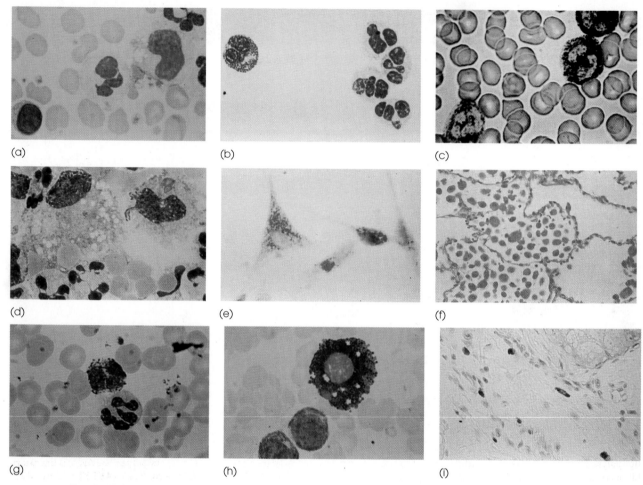

Figure 1.2 Cells involved in innate immunity. (a) Monocyte, showing "horseshoe-shaped" nucleus and moderately abundant pale cytoplasm. Note the three multilobed polymorphonuclear neutrophils and the small lymphocyte (bottom left) (Romanowsky). (b) Four polymorphonuclear neutrophils and one eosinophil. The multilobed nuclei and the cytoplasmic granules are clearly shown, those of the eosinophil being heavily stained. (c) Polymorphonuclear neutrophil showing cytoplasmic granules stained for alkaline phosphatase. (d) Inflammatory cells from the site of a brain hemorrhage showing the large active macrophage in the center with phagocytosed red cells and prominent vacuoles. To the right is a monocyte with horseshoe-shaped nucleus and cytoplasmic bilirubin crystals (hematoidin). Several multilobed neutrophils are clearly delineated (Giemsa). (e) Macrophages in monolayer cultures after phagocytosis of mycobacteria (stained red) (Carbol-Fuchsin counterstained with Malachite Green.) (f) Numerous plump alveolar macrophages within air spaces in the lung. (g) Basophil with heavily staining granules compared with a neutrophil (below). (h) Mast cell from bone marrow. Round central nucleus surrounded by large darkly staining granules. Two small red cell precursors are shown at the bottom (Romanowsky). (i) Tissue mast cells in skin stained with Toluidine Blue. The intracellular granules are metachromatic and stain reddish purple. (The slides for (a), (c), (d), (g) and (h) were very kindly provided by Mr M. Watts. (b) was kindly supplied by Professor J.J. Owen; (e) by Professors P. Lydyard and G. Rook; (f) by Dr Meryl Griffiths and (i) by Professor N. Woolf.)

Pattern recognition receptors (PRRs) on phagocytic cells recognize and are activated by pathogen-associated molecular patterns (PAMPs)

Phagocytes must have mechanisms to enable them to distinguish friendly self-components from unfriendly and potentially dangerous microbial agents. Phagocytic cells have therefore evolved a system of receptors called **pattern recognition receptors** (PRRs) capable of recognizing PAMPs expressed on the surface of infectious agents. These PAMPs are essentially polysaccharides and polynucleotides that differ minimally from one pathogen to another but are not found in the host. By and large the PRRs are lectin-like and bind multivalently with considerable specificity to exposed microbial surface sugars. Engagement of the PRR generates a signal through a NFκB (nuclear factor-kappa B) transcription factor pathway which alerts the cell to danger and initiates the phagocytic process.

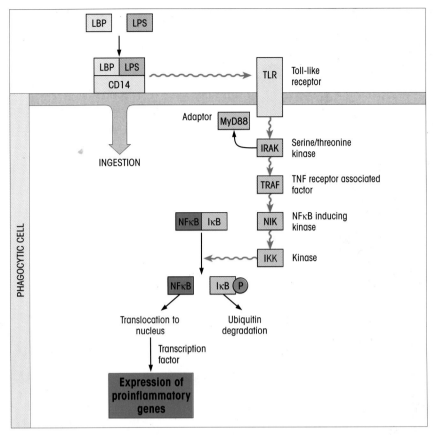

Figure 1.3 Activation of a phagocytic cell by a Gram-negative lipopolysaccharide (LPS) (endotoxin) danger signal. Circulating LPS is complexed by LPS-binding protein (LBP) and captured by the CD14 surface scavenging receptor. This signals internalization of the complex and activates the Toll-like receptor (TLR), which then initiates a phosphorylation cascade mediated by different kinase enzymes. As a result the transcription factor nuclear factor-kappa B (NFκB) is released from its inhibitor IκB and translocates to the nucleus, where it upregulates genes encoding defensive factors such as tumor necrosis factor (TNF), antibiotic peptides and the nicotinamide adenine dinucleotide phosphate (NADPH) oxidase which generates reactive oxygen intermediates (ROIs). The TLR appears to control the type of defensive response to different microbes. Thus TLR4 engineers the response to Gram-negative bacteria and LPS while TLR2 plays a key role in yeast and Gram-positive infections.

Toll-like receptors (TLRs) recognize PAMPs and cause cytokine release

Toll-like receptors are a family of at least 10 transmembrane proteins that recognize various microbial products. For example TLR2 recognizes Gram-positive bacterial peptidoglycan, TLR4 is specialized for the recognition of Gram-negative bacterial lipopolysaccharide (LPS) (endotoxin) and TLR3 and TLR5 are important in the recognition of virus derived double-stranded RNA. When the TLRs are activated they trigger a biochemical cascade with activation of NFκB and ultimately synthesis of proinflammatory cytokines and other antimicrobial peptides that lead to the development of adaptive immunity (figure 1.3).

Microbes are engulfed by phagocytosis

Before phagocytosis can occur, the microbe must first adhere to the surface of the polymorph or macrophage through recognition of a PAMP. The resulting signal initiates the ingestion phase by activating an actin–myosin contractile system which results in pseudopods being extended around the particle (figures 1.4 & 1.5a). As adjacent receptors sequentially attach to the surface of the microbe, the plasma membrane is pulled around the particle just like a "zipper" until it is completely enclosed in a vacuole called a phagosome (figures 1.4 & 1.5b). Within 1 min the cytoplasmic granules fuse with the phagosome and discharge their contents around the imprisoned microorganism (figure 1.5c), which is now

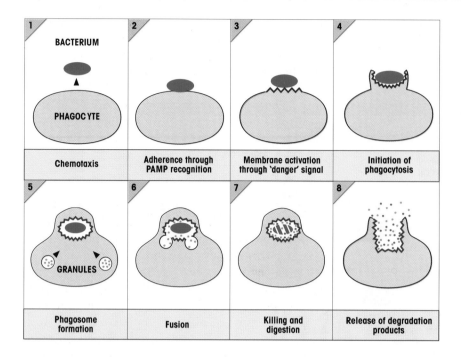

Figure 1.4 Phagocytosis and killing of a bacterium.

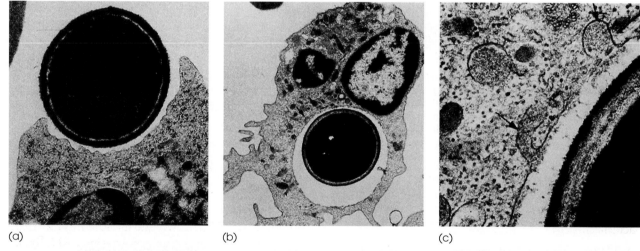

(a)   (b)   (c)

Figure 1.5 Adherence and phagocytosis. (a) Phagocytosis of *Candida albicans* by a polymorphonuclear neutrophil. Adherence to the surface initiates enclosure of the fungal particle within arms of cytoplasm (×15000). (b) Phagolysosome formation by a neutrophil 30 min after ingestion of *C. albicans*. The cytoplasm is already partly degranulated and two lysosomal granules (arrowed) are fusing with the phagocytic vacuole. Two lobes of the nucleus are evident (×5000). (c) Higher magnification of (b) showing fusing granules discharging their contents into the phagocytic vacuole (arrowed) (×33000). (Courtesy of Dr H. Valdimarsson.)

subject to a formidable battery of microbicidal mechanisms.

Killing by reactive oxygen intermediates (ROIs)

Trouble starts for the invader from the moment phagocytosis is initiated. There is a dramatic increase in activity of the hexose monophosphate shunt gener-ating reduced nicotinamide adenine dinucleotide phosphate (NADPH). Electrons pass from the NADPH to a unique plasma membrane **cytochrome (cyt b_{558})**, which reduces molecular oxygen directly to superoxide anion (figure 1.6). Thus, the key reaction catalysed by this NADPH oxidase, which initiates the formation of ROIs, is:

$$NADPH + O_2 \xrightarrow{\text{oxidase}} NADP^+ + \cdot O_2^- \text{ (superoxide anion)}$$

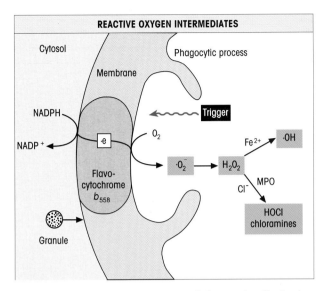

REACTIVE OXYGEN INTERMEDIATES

Figure 1.6 Microbicidal mechanisms of phagocytic cells. Production of reactive oxygen intermediates (ROIs). Electrons from nicotinamide adenine dinucleotide phosphate (NADPH) are transferred by the flavocytochrome oxidase enzyme to molecular oxygen to form the microbicidal molecular species shown in the boxes.

The superoxide anion undergoes conversion to hydrogen peroxide under the influence of superoxide dismutase, and subsequently to hydroxyl radicals ·OH. Each of these products has remarkable chemical reactivity with a wide range of molecular targets making them formidable microbicidal agents; ·OH in particular is one of the most reactive free radicals known. Furthermore, the combination of peroxide, myeloperoxidase (MPO) and halide ions constitutes a potent halogenating system capable of killing both bacteria and viruses (figure 1.6).

Other killing mechanisms

Nitric oxide (NO) can be formed by an inducible NO synthase (iNOS) in many cells of the body. In macrophages and human neutrophils it generates a powerful antimicrobial system. Whereas NADPH oxidase is dedicated to the killing of extracellular organisms taken into phagosomes by phagocytosis, the NO mechanism can operate against microbes that invade the cytosol. It is not surprising therefore that iNOS capability is present in many nonphagocytic cells that may be infected by viruses and other parasites.

If microorganisms are not destroyed by these systems, they will be subjected to a family of peptides called defensins, which reach very high levels within the phagosome and act as disinfectants against

a wide variety of bacteria, fungi and enveloped viruses. Further damage is inflicted on the bacterial membranes by neutral proteinase (cathepsin G) action and by the bactericidal or bacteriostatic factors, lysozyme and lactoferrin. Finally, the killed organisms are digested by hydrolytic enzymes and the degradation products released to the exterior (figure 1.4).

COMPLEMENT FACILITATES PHAGOCYTOSIS

Complement and its activation

Complement is the name given to a complex series of over 30 proteins found in plasma and on cell surfaces which, along with blood clotting, fibrinolysis and kinin formation, forms one of the triggered enzyme systems found in plasma. These systems characteristically produce a rapid, highly amplified response to a trigger stimulus mediated by a cascade phenomenon where the product of one reaction is the enzymic catalyst of the next. The activated or the split products of the cascade have a variety of defensive functions and the complement proteins can therefore be regarded as a crucial part of the innate immune system.

Some of the complement components are designated by the letter "C" followed by a number which is related more to the chronology of its discovery than to its position in the reaction sequence. The most abundant and the most pivotal component is C3.

C3 continuously undergoes slow spontaneous cleavage

Under normal circumstances, small amounts of C3 are continuously broken down into the split product C3b, or a functionally similar molecule designated C3bi. In the presence of Mg^{2+} this can complex with another complement component, factor B, which then undergoes cleavage by a normal plasma enzyme (factor D) to generate $C3b\overline{Bb}$. Note that conventionally a bar over a complex denotes enzymic activity, and that on cleavage of a complement component the larger product is generally given the suffix "b" and the smaller the suffix "a."

$C3b\overline{Bb}$ has an important new enzymic activity: it is a C3 convertase which can now split large amounts of C3 to give C3a and C3b. We will shortly discuss the important biological consequences of C3 cleavage in relation to microbial defenses, but under normal conditions there must be some mechanism to restrain this process to a "tick-over" level since it can also give rise to even more $C3b\overline{Bb}$. That is, we are dealing with a potentially

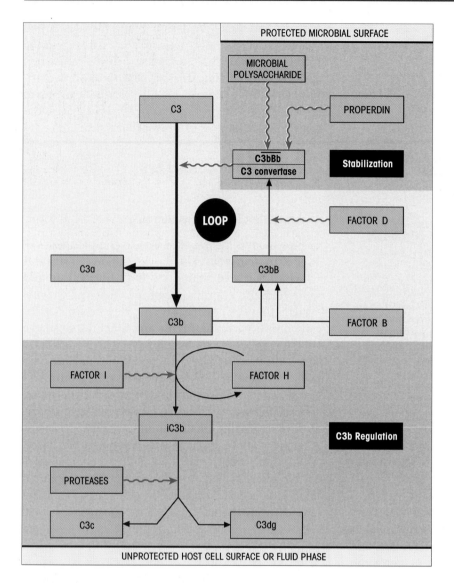

Figure 1.7 Microbial activation of the alternative complement pathway loop by stabilization of the C3 convertase (C3bBb), and its control by factors H and I. When bound to the surface of a host cell or in the fluid phase, the C3b in the convertase is said to be "unprotected" in that its affinity for factor H is much greater than for factor B and is therefore susceptible to breakdown by factors H and I. On a microbial surface, C3b binds factor B more strongly than factor H and is therefore "protected" from or "stabilized" against cleavage—even more so when subsequently bound by properdin. Although in phylogenetic terms this is the oldest complement pathway, it was discovered after a separate pathway to be discussed in the next chapter, and so has the confusing designation "alternative." ⤳ represents an activation process. The horizontal bar above a component designates its activation.

runaway **positive-feedback** or **amplification loop** (figure 1.7). As with all potentially explosive triggered cascades, there are powerful regulatory proteins in the form of factor H and factor I which control this feedback loop.

During infection C3 convertase is stabilized and the alternative complement pathway is activated

A number of microorganisms can activate the C3bBb convertase to generate large amounts of C3 cleavage products by stabilizing the enzyme on their (carbohydrate) surfaces. This protects the C3b from factor H and allows large quantities of C3bBb to build up and cleave C3. Another protein, properdin, acts subsequently on the bound convertase to stabilize it even

further. This series of reactions provoked directly by microbes leads to the clustering of large numbers of C3b molecules on the microorganism and has been called the **alternative pathway** of complement activation (figure 1.7).

Complement can be activated when carbohydrates on bacterial surfaces combine with a serum protein called mannose-binding lectin (MBL)

Mannose-binding lectin is found at low levels in normal serum and binds to mannose and other carbohydrates on bacterial surfaces. This initiates a series of reactions which culminate in complement activation. Mannose-binding lectin activates complement by interacting with two serine proteases

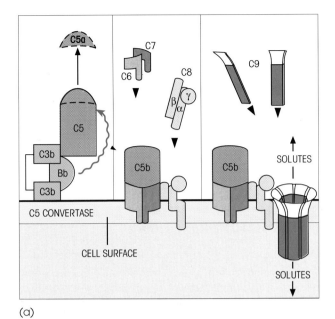

(a)

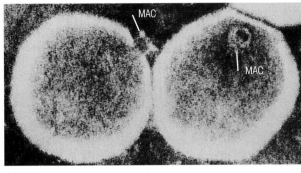

(b)

Figure 1.8 Post-C3 pathway generating C5a and the C5b–9 membrane attack complex (MAC). (a) Cartoon of molecular assembly. (b) Electron micrograph of a membrane C5b–9 complex incorporated into liposomal membranes clearly showing the annular structure. The cylindrical complex is seen from the side inserted into the membrane of the liposome on the left, and end-on in that on the right. (Courtesy of Professor J. Tranum-Jensen and Dr S. Bhakdi.)

called MASP1 and MASP2. It is known that MASP2 cleaves and activates C4 and C2, generating a C3 convertase called C4b2a which we shall discuss in Chapter 2. Activation of C3 initiates the alternative pathway loop and the formation of the membrane-attack complex.

The post-C3 pathway generates a membrane attack complex (MAC)

Recruitment of a further C3b molecule into the C3bBb enzymic complex generates a C5 convertase. This activates C5 by proteolytic cleavage releasing a small polypeptide, C5a, and leaving the large C5b fragment loosely bound to C3b. Sequential attachment of C6 and C7 to C5b forms a complex with a transient membrane binding site and an affinity for C8. The C8 sits in the membrane and directs the conformational changes in C9 which transform it into an amphipathic molecule capable of insertion into the lipid bilayer and polymerization to an annular MAC (figures 1.8 & 2.3). This forms a transmembrane channel fully permeable to electrolytes and water. Due to the high internal colloid osmotic pressure of cells, there is a net influx of Na+ and water, leading to cell lysis.

Complement has a range of defensive biological functions

1 C3b adheres to complement receptors

Phagocytic cells have receptors for C3b (CR1) and C3bi

(CR3) which facilitate the adherence of C3b-coated microorganisms to the cell surface and their subsequent phagocytosis. This process is called opsonization and is perhaps the most important function resulting from complement activation.

2 Biologically active fragments are released

C3a and C5a, the small peptides split from the parent molecules during complement activation, have several important actions. Both are **anaphylatoxins** in that they are capable of triggering the release of host defence mediators such as histamine, leukotriene B4 and tumor necrosis factor (TNF) from mast cells (figures 1.2i, 1.9 & 1.10) and their circulating counterparts the basophils. C5a acts directly on neutrophils, and both C3a and C5a on eosinophils (described later in this chapter), to stimulate the respiratory burst associated with production of ROIs and to enhance the expression of surface receptors for C3b. Importantly, C5a is also a potent neutrophil chemotactic agent. Both C3a and C5a have a striking ability to act directly on the capillary endothelium to produce vasodilatation and increased permeability, an effect that seems to be prolonged by leukotriene B4 released from activated mast cells, neutrophils and macrophages.

3 The terminal complex can induce membrane lesions

As described above, the insertion of the MAC into a membrane may bring about cell lysis.

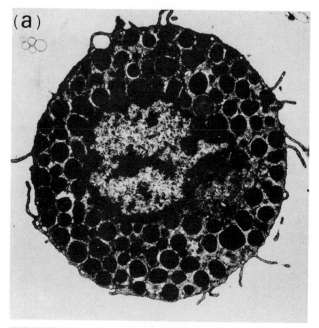

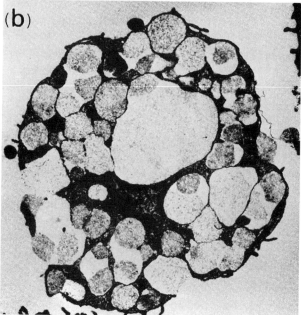

Figure 1.9 The mast cell. (a) A resting cell with many membrane-bound granules containing preformed mediators. (b) A triggered mast cell. Note that the granules have released their contents and are morphologically altered, being larger and less electron dense. Although most of the altered granules remain within the circumference of the cell, they are open to the extracellular space (electron micrographs ×5400). (Reproduced from D. Lawson, C. Fewtrell, B. Gomperts and M.C. Raff (1975) *Journal of Experimental Medicine* **142**, 391–402. Copyright permission of The Rockefeller University Press.)

4   Complement plays a role in the induction of antibody responses

As shall be described in detail later, B-cells proliferate and produce antibody when antigen binds to its surface receptors. This activation is modulated by co-receptors, including one for C3b. Therefore, when a B-cell is activated in the presence of C3b, the threshold for activation is lowered, and much less antigen is required to activate the B-cell.

COMPLEMENT CAN MEDIATE AN ACUTE INFLAMMATORY REACTION

We can now put together an effectively orchestrated defensive scenario initiated by activation of the alternative complement pathway (figure 1.10).

In the first act, C3bBb is stabilized on the surface of the microbe and cleaves large amounts of C3. The C3a fragment is released but C3b molecules bind copiously to the microbe. C3bBb activates the next step in the sequence to generate C5a and the MAC.

The next act sees the proinflammatory peptides, C3a and C5a (anaphylatoxins), together with the mediators they trigger from the mast cell, recruiting polymorphonuclear neutrophils and further plasma complement components to the site of microbial invasion. Complement activation also causes the expression of the adhesion molecules P-selectin and ICAM-1 (intercellular adhesion molecule-1) on endothelial cells. Under the influence of the chemotaxins, neutrophils slow down and the surface adhesion molecules they are stimulated to express cause them to marginate to the walls of the capillaries. Here they first adhere to the endothelial cells, then pass through gaps between these cells (diapedesis), and then move up the concentration gradient of chemotactic factors until they come face to face with the C3b-coated microbe. C5a, which is at a relatively high concentration in the chemotactic gradient, activates the respiratory burst in the neutrophils, with subsequent generation of toxic oxygen radicals and other phagocytic bactericidal mechanisms.

The processes of capillary dilatation (redness), exudation of plasma proteins and also of fluid (edema) due to hydrostatic and osmotic pressure changes, and accumulation of neutrophils are collectively termed the **acute inflammatory response**.

Macrophages can also do it

Tissue macrophages also play a crucial role in acute inflammatory reactions. They may be activated by the

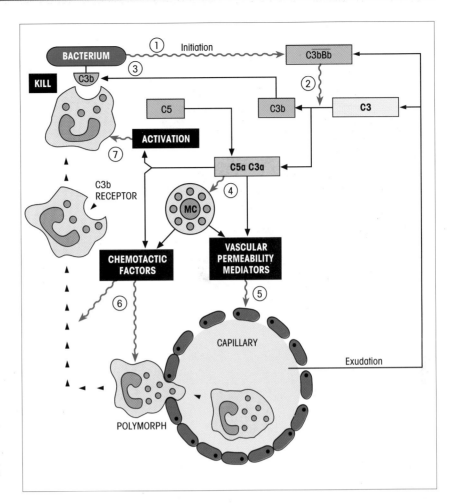

Figure 1.10 The defensive strategy of the acute inflammatory reaction initiated by bacterial activation of the alternative C pathway. Directions: ① start with the activation of the C$\overline{3b\overline{Bb}}$ C3 convertase by the bacterium, ② notice the generation of C3b (③ which binds to the bacterium), C3a and C5a, ④ which recruit mast cell mediators; ⑤ follow their effect on capillary dilatation and exudation of plasma proteins and ⑥ their chemotactic attraction of neutrophils to the C3b-coated bacterium and triumph in ⑦ the adherence and final activation of neutrophils for the kill.

direct action of C5a or certain bacterial toxins such as the LPSs acting on the TLRs, or by the phagocytosis of C3b-opsonized microbes. Following activation, the macrophages will secrete a variety of soluble mediators which amplify the acute inflammatory response (figure 1.11). These include cytokines such as interleukin-1 (IL-1) and TNF, which upregulate the expression of adhesion molecules for neutrophils on the surface of endothelial cells, increase capillary permeability and promote the chemotaxis and activation of the polymorphonuclear neutrophils themselves. Thus, under the stimulus of complement activation, the macrophage provides a pattern of cellular events which reinforces acute inflammation.

HUMORAL MECHANISMS PROVIDE A SECOND DEFENSIVE STRATEGY

Turning now to those defense systems which are mediated entirely by soluble factors, we recollect that many microbes activate the complement system and may be lysed by the insertion of the MAC. The spread of infection may be limited by enzymes released through tissue injury which activate the clotting system. Of the soluble bactericidal substances elaborated by the body, perhaps the most abundant and widespread is the enzyme lysozyme, a muramidase which splits the exposed peptidoglycan wall of susceptible bacteria. Interferons are a family of broad-spectrum antiviral agents induced by viruses and act to limit proliferation and spread of the infection. Interferon α (IFNα) is produced particularly by leukocytes, and interferon β (IFNβ) especially by fibroblasts, although all nucleated cells can probably synthesize these molecules. Lastly, we may mention the two lung surfactant proteins SP-A and SP-D which, in conjunction with various lipids, lower the surface tension of the epithelial lining cells of the lung to keep the airways patent. They belong to a totally different structural group of molecules termed collectins, which contribute to innate immunity through binding of their lectin-like domains to carbohydrates on microbes and their

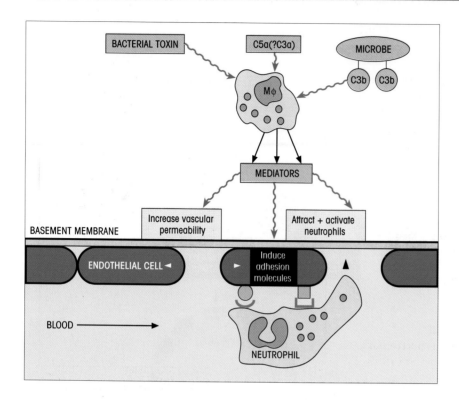

Figure 1.11 Stimulation by complement components and bacterial toxins such as lipopolysaccharide (LPS) induces macrophage secretion of mediators of an acute inflammatory response. Blood neutrophils stick to the adhesion molecules on the endothelial cell and use this to provide traction as they force their way between the cells, through the basement membrane (with the help of secreted elastase) and up the chemotactic gradient.

collagenous stem to cognate receptors on phagocytic cells, thereby facilitating the ingestion and killing of the infectious agents.

Acute phase proteins increase in response to infection

During an infection, microbial products such as endotoxins (LPS) activate macrophages and other cells to release various cytokines including IL-1, which is an endogenous pyrogen (incidentally capable of improving our general defenses by raising the body temperature), TNF and IL-6. These in turn act on the liver to increase the synthesis and secretion of a number of plasma proteins collectively termed acute phase proteins. These include C-reactive protein (CRP, the plasma concentration of which may increase 1000-fold), serum amyloid P component and MBL (Table 1.1). We have previously described the role that MBL plays in activating the complement system. Other acute phase proteins showing a more modest rise in concentration include α_1-antitrypsin, fibrinogen, ceruloplasmin, C9 and factor B. Overall it seems likely that the acute phase response achieves a beneficial effect through enhancing host resistance, minimizing tissue injury and promoting the resolution and repair of the inflammatory lesion. For example, CRP can bind to numerous

Table 1.1 Acute phase proteins.

Acute phase reactant	Role
Dramatic increases in concentration:	
C-reactive protein	Fixes complement, opsonizes
Mannose binding lectin	Fixes complement, opsonizes
α_1-acid glycoprotein	Transport protein
Serum amyloid P component	Amyloid component precursor
Moderate increases in concentration:	
α_1-proteinase inhibitors	Inhibit bacterial proteases
α_1-antichymotrypsin	Inhibit bacterial proteases
C3, C9, factor B	Increase complement function
Ceruloplasmin	$\cdot O_2^-$ scavenger
Fibrinogen	Coagulation
Angiotensin	Blood pressure
Haptoglobin	Bind hemoglobin
Fibronectin	Cell attachment

microorganisms forming a complex that may activate the complement pathway (by the classical pathway, not the alternative pathway with which we are at present familiar). This results in the deposition of C3b on the surface of the microbe which thus becomes opsonized (i.e., "made ready for the table") for adherence to phagocytes. Measurement of CRP is a useful laboratory test to assess the activity of inflammatory disease.

EXTRACELLULAR KILLING

Natural killer (NK) cells are part of the innate immune system

Viruses lack the apparatus for self-renewal so it is essential for them to penetrate the cells of the infected host in order to take over its replicative machinery. It is clearly in the interest of the host to find a way to kill such infected cells before the virus has had a chance to reproduce. **Natural killer cells** appear to do just that.

Natural killer cells are large granular lymphocytes (figure 2.4a) with a characteristic morphology. They possess activating receptors which recognize structures on glycoproteins on the surface of virally infected cells or on tumor cells, and which bring killer and target into close apposition (figure 1.12). Many of the ligands for the activating receptors can also be present on noninfected normal cells, and therefore the NK cells also possess inhibitory receptors to prevent killing of normal cells. These inhibitory receptors, which override the signals from the activating receptors, recognise ubiquitous molecules such as the major histocompatibility complex (MHC) class I glycoprotein normally found on the surface of all nucleated cells. However, virally infected or tumor cells often lose expression of MHC class I. Thus, only in the absence of MHC class I is the killing of the target cell allowed to proceed (see figure 4.4). Activation of the NK cell ensues and leads to polarization of granules between nucleus and target within minutes and extracellular release of their contents into the space between the two cells. This is followed by target cell death.

The most important of these granule contents is a **perforin** or cytolysin bearing some structural homology to C9. Like that protein, but without any help other than from Ca^{2+}, it can insert itself into the membrane of the target forming a transmembrane pore with an annular structure, comparable to the complement MAC (figure 1.8). In addition to perforin, the granules contain lymphotoxin α and a family of serine proteases termed granzymes, one of which, granzyme B, can

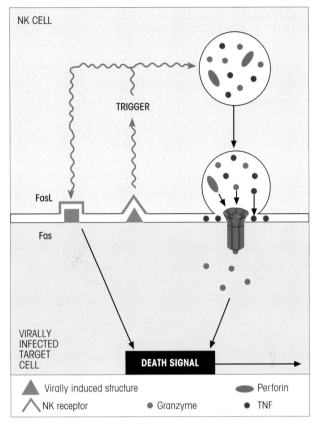

Figure 1.12 Extracellular killing of virally infected cell by natural killer (NK) cell. Binding of the NK receptors to the surface of the virally infected cell triggers the extracellular release of perforin molecules from the granules. These polymerize to form transmembrane channels which may facilitate lysis of the target by permitting entry of granzymes, tumor necrosis factor (TNF) and other potentially cytotoxic factors derived from the granules. (Model resembling that proposed by D. Hudig, G.R. Ewoldt and S.L. Woodward in (1993) *Current Opinion in Immunology* **5**, 90–6.) Engagement of the NK receptor also activates a parallel killing mechanism mediated through the binding of the FasL (Fas-ligand) on the effector to the target cell Fas receptor thereby delivering a signal for apoptosis.

function as an NK cytotoxic factor by inducing **apoptosis** (programmed cell death) in the target cell. Very rapid nuclear fragmentation effected by a Ca-dependent endonuclease that acts on the vulnerable DNA between nucleosomes can be detected.

An alternative recognition system for NK-cell-mediated killing can involve engagement of upregulated Fas receptor molecules on the target cell surface by the FasL (Fas-ligand) on the effector NK cell, a process which also induces an apoptotic signal in the unlucky target. Tumor necrosis family members, interacting with TNF receptors on target cells can also mediate cytotoxicity. One member of the family that is expressed by activated NK cells is TRAIL (tumor necrosis factor-related apoptosis-inducing ligand).

Natural killer cells also produce cytokines which regulate inflammation and acquired immune function

Not only do NK cells have the ability to lyse virally infected and tumor cells, but they also produce a wide range of cytokines once they are activated. These include cytokines such as IL-1 and TNF, which play an important role in inflammation, and granulocyte-macrophage colony-stimulating factor (GM-CSF), interferon γ (IFNγ) and transforming growth factor-β (TGFβ), which modulate the acquired immune response (see Chapter 2). Natural killer cells also express costimulatory molecules such as CD40L (CD40-ligand) and have been shown to regulate B-cell function when they are activated.

Eosinophils

Large parasites such as helminths (worms) cannot physically be phagocytosed and extracellular killing by eosinophils would seem to have evolved to help cope with this situation. Eosinophils, when released from the bone marrow, circulate in the peripheral blood and then traffic to peripheral tissue especially to the lung and the gut. Their prominent location in these sites suggests that they play an important role in host defence surveillance of mucosal surfaces. Eosinophils have distinctive granules which stain avidly with acid dyes (figure 1.2b). They have surface receptors for cytokines, chemokines, adhesion molecules and complement components, and on activation produce an impressive respiratory burst with concomitant generation of active oxygen metabolites and proinflammatory cytokines.

Most helminths can activate the alternative complement pathway, but although resistant to C9 attack, their coating with C3b allows adherence of eosinophils through the eosinophil C3b receptors. If this contact should lead to activation, the eosinophil will launch its extracellular attack, which includes the release of major basic protein (MBP) present in the eosinophil granules which damages the parasite membrane.

REVISION

A wide range of innate immune mechanisms operate which do not improve with repeated exposure to infection.

Barriers against infection
• Microorganisms are kept out of the body by the skin, the secretion of mucus, ciliary action, the lavaging and antibacterial action of fluids and microbial antagonism.
• If penetration occurs, bacteria are destroyed by soluble factors such as lysozyme and by phagocytosis which is followed by intracellular digestion.
• Phagocytic cells kill microorganisms.
• The main phagocytic cells are polymorphonuclear neutrophils and mononuclear macrophages. Organisms adhere via their pathogen-associated molecular patterns (PAMPs) to pattern recognition receptors (PRRs) on the phagocytic cell surface.
• Toll-like receptors (TLRs) are transmembrane proteins that recognize bacterial products. When activated they trigger the release of proinflammatory cytokines.

• Binding to PRRs activates the engulfment process and the microorganism is taken inside the cell where it fuses with cytoplasmic granules.
• A formidable array of microbicidal mechanisms then come into play including the conversion of oxygen to reactive oxygen intermediates (ROIs), the synthesis of nitric oxide and the release of multiple oxygen-independent factors from the granules.
• The complement system, a multicomponent triggered enzyme cascade, is used to attract phagocytic cells to the microbes and engulf them.
• The most abundant component, C3, is split by a convertase enzyme to form C3b, which binds the adjacent microorganisms.
• Mannose-binding lectin (MBL) binds to mannose on the surface of microorganisms and initiates complement activation by binding the proteases MASP1 and MASP2.
• Once C3 is split the next component, C5, is activated yielding a small peptide, C5a. The residual C5b binds to the surface of the organism and assembles the terminal components C6–9 into a membrane attack complex

(MAC), which is freely permeable to solutes and can lead to osmotic lysis of the offending pathogen.

Complement has a range of defensive functions

- C3b coated organisms bind to C3b receptor (CR1) on phagocytic cells and are more readily phagocytosed.
- C5a is highly chemotactic for, and can activate, neutrophils. Both C3a and C5a are potent chemotactic and activating agents for eosinophils and they both greatly increase capillary permeability.
- C3a and C5a act on mast cells causing the release of further mediators such as histamine, leukotriene B4 and tumor necrosis factor (TNF) with effects on capillary permeability and adhesiveness, and neutrophil chemotaxis; they also activate neutrophils.
- Insertion of the MAC into an organism brings about cell lysis.
- C3b plays a role in facilitating antibody production by B-cells.

The complement-mediated acute inflammatory reaction

- Following the activation of complement with the ensuing attraction and stimulation of neutrophils, the activated phagocytes bind to the C3b-coated microbes by their surface C3b receptors and may then ingest them. The influx of polymorphs and the increase in vascular permeability constitute the potent antimicrobial **acute inflammatory response**.
- Complement activation induces endothelial cells to express adhesion molecules which attach to leukocytes and cause them to move between endothelial cells into the area of the microbes.
- Phagocytic cells are activated by C5a to ingest and kill invading microbes.
- Inflammation can also be initiated by tissue macrophages, which can be activated by C5a or by bacterial products such as endotoxin acting on the TLRs. These cells secrete cytokines including interleukin-1 (IL-1) and TNF which increase the adhesiveness of endothelial cells thereby bringing more cells to the site of inflammation.

Humoral mechanisms provide a second defensive strategy

- In addition to lysozyme, defensins and the complement system, other humoral defenses involve the acute phase proteins such as C-reactive protein and mannose-binding ligand whose synthesis is greatly augmented by infection.
- Recovery from viral infections can be effected by the interferons, which block viral replication.
- Collectins bind to carbohydrates on organisms and also to receptors on phagocytic cells thereby facilitating phagocytosis.

Acute phase proteins increase during infection

- Cytokines such as IL-1 and TNF, released during acute inflammation, act on the liver that synthesises plasma proteins called acute phase proteins.
- These have a beneficial effect on host defence.
- Measurement of C-reactive protein (CRP) is useful to assess the activity of inflammatory processes.

Extracellular killing

- Natural killer (NK) cells possess killer activating receptors recognizing glycoproteins on the surface of the virally infected cell or tumor cell, and dominant inhibitory receptors recognizing major histocompatibility complex (MHC) class I on normal cells.
- Virally infected cells can be destroyed by NK cells using programmed cell death (apoptosis) through a perforin/granzyme pathway, or by FasL (Fas-ligand) on the NK cell engaging Fas on the target cell.
- Extracellular killing by C3b-bound eosinophils may be responsible for the failure of many large parasites to establish a foothold in potential hosts.

See the accompanying website (**www.roitt.com**) for multiple choice questions

FURTHER READING

Beutler, B. & Hoffmann, J. (eds) (2004) Section on innate immunity. *Current Opinion in Immunology*, **16**, 1–62.

Gregory, S.H. & Wing, E.J. (1998) Neutrophil–Kupffer cell interaction in host defenses to systemic infections. *Immunology Today*, **19**, 507–10.

Mollinedo, F., Borregaard, N. & Boxer, L.A. (1999) Novel trends in neutrophil structure, function and development. *Immunology Today*, **20**, 535–7.

Nature Encyclopedia of Life Sciences. http://www.els.net (constantly updated web-based resource, includes numerous immunology review articles at both introductory and advanced levels).

Prussin, C. & Metcalfe, D. (2003) IgE, mast cells, basophils, and eosinophils. *Journal of Allergy and Clinical Immunology*, **111**, S486–94.

Sabroe, I., Read, R.C., Whyte, M.K.B. *et al.* (2003) Toll-like receptors in health and disease: Complex questions remain. *Journal of Immunology*, **171**, 1630–5.

Walport, M.J. (2001) Advances in immunology: Complement (second of two parts). *New England Journal of Medicine*, **344**, 1140–4.

Specific acquired immunity

THE NEED FOR SPECIFIC IMMUNE MECHANISMS

Our microbial adversaries have tremendous opportunities through mutation to evolve strategies which evade our innate immune defenses, and many organisms may shape their exteriors so as to avoid complement activation completely. The body obviously needed to "devise" defense mechanisms which could be dovetailed individually to each of these organisms no matter how many there were. In other words a very large number of **specific immune defenses** needed to be at the body's disposal. Quite a tall order!

ANTIBODY—THE SPECIFIC ADAPTER

Evolutionary processes came up with what can only be described as a brilliant solution. This was to fashion an adapter molecule which was intrinsically capable not only of activating the complement system *and* of attaching to and stimulating phagocytic cells, but also of sticking to the offending microbe. The adapter thus had three main regions; two concerned with communicating with complement and the phagocytes (the biological functions) and one devoted to binding to an individual microorganism (the external recognition function). This latter portion would be complementary in shape to some microorganism to which it could then bind reasonably firmly. Although the part of the adapter with biological function would be constant, a special recognition portion would be needed for each of the hundreds and thousands of different organisms. The adapter is of course the molecule we know affectionately as **antibody** (figure 2.1).

Antigen–antibody complexes initiate a different complement pathway ("classical")

One of the important functions of antibody when bound to a microbe is to activate the **classical complement sequence**. This occurs when the antigen–antibody complex binds a protein called C1q, which is the first molecule in the classical complement sequence. C1q consists of a central collagen-like stem branching into six peptide chains each tipped by an antibody-binding subunit (resembling the blooms on a bouquet of flowers). Changes in C1q consequent upon binding the antigen–antibody complex bring about the sequential activation of proteolytic activity in two other molecules, C1r and then C1s. This forms a Ca^{2+}-stabilized trimolecular C1 complex which dutifully plays its role in an amplifying cascade by acting on components C4 and C2 to generate many molecules of $\overline{C4b2a}$, a new **C3-splitting enzyme** (figure 2.2).

The next component in the chain, C4 (unfortunately components were numbered before the sequence was established), now binds to C1 and is cleaved enzymically by $C\overline{1s}$. As expected in a multienzyme cascade, several molecules of C4 undergo cleavage into two fragments, C4a and C4b. Note that C4a, like C5a and C3a, has anaphylatoxin activity, although feeble, and C4b resembles C3b in its opsonic activity. In the pres-

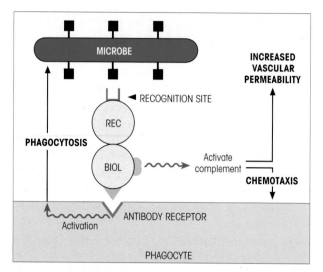

Figure 2.1 The antibody adapter molecule. The constant part with biological function (BIOL) activates complement and the phagocyte. The portion with the recognition unit for the foreign microbe (REC) varies from one antibody to another.

ence of Mg^{2+}, C2 can complex with the C$\overline{4b}$ to become a new substrate for the C$\overline{1s}$; the resulting product, C$\overline{4b2a}$, now has the vital C3 convertase activity required to cleave C3.

This classical pathway C3 convertase has the same specificity as the C$\overline{3bBb}$ generated by the alternative pathway, likewise producing the same C3a and C3b fragments. Activation of a single C1 complex can bring about the proteolysis of literally thousands of C3 molecules. From then on things march along exactly in parallel to the post-C3 pathway, with one molecule of C3b added to the C$\overline{4b2a}$; to make it into a C5-splitting enzyme with eventual production of the **membrane attack complex** (figures 1.8 & 2.3). Just as the alternative pathway C3 convertase is controlled by Factors H and I, so the breakdown of C$\overline{4b2a}$ is brought about by either a C4-binding protein (C4bp) or a cell surface C3b receptor called CR1.

The similarities between the two pathways are set out in figure 2.2 and show how antibody can supplement and even improve on the ability of the innate immune system to initiate **acute inflammatory reactions**.

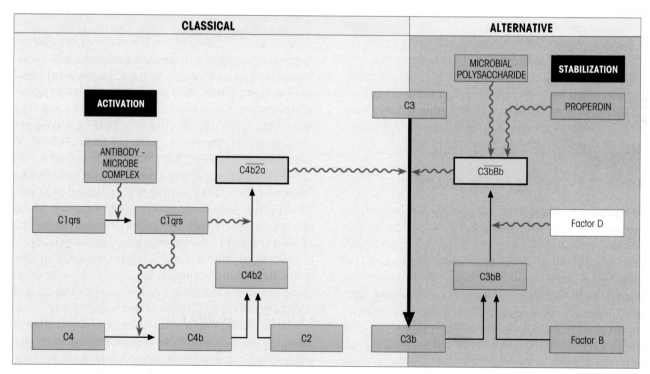

Figure 2.2 Comparison of the alternative and classical complement pathways. The classical pathway is antibody dependent, the alternative pathway is not. The molecular units with protease activity are highlighted. The mannose-binding lectin (MBL) pathway for complement activation (see p. 8) is not shown in this figure.

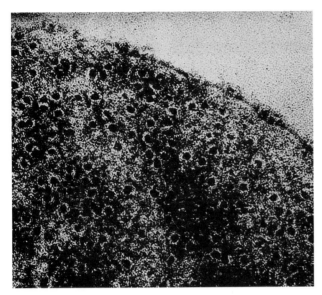

Figure 2.3 Multiple lesions in cell wall of *Escherichia coli* bacterium caused by interaction with immunoglobulin M (IgM) antibody and complement. (Human antibodies are divided into five main classes: IgM, IgG, IgA, IgE and IgD, which differ in the specialization of their "rear ends" for different biological functions such as complement activation or mast cell sensitization.) Each lesion is caused by a single IgM molecule and shows as a "dark pit" due to penetration by the "negative stain." This is somewhat of an illusion since in reality these "pits" are like volcano craters standing proud of the surface, and are each single "membrane attack" complexes (cf. figure 1.8) (×400 000). (Kindly supplied by Drs R. Dourmashkin and J.H. Humphrey.)

CELLULAR BASIS OF ANTIBODY PRODUCTION

Antigen selects the lymphocytes that make antibody

The majority of resting lymphocytes are small cells with a darkly staining nucleus due to condensed chromatin and relatively little cytoplasm containing the odd mitochondrion required for basic energy provision (figure 2.4a). Each lymphocyte of a subset called the **B-lymphocytes**—because they differentiate in the *bone marrow*—is programmed to make one, and only one, specificity of antibody and it places these antibodies on its outer surface to act as receptors for the relevant antigen. These receptors can be detected by using fluorescent probes. In figure 2.4c one can see the molecules of antibody on the surface of a human B-lymphocyte stained with a fluorescent rabbit antiserum raised against a preparation of human

antibodies. Each lymphocyte has of the order of 10^5 identical antibody molecules on its surface.

The molecules in the microorganisms that evoke and react with antibodies are called **antigens** (**gener**ates **anti**bodies). When an antigen enters the body, it is confronted by a dazzling array of lymphocytes all bearing different antibodies each with its own individual recognition site. The antigen will only bind to those receptors with which it makes a good fit. Lymphocytes whose receptors have bound antigen receive a triggering signal causing them to enlarge, proliferate (figure 2.4b) and develop into antibody-forming plasma cells (figures 2.4d & 2.5). Since the lymphocytes are programmed to make only one antibody specificity, that secreted by the plasma cell will be identical with that originally acting as the lymphocyte receptor, i.e. it will bind well to the antigen. In this way, antigen selects for the antibodies that recognize it most effectively (figure 2.6).

The need for clonal expansion means humoral immunity must be acquired

Because we can make hundreds of thousands, maybe even millions, of different antibody molecules, it is not feasible for us to have too many lymphocytes producing each type of antibody; there just would not be enough room in the body to accommodate them. To compensate for this, lymphocytes that are triggered by contact with antigen undergo successive waves of proliferation (figure 2.4b) to build up a large clone of plasma cells which will be making antibody of the kind for which the parent lymphocyte was programmed. By this system of **clonal selection**, large enough concentrations of antibody can be produced to combat infection effectively (figure 2.6).

Because it takes time for the proliferating clone to build up its numbers sufficiently, it is usually several days before antibodies are detectable in the serum following primary contact with antigen. The newly formed antibodies are a consequence of antigen exposure and it is for this reason that we speak of the **acquired immune response**.

ACQUIRED MEMORY

When we make an antibody response to a given infectious agent, by definition that microorganism must exist in our environment and we are likely to meet it again. It would make sense then for the immune mechanisms alerted by the first contact with antigen to leave

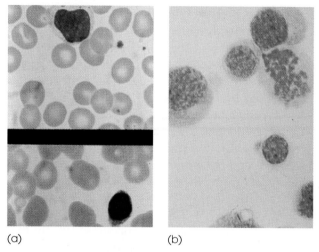

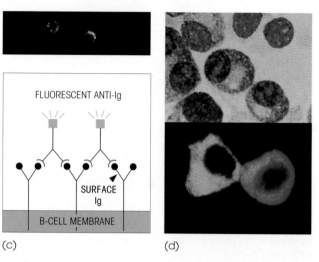

(a)   (b)   (c)   (d)

Figure 2.4 Cells involved in the acquired immune response. (a) Small lymphocytes. Condensed chromatin gives rise to heavy staining of the nucleus. The bottom cell is a typical resting agranular T-cell with a thin rim of cytoplasm. The upper nucleated cell is a large granular lymphocyte (LGL); it has more cytoplasm and azurophilic granules are evident. B-lymphocytes range from small to intermediate in size and lack granules (Giemsa). (b) Transformed lymphocytes (lymphoblasts) following stimulation of lymphocytes in culture with a polyclonal activator. The large lymphoblasts with their relatively high ratio of cytoplasm to nucleus may be compared in size with the isolated small lymphocyte. One cell is in mitosis (May–Grünwald–Giemsa). (c) Immunofluorescent staining of B-lymphocyte surface immunoglobulin (Ig) using fluorescein-conjugated (■) anti-Ig. Provided the reaction is carried out in the cold to prevent pinocytosis, the labeled antibody cannot penetrate to the interior of the viable lymphocytes and reacts only with surface components. Patches of aggregated surface Ig (sIg) are seen which are beginning to form a cap in the right-hand lymphocyte. During cap formation, submembranous myosin becomes redistributed in association with the sIg and induces locomotion of the previously sessile cell in a direction away from the cap. (d) (*upper*) Plasma cells. The nucleus is eccentric. The cytoplasm is strongly basophilic due to high RNA content. The juxtanuclear lightly stained zone corresponds with the Golgi region (May–Grünwald–Giemsa). (*lower*) Plasma cells stained to show intracellular Ig using a fluorescein-labeled anti-IgG (green) and a rhodamine-conjugated anti-IgM (red). (Material for (a) was kindly supplied by Mr M. Watts, (b) and (c) by Professor P. Lydyard, and (d) by Professor C. Grossi.)

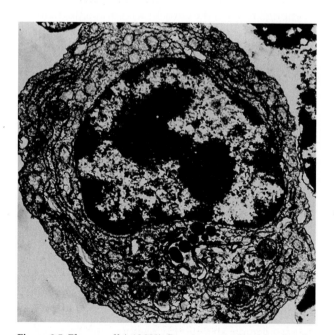

Figure 2.5 Plasma cell (×10 000). Prominent rough-surfaced endoplasmic reticulum associated with the synthesis and secretion of immunoglobulin (Ig).

behind some memory system which would enable the response to any subsequent exposure to be faster and greater in magnitude.

Our experience of many common infections tells us that this must be so. We rarely suffer twice from such diseases as measles, mumps, chickenpox, whooping cough and so forth. The first contact clearly imprints some information, and imparts some **memory** so that the body is effectively prepared to repel any later invasion by that organism and a state of immunity is established.

Secondary antibody responses are better

By following the production of antibody on the first and second contacts with antigen we can see the basis for the development of immunity. For example, when we immunize a child with a bacterial product such as tetanus toxoid, several days elapse before antibodies can be detected in the blood; these reach a peak and then fall (figure 2.7). If at a later stage we give a second injection of toxoid, the course of events is dramatically altered. Within 2–3 days the antibody level in the blood rises steeply to reach much higher values than were observed in the **primary response**. This **secondary**

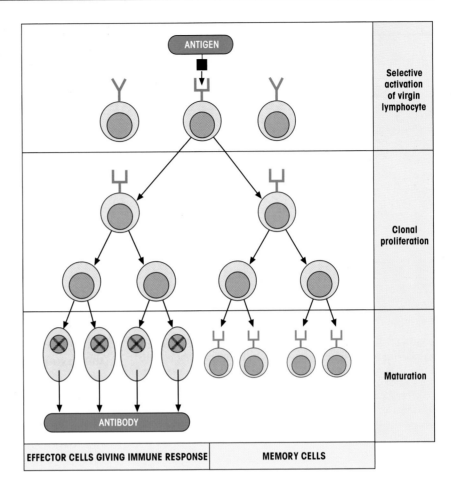

Figure 2.6 The cellular basis for the generation of effector and memory cells by clonal selection after primary contact with antigen. The cell selected by antigen undergoes many divisions during the clonal proliferation and the progeny mature to give an expanded population of antibody-forming cells. A fraction of the progeny of the original antigen-reactive lymphocytes becomes memory cells. Others mature into effector cells of either humoral, i.e. antibody-mediated, or cell-mediated immunity. Memory cells require fewer cycles before they develop into effectors and this shortens the reaction time for the secondary response. The expanded clone of cells with memory for the original antigen provides the basis for the greater secondary response relative to the primary immune response.

response then is characterized by a more rapid and more abundant production of antibody resulting from the "tuning up" or priming of the antibody-forming system.

The higher response given by a primed lymphocyte population can be ascribed mainly to an expansion of the numbers of cells capable of being stimulated by the antigen, although we shall see later that there are also some qualitative differences in these memory cells.

ACQUIRED IMMUNITY HAS ANTIGEN SPECIFICITY

Discrimination between different antigens

The establishment of memory or immunity to one organism does not confer protection against another unrelated organism. After an attack of measles we are immune to further infection but are susceptible to other agents such as the polio or mumps viruses. Acquired immunity therefore shows **specificity** and the immune system can differentiate specifically between the two organisms. The basis for this lies of course in the ability of the recognition sites of the antibody molecules to distinguish between antigens.

Discrimination between self and nonself

This ability to recognize one antigen and distinguish it from another goes even further. The individual must also recognize what is foreign, i.e. what is "nonself." The failure to discriminate between **self** and **nonself** could lead to the synthesis of antibodies directed against components of the subject's own body (**autoantibodies**), resulting in autoimmune disease. The body must therefore develop mechanisms whereby "self" and "nonself" can be distinguished. As we shall see later, those circulating body components that are able to reach the developing lymphoid system in the perinatal period will thereafter be regarded as "self." A permanent unresponsiveness or **tolerance** to the antigens on these tissues is then created, so that as immunologic maturity is reached, self-reacting lymphocytes are suppressed or tolerized. It should be

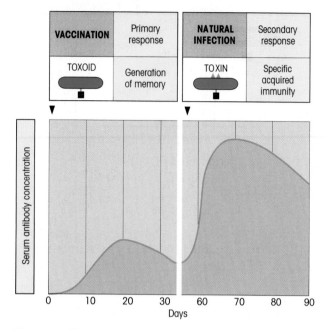

Figure 2.7 The basis of vaccination is illustrated by the response to tetanus toxoid. The toxoid is formed by treatment of the bacterial toxin with formaldehyde which destroys its toxicity (associated with ▲▲) but retains antigenicity. The antibody response on the second contact with antigen is more rapid and more intense. Thus, exposure to toxin in a subsequent natural infection boosts the memory cells, rapidly producing high levels of neutralizing protective antibody.

pointed out at this stage that self-tolerance is not absolute and potentially harmful anti-self lymphocytes do exist in all of us.

VACCINATION DEPENDS ON ACQUIRED MEMORY

Nearly 200 years ago, Edward Jenner carried out the remarkable studies which mark the beginning of immunology as a systematic subject. Noting the pretty pox-free skin of the milkmaids, he reasoned that deliberate exposure to the poxvirus of the cow, which is not virulent for the human, might confer protection against the related human smallpox organism. Accordingly, he inoculated a small boy with cowpox and was delighted—and presumably relieved—to observe that the child was now protected against a subsequent exposure to smallpox. By injecting a harmless form of a disease organism, Jenner had utilized the specificity and memory of the acquired immune response to lay the foundations for modern **vaccination** (Latin *vacca*, cow).

The essential strategy is to prepare an innocuous form of the infectious organism or its toxins, which still substantially retains the antigens responsible for

establishing protective immunity. This has been done by using killed or live attenuated organisms, purified microbial components or chemically modified antigens (figure 2.7).

CELL-MEDIATED IMMUNITY PROTECTS AGAINST INTRACELLULAR ORGANISMS

Many microorganisms live inside host cells where it is impossible for humoral antibody to reach them. Obligate intracellular parasites such as viruses have to replicate inside cells. Facultative intracellular parasites such as *Mycobacteria* and *Leishmania* can replicate within cells, particularly macrophages, but do not have to; they like the intracellular life because of the protection it affords. A totally separate acquired immunity system has evolved to deal with intracellular organisms. It is based on a distinct lymphocyte subpopulation called **T-cells** (figure 2.4a), designated thus because, unlike the B-lymphocytes, they differentiate within the **thymus gland**. Because they are specialized to operate against cells bearing intracellular organisms, T-cells only recognize antigen derived from these microbes when it is on the surface of a cell. Accordingly, the **T-cell surface receptors**, which are similar (but not identical) to the antibody molecules used by B-lymphocytes, recognize antigen plus a surface marker that informs the T-lymphocyte that it is making contact with another cell. These cell markers belong to an important group of molecules known as the **major histocompatibility complex (MHC)**, identified originally through their ability to evoke powerful transplantation reactions in other members of the same species.

Cytokine-producing T-cells help macrophages to kill intracellular parasites

Intracellular organisms only survive inside macrophages through their ability to subvert the innate killing mechanisms of these cells. Nonetheless, they cannot prevent the macrophage from processing small antigenic fragments (possibly of organisms that have spontaneously died) and moving them to their cell surface. A subpopulation of T-lymphocytes called **T-helper cells**, if primed to that antigen, will recognize and bind to the combination of antigen with so-called class II MHC molecules on the macrophage surface and produce a variety of soluble factors termed **cytokines**, which include the interleukins (interleukin-2, etc; see p. 84). Different cytokines can be made by various cell types and generally act at a short range on neighboring cells. Some T-cell cytokines help B-cells to make antibodies while others such as

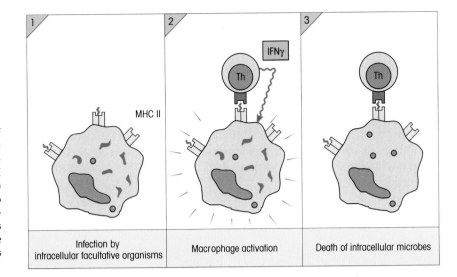

Figure 2.8 Intracellular killing of microorganisms by macrophages. (1) Surface antigen ($) derived from the intracellular microbes is complexed with class II major histocompatibility complex (MHC) molecules (⊔). (2) The T-helper binds to this surface complex and is triggered to release the cytokine interferon γ (IFNγ). This activates microbicidal mechanisms in the macrophage. (3) The infectious agent meets a timely death.

interferon γ (IFNγ) act as **macrophage activating factors**, which switch on the previously subverted microbicidal mechanisms of the macrophage and bring about the death of the intracellular microorganisms (figure 2.8).

Virally infected cells can be killed by antibody-dependent cellular cytotoxicity (ADCC) and by cytotoxic T-cells

We have already discussed the advantage to the host of killing virally infected cells before the virus begins to replicate and have seen that **natural killer (NK) cells** can subserve a cytotoxic function. However, NK cells have a limited range of specificities using their lectin-like and other activating receptors and in order to improve their efficacy, this range needs to be expanded.

One way in which this can be achieved is by coating the target cell with antibodies specific for the virally coded surface antigens because NK cells have Fcγ receptors for the constant part of the antibody molecule, rather like phagocytic cells. Thus antibodies will bring the NK cell very close to the target by forming a bridge, and the NK cell being activated by the complexed antibody molecules is able to kill the virally infected cell by its extracellular mechanisms (figure 2.9). This system is termed **antibody-dependent cellular cytotoxicity (ADCC)**.

Virally infected cells can also be controlled by a subset of T-lymphocytes called **cytotoxic T-cells**. These, like the T-helpers, have a very wide range of antigen specificities because they clonally express a large number of different T-cell receptors. Again, each lymphocyte is programmed to make only one receptor and,

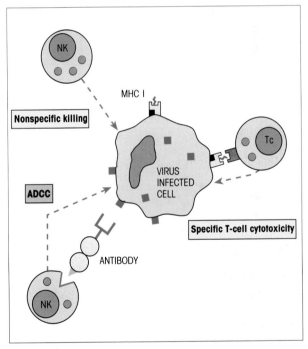

Figure 2.9 Killing virally infected cells. The nonspecific killing mechanism of the natural killer (NK) cell can be focused on the target by antibody to produce antibody-dependent cellular cytotoxicity (ADCC). The cytotoxic T-cell homes onto its target specifically through receptor recognition of surface antigen in association with class I major histocompatibility complex (MHC) molecules.

again like the T-helper cell, recognizes antigen only in association with a cell marker, in this case the class I MHC molecule (figure 2.9). Through this recognition of surface antigen, the cytotoxic cell comes into intimate contact with its target and administers the "kiss of apoptotic death."

In an entirely analogous fashion to the B-cell, T-cells are selected and activated by combination with antigen. They are then expanded by clonal proliferation and mature to give T-helper and T-cytotoxic cells, together with an enlarged population of memory cells. Thus both T- and B-cells provide **specific acquired immunity** which extends the range of effectiveness of innate immunity and confers the valuable advantage of memory, i.e. a first infection prepares us to withstand further contact with the same microorganism.

IMMUNOPATHOLOGY

The immune system is clearly "a good thing," but under certain circumstances it can cause damage to the host. Thus, where there is an especially heightened response or persistent exposure to exogenous antigens, tissue-damaging or **hypersensitivity** reactions may result. Examples are an allergy to grass pollens, blood dyscrasias associated with certain drugs, immune complex glomerulonephritis occurring after streptococcal infection, and chronic granulomas produced during tuberculosis or schistosomiasis.

In other cases, hypersensitivity to autoantigens may arise through a breakdown in the mechanisms which control self-tolerance resulting in a wide variety of **autoimmune diseases** such as Graves' disease, myasthenia gravis and many of the rheumatologic disorders.

Another immunopathologic reaction of some consequence is **transplant rejection**, where the MHC antigens on the donor graft may well provoke a fierce reaction. Lastly, one should consider the by no means infrequent occurrence of inadequate functioning of the immune system—**immunodeficiency**.

REVISION

Antibody—the specific adapter

- The antibody molecule evolved as a specific adapter to attach to microorganisms which either fail to activate the alternative complement pathway or prevent activation of the phagocytic cells.
- The antibody fixes to the antigen by its specific recognition site and its constant structure regions activate complement through the classical pathway (binding C1 and generating a $\overline{C4b2a}$; convertase to split C3) and phagocytes through their antibody receptors.

Cellular basis of antibody production

- Antibodies are made by plasma cells derived from B-lymphocytes; each of which is programmed to make only one antibody specificity, which is placed on the cell surface as a receptor.
- Antigen binds to the cell with a complementary antibody, causing cell activation, clonal proliferation and finally maturation to antibody-forming cells and memory cells. Thus, the antigen brings about clonal selection of the cells making antibody to itself.

Acquired memory and vaccination

- The increase in memory cells after priming means that the acquired secondary response is faster and greater, providing the basis for vaccination using a harmless form of the infective agent for the initial immunization.

Acquired immunity has antigen specificity

- Antibodies differentiate between antigens because recognition is based on molecular shape complementarity. Thus, memory induced by one antigen will not extend to another unrelated antigen.
- The immune system differentiates self components from foreign antigens by making immature self-reacting lymphocytes unresponsive through contact with host molecules; lymphocytes reacting with foreign antigens are unaffected since they only make contact after reaching maturity.

Cell-mediated immunity protects against intracellular organisms

- Another class of lymphocyte, the T-cell, is concerned with control of intracellular infections. Like the B-cell, each T-cell has its individual antigen receptor (although it differs structurally from antibody) which recognizes antigen and the cells undergo clonal expansion to form effector and memory cells providing specific acquired immunity.
- The T-cell recognizes cell surface antigens in association with molecules of the major histocompatibility complex (MHC).
- T-helper cells that see antigen with class II MHC on the surface of macrophages release cytokines, which in some cases can help B-cells to make antibody and in other cases activate macrophages and enable them to kill intracellular parasites.

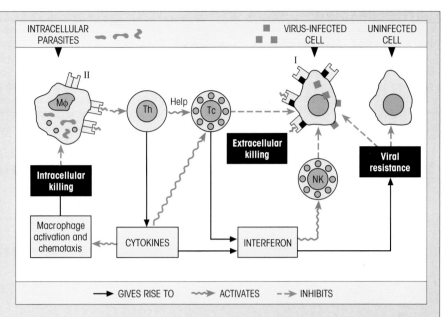

Figure 2.10 T-cells link with the innate immune system to resist intracellular infection. Class I (▯) and class II (▯) major histocompatibility complex (MHC) molecules are important for T-cell recognition of surface antigen. The T-helper (Th) cells cooperate in the development of cytotoxic T-cells (Tc) from precursors. The macrophage (Mφ) microbicidal mechanisms are switched on by macrophage-activating cytokines. Interferon inhibits viral replication and stimulates natural killer (NK) cells which together with Tc kill virus-infected cells.

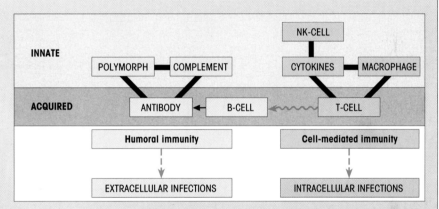

Figure 2.11 The two pathways linking innate and acquired immunity which provide the basis for humoral and cell-mediated immunity, respectively.

• Cytotoxic T-cells have the ability to recognize specific antigen plus class I MHC on the surface of virally infected cells, which are killed before the virus replicates. They also release interferon γ, which can make surrounding cells resistant to viral spread (figure 2.10).

• Natural killer (NK) cells have lectin-like "non-specific" receptors for cells infected by viruses but do not have antigen-specific receptors; however, they can recognize antibody-coated virally infected cells through their Fcγ receptors and kill the target by antibody-dependent cellular cytotoxicity (ADCC).

• Although the innate mechanisms do not improve with repeated exposure to infection as do the acquired, they play a vital role since they are intimately linked to the acquired systems by **two different pathways** which all but **encapsulate the whole of immunology**. Antibody, complement and polymorphs give protection against most extracellular organisms, while T-cells, soluble cytokines, macrophages and NK cells deal with intracellular infections (figure 2.11).

Immunopathology

• Immunopathologically mediated tissue damage to the host can occur as a result of:

(a) inappropriate hypersensitivity reactions to exogenous antigens;

(b) loss of tolerance to self giving autoimmune disease;

(c) reaction to foreign grafts.

• Immunodeficiency leaves the individual susceptible to infection.

See the accompanying website (**www.roitt.com**) for multiple choice questions

FURTHER READING

Alt, F. & Marrack, P. (eds) *Current Opinion in Immunology*. Current Science, London. (Six issues published a year.)

Mackay, I. & Rosen, F.S. (eds). Series of articles entitled Advances in immunology. *New England Journal of Medicine* (2000) **343**, 37–49, 108–17, 702–9, 1020–34, 1313–24, 1703–14; (2001) **344**, 30–7, 350–62, 655–64; **345**, 340–50.

Roitt, I.M. & Delves, P.J. (eds) (1998) *Encyclopedia of Immunology*, 2nd edn. Academic Press, London. (Covers virtually all aspects of the subject and describes immune responses to most infections.)

Schwaeble, W.J. & Reid, K.B.M. (1999) Does properdin crosslink the cellular and the humoral immune response? *Immunology Today*, **20**, 17–21.

The Immunologist. Hogrefe & Huber, Seattle. (Official organ of the International Union of Immunological Society—IUIS. Excellent, didactic and compact articles on current trends in immunology.)

Trends in Immunology. Elsevier Science, Amsterdam. (The immunologist's "newspaper": Excellent.)

Website www.roitt.com (linked to *Roitt's Essential Immunology* and this book). Animated immunology tutorials, over 400 multiple-choice questions with teaching comments on every answer, further reading, downloadable figures.

Antibodies

THE BASIC STRUCTURE IS A FOUR-PEPTIDE UNIT

The antibody molecule is made up of two identical heavy and two identical light chains held together by interchain disulfide bonds. These chains can be separated by reduction of the S–S bonds and acidification. In the most abundant type of antibody, **immunoglobulin G (IgG)**, the exposed hinge region is extended in structure due to the high proline content and is therefore vulnerable to proteolytic attack. Therefore the molecule is split by papain to yield two identical **Fab** fragments, each with a single combining site for antigen, and a third fragment, **Fc**, which lacks the ability to bind antigen. Pepsin strikes at a different point and cleaves the Fc from the remainder of the molecule to leave a large fragment, which is formulated as F(ab')$_2$ since it is still divalent with respect to antigen binding just like the parent antibody (figure 3.1).

AMINO ACID SEQUENCES REVEAL VARIATIONS IN IMMUNOGLOBULIN (Ig) STRUCTURE

For good reasons, the antibody population in any given individual is incredibly heterogeneous, with maybe 10^9 or more different Ig molecules in normal serum. This meant that determination of amino acid sequences was utterly useless until it proved possible to obtain the homogeneous product of a single clone. The opportunity to do this first came from the study of **myeloma proteins**.

In the human disease known as multiple myeloma, one cell making one particular individual Ig divides over and over again in the uncontrolled way a cancer cell does, without regard for the overall requirement of the host. The patient then possesses enormous numbers of identical cells derived as a clone from the original cell and they all synthesize the same Ig — the myeloma protein, or M-protein, which appears in the serum, sometimes in very high concentrations. By purification of the myeloma protein we can obtain a preparation of an Ig with a unique structure. **Monoclonal antibodies** can also be obtained by fusing individual antibody-forming cells with a B-cell tumor to produce a constantly dividing clone of cells dedicated to making the one antibody.

The sequencing of a number of such proteins has revealed that the N-terminal portions of both heavy and light chains show considerable variability, whereas the remaining parts of the chains are relatively constant, being grouped into a restricted number of structures. It is conventional to speak of variable and constant regions of both heavy and light chains (figure 3.2).

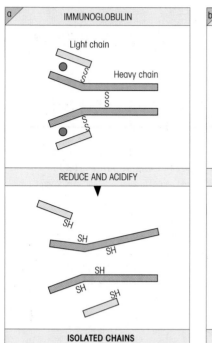

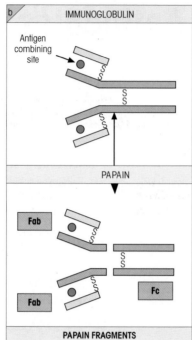

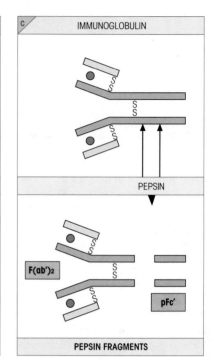

Figure 3.1 The antibody basic unit consisting of two identical heavy and two identical light chains held together by interchain disulfide bonds, can be broken down into its constituent peptide chains and to proteolytic fragments, the pepsin F(ab')₂ retaining two binding sites for antigen and the papain Fab with one. After papain digestion the Fc fragment representing the C-terminal half of the Ig molecule is formed and is held together by disulphide and noncovalent bonds. The portion of the heavy chain in the Fab fragment is given the symbol Fd. The N-terminal residue is on the left for each chain.

Certain sequences in the variable regions show quite remarkable diversity, and systematic analysis localizes these hypervariable sequences to three segments on the light chain and three on the heavy chain (figure 3.3).

IMMUNOGLOBULIN GENES

Immunoglobulins are encoded by multiple gene segments

Clusters of genes on three different chromosomes code for κ light chains, λ light chains and heavy chains respectively. Since a wide range of antibodies with differing amino acid sequences can be produced, there must be corresponding nucleotide sequences to encode them. However, the complete gene encoding each heavy and light chain is not present as such in the germ line DNA, but is created during early development of the B-cell by the joining together of mini segments of the gene. Take the human κ light chain, for example; the variable region is encoded by two gene segments, a large V_κ and a small J_κ, while a single gene encodes the constant region (figure 3.4). There is a cluster of some 40 or more variable (V) genes and just five joining (J) genes. In the immature B-cell, a translocation event leads to the joining of one of the V_κ genes to one of the J_κ segments. Each V segment has its own leader sequence and a number of upstream promoter sites including a characteristic octamer sequence, to which transcription factors bind. When the immunoglobulin gene is transcribed, splicing of the nuclear RNA brings the $V_\kappa J_\kappa$ sequence into contiguity with the constant region C_κ sequence, the whole being read off as a continuous κ chain peptide within the endoplasmic reticulum.

The same general principles apply to the arrangement of λ light chains with about 30 V gene segments and four J segments, and the heavy chain genes. The latter constellation shows additional features: the different constant region genes form a single cluster and there is a group of around 25 highly variable D segments located between the 50 or so V genes and six J genes (figure 3.5). The D segment, together with its junctions to the V and J segments, encodes almost the entire third hypervariable region, the first two being encoded entirely within the V sequence.

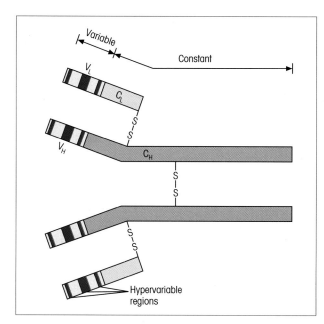

Figure 3.2 **Amino acid sequence variability in the antibody molecule.** The terms "V region" and "C region" are used to designate the variable and constant regions respectively; "V_L" and "C_L" are generic terms for these regions on the light chain and "V_H" and "C_H" specify variable and constant regions on the heavy chain. Certain segments of the variable region are hypervariable but adjacent framework regions are more conserved. As stressed previously, each pair of heavy chains is identical, as is each pair of light chains.

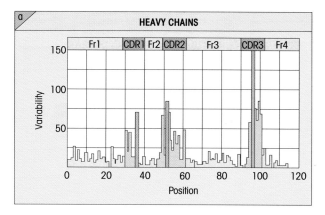

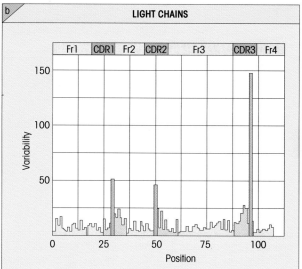

Figure 3.3 **Wu and Kabat plot of amino acid variability in the variable region of immunoglobulin (Ig) heavy and light chains.** The sequences of chains from a large number of myeloma monoclonal proteins are compared and variability at each position is computed as the number of different amino acids found divided by the frequency of the most common amino acid. Obviously, the higher the number the greater the variability; for a residue at which all 20 amino acids occur randomly, the number will be 400 (20/0.05) and at a completely invariant residue, the figure will be 1 (1/1). The three hypervariable regions (darker blue) in the (a) heavy and (b) light chains, usually referred to as complementarity-determining regions (CDRs), are clearly defined. The intervening peptide sequences (gray) are termed framework regions (Fr1–4). (Courtesy of Professor E.A. Kabat.)

A special mechanism effects *VDJ* recombination

In essence, the translocation involves the mutual recognition of conserved heptamer–spacer–nonamer recombination signal sequences (RSS) which flank each germ line *V, D* and *J* segment. The products of the recombination activating genes *RAG-1* and *RAG-2* catalyse the introduction of double-strand breaks between the elements to be joined and their respective flanking sequences. At this stage, nucleotides may either be deleted or inserted between the *VD, DJ* or *VJ* joining elements before they are ultimately ligated.

STRUCTURAL VARIANTS OF THE BASIC Ig MOLECULE

Isotypes

Based upon the structure of their heavy chain constant regions, Igs are divided into major groups termed **classes,** which may be further subdivided into **subclasses**. In the human, there are five classes: IgG, IgA, IgM, IgD and IgE. Since all the heavy chain constant re-

gion (C_H) structures that give rise to classes and subclasses are expressed together in the serum of a normal subject, they are termed **isotypic variants** (table 3.1). Likewise, the light chain constant regions (C_L) exist in isotypic forms known as κ and λ which are associated with all heavy chain isotypes. Because the light chains in a given antibody are identical, Igs are either κ or λ but never mixed (unless specially engineered in the

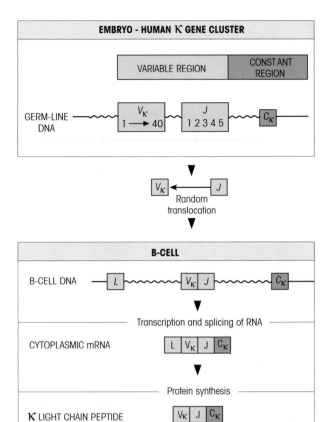

Figure 3.4 Genetic basis for synthesis of human κ chains. The $V_κ$ genes are arranged in a series of families or sets of a closely related sequence. Each $V_κ$ gene has its own leader sequence (*L*). As the cell becomes immunocompetent, the variable region is formed by the random combination of a $V_κ$ gene with a joining segment *J*, a translocation process facilitated by base sequences in the intron following the 3' end of the $V_κ$ segment pairing up with sequences in the intron 5' to *J*. The final joining occurs when the intervening intron sequence is spliced out of the RNA transcript. By convention, the genes are represented in italics and the antigens they encode in normal type.

laboratory). Thus IgG exists as IgGκ or IgGλ, IgM as IgMκ or IgMλ, and so on.

Allotypes

This type of variation depends upon the existence of allelic forms (encoded by alleles or alternative genes at a single locus) which therefore provide genetic markers (table 3.1). In somewhat the same way as the red cells in genetically different individuals can differ in terms of the blood group antigen system ABO, so the Ig heavy chains differ in the expression of their allotypic groups. Typical allotypes are the **Gm specificities** on IgG (Gm = *marker* on IgG). Allotypic differences at a given Gm locus usually involve one or two amino acids in the peptide chain. Take, for example, the G1m(a) locus on IgG1. An individual with this allotype would have the peptide sequence Asp . Glu . Leu . Thr . Lys on each of their IgG1 molecules. Another person whose IgG1 was a-negative would have the sequence Glu . Glu . Met . Thr . Lys, i.e. two amino acids different. To date, 25 Gm groups have been found on the γ-heavy chains and a further three on the κ constant region.

Idiotypes

It is possible to obtain antibodies that recognize the isotypic and allotypic variants described above. Similarly one can also raise antisera that are specific for individual antibody molecules and discriminate between one monoclonal antibody and another independently of isotypic or allotypic structures. Such antisera define the individual determinants characteristic of each antibody, collectively termed the **idiotype**. Not surprisingly, it turns out that the idiotypic determinants are located in the variable part of the antibody associated with the hypervariable regions. The reader will (or should) be startled to learn that it is possible to raise autoanti-idiotypic sera since this means that individuals can make antibodies to their own idiotypes. Some T-cell receptors are also capable of recognizing idiotypes.

IMMUNOGLOBULINS ARE FOLDED INTO GLOBULAR DOMAINS WHICH SUBSERVE DIFFERENT FUNCTIONS

Immunoglobulin domains have a characteristic structure

In addition to the *interchain* disulfide bonds, which bridge heavy and light chains, there are internal, *intrachain* disulfide links, which form loops in the peptide chain. These loops are compactly folded to form globular **domains** which have a characteristic β-pleated sheet protein structure.

Significantly, the hypervariable sequences appear at one end of the variable domain where they form parts of the β-turn loops and are clustered close to each other in space (figure 3.6).

The variable domain binds antigen

The clustering of the hypervariable loops at the tips of the variable regions where the antigen binding site is localized makes them the obvious candidates to subserve the function of antigen recognition (figures 3.6 &

Table 3.1 Summary of immunoglobulin (Ig) variants.

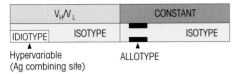

TYPE OF VARIATION	DISTRIBUTION	VARIANT	LOCATION	EXAMPLES
ISOTYPIC	All variants present in serum of a normal individual	Classes Subclasses Types Subgroups Subgroups	C_H C_H C_L C_L V_H/V_L	IgM, IgE IgA1, IgA2 κ, λ $\lambda Oz^+, \lambda Oz^-$ $V_{\kappa I}\ V_{\kappa II}\ V_{\kappa III}$ $V_{HI}\ V_{HII}\ V_{HIII}$
ALLOTYPIC	Alternative forms: genetically controlled so not present in all individuals	Allotypes	Mainly C_H/C_L sometimes V_H/V_L	Gm groups (human) b4, b5, b6, b9 (rabbit light chains) Igh-1^a, Igh-1^b (mouse γ_{2a} heavy chains)
IDIOTYPIC	Individually specific to each immunoglobulin molecule	Idiotypes	Variable regions	Probably one or more hypervariable regions forming the antigen-combining site

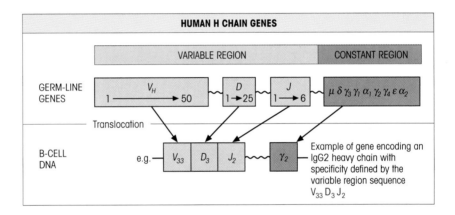

Figure 3.5 Human *V*-region genes shuffled by translocation to generate the single heavy chain specificity characteristic of each B-cell. Note the additional *D* (diversity)-segment minigenes.

3.7). X-ray crystallographic analysis of complexes formed between the Fab fragments of monoclonal antibodies and their respective antigens has confirmed this. The sequence heterogeneity of the three heavy and three light chain hypervariable loops ensures tremendous diversity in combining specificity for antigen through variation in the shape and nature of the surface they create. Thus, each hypervariable region may be looked upon as an independent structure contributing to the complementarity of the binding site for antigen, and one speaks of **complementarity-determining regions (CDRs)**.

Constant region domains determine secondary biological function

The classes of antibody differ from each other in many respects: in their half-life, their distribution throughout the body, their ability to fix complement and their binding to cell surface Fc receptors. Since the classes all have the same κ and λ light chains, and heavy and light variable region domains, these differences must lie in the heavy chain constant regions.

A model of the IgG molecule is presented in figure 3.8. It shows the spatial disposition and interaction of the domains in IgG and ascribes the various biological functions to the relevant structures. In principle, the V-region domains form the recognition unit and the C-region domains mediate the secondary biological functions.

IMMUNOGLOBULIN CLASSES AND SUBCLASSES

The physical and biological characteristics of the five major Ig classes in the human are summarized in tables 3.2 and 3.3. The following comments are intended to supplement this information.

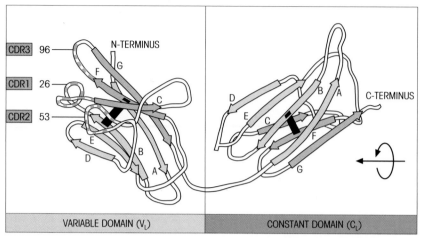

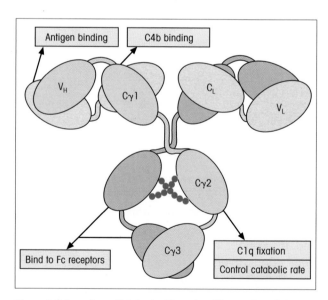

Figure 3.6 Immunoglobulin (Ig) domain structure. Structure of the globular domains of a light chain (from X-ray crystallographic studies of a Bence-Jones protein by Schiffer, M., Girling, R.L., Ely, R.R. *et al.* (1973) *Biochemistry* **12**, 4620. Copyright American Chemical Society.). One surface of each domain is composed essentially of four chains (light blue arrows) arranged in an antiparallel β-pleated structure stabilized by interchain H bonds between the amide CO· and NH· groups running along the peptide backbone, and the other surface of three such strands (darker blue arrows); the black bar represents the intrachain disulfide bond. This overall structure is characteristic of all Ig domains. Of particular interest is the location of the hypervariable regions (▪ ▪ ▪ ▪) in three separate loops which are closely disposed relative to each other and form the light chain contribution to the antigen binding site. One numbered residue from each complementarity determinant is identified.

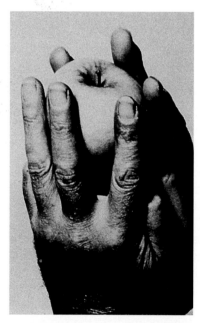

Figure 3.7 The binding site. A simulated combining site for the reactive surface of a single antigenic epitope (such as a hapten, cf. figure 5.1) formed by apposing the three middle fingers of each hand, each finger representing a hypervariable loop. With protein epitopes the area of contact is usually greater and tends to involve more superficial residues (cf. figure 5.3). (Photograph by B.N.A. Rice; inspired by A. Munro!)

Figure 3.8 Location of biological function. The combined Cγ2 and Cγ3 domains bind to Fc receptors on phagocytic cells, natural killer (NK) cells and placental syncytiotrophoblast, and also to staphylococcal protein A. (Note the immunoglobulin G (IgG) heavy chain is designated γ and the constant region domains Cγ1, Cγ2 and Cγ3.)

Table 3.2 Physical properties of major human immunoglobulin (Ig) classes.

DESIGNATION	IgG	IgA	IgM	IgD	IgE
Sedimentation coefficient	7S	7S,9S,11S*	19S	7S	8S
Molecular weight	150 000	160 000 and dimer	970 000	175 000	190 000
Number of basic four-peptide units	1	1,2*	5	1	1
Heavy chains	γ	α	μ	δ	ε
Light chains	κ or λ	κ or λ	κ or λ	κ or λ	κ or λ
Molecular formula†	$\gamma_2\kappa_2, \gamma_2\lambda_2$	$(\alpha_2\kappa_2)_{1-2}$ $(\alpha_2\lambda_2)_{1-2}$ $(\alpha_2\kappa_2)_2 S^*$ $(\alpha_2\lambda_2)_2 S^*$	$(\mu_2\kappa_2)_5$ $(\mu_2\lambda_2)_5$	$\delta_2\kappa_2$ $\delta_2\lambda_2$?	$\varepsilon_2\kappa_2, \varepsilon_2\lambda_2$
Valency for antigen binding	2	2,4	5(10)	2	2
Concentration range in normal serum	8-16 mg/ml	1.4-4 mg/ml	0.5-2 mg/ml	0.003-0.04 mg/ml	17-450 ng/ml‡
% Total immunoglobin	75	15	5-10	0-1	0.002
% Carbohydrate content	3	8	12	9	12

*7S monomer, 9S dimer, and 11S dimer in external secretions which carries the secretory component (S).
†IgA dimer and IgM contain J chain.
‡ng = 10^{-9} g.

Table 3.3 Biological properties of major immunoglobulin (Ig) classes in the human.

	IgG	IgA	IgM	IgD	IgE
Major characteristics	Most abundant Ig of internal body fluids particularly extravascular where it combats micro-organisms and their toxins	Major Ig in seromucous secretions where it defends external body surfaces	Very effective agglutinator; produced early in immune response – effective first-line defence against bacteremia	Mostly present on lymphocyte surface	Protection of external body surfaces. Recruits anti-microbial agents. Raised in parasitic infections. Responsible for symptoms of atopic allergy
Complement fixation Classical	++	–	+++	–	–
Alternative	–	+	–	–	–
Cross placenta	++	–	–	–	–
Sensitizes mast cells and basophils	–	–	–	–	+++
Binding to macrophages and polymorphs	+++	+	–	–	+

Immunoglobulin G has major but varied roles in extracellular defenses

Its relative abundance, its ability to develop high-affinity binding for antigen and its wide spectrum of secondary biological properties make IgG appear as the prime workhorse of the Ig stable. During the secondary response IgG is probably the major Ig to be synthesized. Immunoglobulin G diffuses more readily than the other Igs into the extravascular body spaces where, as the predominant species, it carries the major burden of neutralizing bacterial toxins and of binding to microorganisms to enhance their phagocytosis.

Activation of the classical complement pathway

Complexes of bacteria or other antigens with IgG antibody trigger the C1 complex when a minimum of two

Fcγ regions in the complex bind C1q. Activation of the next component, C4, produces attachment of C4b to the Cγ1 domain. Thereafter, one observes C3 convertase formation, covalent coupling of C3b to the bacteria and release of C3a and C5a leading to the chemotactic attraction of our friendly polymorphonuclear phagocytic cells. These adhere to the bacteria through surface receptors for complement and the Fc portion of IgG (Fcγ) and then ingest the microorganisms through phagocytosis. In a similar way, the extracellular killing of target cells coated with IgG antibody is mediated largely through recognition of the surface Fcγ by natural killer (NK) cells bearing the appropriate receptors. The thesis that the **biological individuality of different Ig classes is dependent on the heavy chain constant regions, particularly the Fc**, is amply borne out in the activities of IgG. Functions such as its ability to cross the placenta, transport across the intestine in the newborn, complement fixation and binding to various cell types have been shown to be mediated by the Fc part of the molecule.

Opsonization by IgG

All phagocytic cells have the ability to engulf microorganisms, a process which can be considerably enhanced by coating the invaders with IgG antibody. The IgG binds to specific epitopes on the microbe via its Fab fragment and to Fcγ receptors on the phagocytic cells by its Fc portion, allowing the phagocytic cell to attach itself firmly to the microbe and provoking much greater phagocytic activity.

Transplacental passage of IgG

Alone of the Ig classes, IgG possesses the crucially important ability to cross the human placenta so that it can provide a major line of defense for the first few weeks of a baby's life. This may be further reinforced by the transfer of colostral IgG across the gut mucosa in the neonate. These transport processes involve translocation of IgG across the cell barrier by complexing to an Fcγ receptor called FcRn (see below).

The diversity of Fcγ receptors

Since a wide variety of interactions between IgG complexes and different effector cells have been identified, we really should spend a little time looking at the membrane receptors for Fcγ that mediate these phenomena.

Specific Fc receptors may exist for all the classes of antibody, although receptors for IgD and IgM are not particularly well characterized. For IgG a quite extensive family of Fc receptors has emerged, the nine known genes encoding four major groups of receptors FcγRI, FcγRII, FcγRIII and FcγRn (or, more simply, FcRn). Within these groups there are a number of splice variants and inherited polymorphic forms.

FcγRI (CD64) is the major Fcγ receptor constitutively present on monocytes, macrophages and dendritic cells, and induced on neutrophils following their activation by the cytokines interferon γ (IFNγ) and granulocyte colony-stimulating factor (G-CSF). Conversely, FcγRI can be downregulated in response to interleukin-4 (IL-4) and IL-13. Its main roles are in facilitating phagocytosis and antigen presentation and in mediating extracellular killing of target cells coated with IgG antibody, a process referred to as antibody-dependent cellular cytotoxicity (ADCC; p. 23).

FcγRII (CD32) is present on the surface of most types of leukocytes and other cells including endothelial cells. These receptors bind insignificant amounts of monomeric IgG but immune complexes bind really well and are selectively adsorbed to the cell surface.

The two *FcγRIII (CD16)* genes encode the isoforms FcγRIIIA and FcγRIIIB found on most types of leukocytes. With respect to their functions, FcγRIIIA is largely responsible for mediating ADCC by NK cells and the clearance of immune complexes from the circulation by macrophages. FcγRIIIB cross-linking stimulates the production of superoxide by neutrophils.

FcRn is the fourth major type of FcγR. It is not present on leukocytes but instead is found on epithelial cells. It is referred to as FcRn due to its original description as a neonatal receptor, although it is also present in adults. It is involved in transferring maternal circulating IgG across the placenta to the fetus (figure 3.9).

Immunoglobulin A guards the mucosal surfaces

Immunoglobulin A appears selectively in the seromucous secretions such as saliva, tears, nasal fluids, sweat, colostrum, and secretions of the lung, genitourinary and gastrointestinal tracts, where it has the job of defending the exposed external surfaces of the body against attack by microorganisms. Immunoglobulin A is synthesized locally by plasma cells and is dimerized intracellularly together with a cysteine-rich polypeptide called the J chain. The dimeric IgA binds strongly through its J chain to a receptor for polymeric Ig present in the membrane of mucosal epithelial cells. The complex is then actively endocytosed, transported across the cytoplasm and secreted

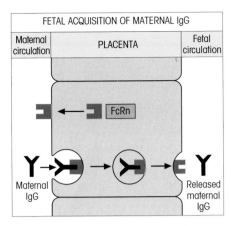

FETAL ACQUISITION OF MATERNAL IgG

Figure 3.9 The epithelial cell surface receptor for immunoglobulin G (IgG) Fc regions. The FcRn receptor is present in the placenta where it fulfills the important task of transferring maternal IgG to the fetal circulation. This will provide important protection prior to the generation of immunocompetence in the fetus. Furthermore, it is self-evident that any infectious agent which might reach the fetus *in utero* will have had to have passed through the mother first, and the fetus will rely upon the mother's immune system to have produced IgG with appropriate binding specificities. This maternal IgG also provides protection for the neonate, because it takes some weeks following birth before the transferred IgG is eventually all catabolized.

into the external body fluids after cleavage of the poly-Ig receptor peptide chain. The fragment of the receptor remaining bound to the IgA is termed secretory component, and the whole molecule is called **secretory IgA** (figure 3.10).

The function of the secretory component may be to protect the IgA hinge from bacterial proteases. It may also serve to anchor IgA to the soluble mucus acting as molecular Teflon to inhibit the adherence of coated microorganisms to the surface of mucosal cells, thereby preventing entry into the body tissues. The secretory IgA will also combine with the numerous soluble antigens of dietary and microbial origin to block their access to the body. Aggregated IgA binds to neutrophils and can also activate the alternative complement pathway. Plasma IgA is predominantly monomeric and, since this form is a relatively poor activator of complement, it seems likely that the body uses it for the direct neutralization of any antigens which breach the epithelial barrier to enter the circulation. However, it has additional functions which are mediated through the FcαR (CD89) for IgA present on monocytes, macrophages, neutrophils, activated eosinophils and on subpopulations of both T- and B-lymphocytes. Following cross-linking, the receptor can activate endocy-

tosis, phagocytosis, inflammatory mediator release and ADCC. Expression of the FcαR on monocytes is strongly upregulated by bacterial lipopolysaccharide.

Immunoglobulin M provides a defense against bacteremia

Often referred to as the macroglobulin antibodies because of their high molecular weight, IgM molecules are polymers of five four-peptide subunits each bearing an extra C_H domain. As with IgA, a single J chain is incorporated into the pentamer. Immunoglobulin M antibodies tend to be of relatively low affinity as measured against single determinants (haptens) but, because of their high valency, they bind with quite respectable avidity to antigens with multiple repeating epitopes. For the same reason, these antibodies are extremely efficient agglutinating and cytolytic agents and, since they appear early in the response to infection and are largely confined to the bloodstream, it is likely that they play a role of particular importance in cases of bacteremia. The isohemagglutinins (anti-A, anti-B) and many of the "natural" antibodies to microorganisms are usually IgM.

Monomeric IgM (i.e. a single four-peptide unit) anchored in the cell membrane is the major antibody receptor used by B-lymphocytes to recognize antigen.

Immunoglobulin D is a cell surface receptor

This class was recognized through the discovery of a myeloma protein which did not have the antigenic specificity of IgG, IgA or IgM, although it reacted with antibodies to Ig light chains and had the basic four-peptide structure. The hinge region is particularly extended and, although protected to some degree by carbohydrate, it may be this feature that makes IgD, among the different Ig classes, uniquely susceptible to proteolytic degradation and accounts for its short half-life in plasma (2.8 days). Nearly all the IgD is present together with IgM on the surface of a proportion of B-lymphocytes, where it seems likely that the two Igs may operate as mutually interacting antigen receptors for the control of lymphocyte activation and suppression.

Immunoglobulin E triggers inflammatory reactions

Only very low concentrations of IgE are present in serum, and only a very small proportion of the plasma cells in the body are synthesizing this Ig. It is not sur-

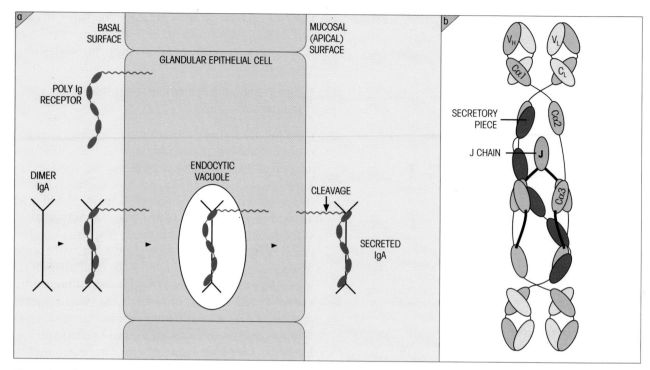

Figure 3.10 Secretory immunoglobulin A (IgA). (a) The mechanism of IgA secretion at the mucosal surface. The mucosal cell synthesizes a receptor for polymeric immunoglobulin which is inserted into the basal membrane. Dimeric IgA binds to this receptor and is transported via an endocytic vacuole to the apical surface. Cleavage of the receptor releases secretory IgA still attached to part of the receptor termed the secretory piece. (b) Schematic view of the structure of secreted IgA.

prising, therefore, that so far only a handful of IgE myelomas have been recognized compared with tens of thousands of IgG paraproteinemias. Immunoglobulin E antibodies remain firmly fixed for an extended period when they are bound with high affinity to the FcεRI receptor on mast cells. Contact with antigen leads to degranulation of the mast cells with release of preformed vasoactive amines and cytokines, and the synthesis of a variety of inflammatory mediators derived from arachidonic acid. This process is responsible for the symptoms of hay fever and of extrinsic asthma when patients with atopic allergy come into contact with the allergen, for example grass pollen.

The main *physiological* role of IgE would appear to be protection of anatomical sites susceptible to trauma and pathogen entry, by local recruitment of plasma factors and effector cells through **triggering an acute inflammatory reaction**. Infectious agents penetrating the IgA defenses would combine with specific IgE on the mast cell surface and trigger the release of vasoactive agents and factors chemotactic for granulocytes, so leading to an influx of plasma IgG, complement, neutrophils and eosinophils.

Another IgE receptor called the low affinity receptor FcεRII or CD23 is present on many different types of hematopoietic cells. Its primary function is to regulate IgE synthesis by B-cells, with a stimulatory role at low concentrations of IgE and an inhibitory role at high concentrations.

Immunoglobulins are further subdivided into subclasses

Antigenic analysis of IgG myelomas revealed further variation and showed that they could be grouped into four isotypic subclasses now termed IgG1, IgG2, IgG3 and IgG4. The differences all lie in the heavy chains, which have been labeled γ1, γ2, γ3 and γ4, respectively. These heavy chains show considerable homology and have certain structures in common with each other — the ones that react with specific anti-IgG antisera — but each has one or more additional structures characteristic of its own subclass arising from differences in primary amino acid composition and in interchain disulfide bridging. These give rise to differences in biological behavior, which are summarized in table 3.4.

Two subclasses of IgA have also been found, of which IgA1 constitutes 80–90% of the total.

Table 3.4 Comparison of human immunoglobulin G (IgG) subclasses.

	IgG1	IgG2	IgG3	IgG4
Serum concentration (mg/ml)	9	3	1	0.5
% Total IgG in normal serum	67	22	7	4
Serum half-life (days)	23	23	8	23
Complement activation (classical pathway)	++	+	+++	±
Binding to monocyte/macrophage Fc receptors	+++	±	+++	+
Ability to cross placenta	+++	±	+++	+++
Spontaneous aggregation	–	–	+++	
Binding to staphyloccal protein A	+++	+++	±	+++
Binding to staphyloccal protein G	+++	+++	+++	+++
Gm allotypes	a,z,f,x	n	b0,b1,b3, g,s,t, etc.	4a,4b

MAKING ANTIBODIES TO ORDER

The monoclonal antibody revolution

First in rodents

A fantastic technological breakthrough was achieved by Milstein and Köhler who devised a technique for the production of "immortal" clones of cells making single antibody specificities by fusing normal antibody-forming cells with an appropriate B-cell tumor line. These so-called "hybridomas" can be grown up either in the ascitic form in mice, when quite prodigious titers of monoclonal antibody can be attained, or propagated in large-scale culture. A major advance of the monoclonal antibody as a reagent is that it provides a single standard material for all laboratories throughout the world and can be used in many different applications. They include the enumeration and separation of individual cell types with specific surface markers (lymphocyte subpopulations, neural cells, etc.), cell depletion, cancer diagnosis, imaging, immunoassay, purification of antigen from complex mixtures, serotyping of microorganisms, immunologic intervention with passive antibody, therapeutic neutralization of inflammatory cytokines and "magic bullet" therapy with cytotoxic agents coupled to antitumor-specific antibody.

Human monoclonals can be made

Mouse monoclonals injected into human subjects for therapeutic purposes are highly immunogenic and may lead to immune-complex mediated disease. It would be useful to remove the xenogeneic (foreign) portions of the monoclonal antibody and replace those portions with human Ig structures using recombinant DNA technology. Chimeric constructs, in which the V_H and V_L mouse domains are spliced onto human C_H and C_L genes (figure 3.11a), are far less immunogenic in humans. Such antibodies can now be produced in "humanized" mice immunized by conventional antigens. One initiative involved the replacement of the mouse $C\gamma1$ gene by its human counterpart in embryonic stem cells. The resulting mutant mice were crossed with animals expressing human in place of murine C_κ chains and mice homozygous for both mutants produced humanized IgG1κ antibodies

Yet another approach is to graft the six CDRs of a high-affinity rodent monoclonal onto a completely human Ig framework without loss of specific reactivity (figure 3.11b). This is not a trivial exercise, however, and the objective of fusing human B-cells to make hybridomas is still appealing. A major restriction arises because the peripheral blood B-cells, which are the only B-cells readily available in the human, are not normally regarded as a good source of antibody-forming cells. Using the various approaches described above, large numbers of human monoclonals have been established and several are undergoing clinical trials; one can cite an antibody to the TRAIL (tumor necrosis factor-related apoptosis-inducing ligand) receptor on tumor cells as an anti-cancer agent, the Trabio™ antibody to transforming growth factor-β aimed at preventing scarring following eye surgery, the ABthrax™ antibody against a *Bacillus anthracis* protective antigen for the prevention and treatment of anthrax infection, and highly potent monoclonals for protection against varicella zoster and cytomegalovirus.

Engineering antibodies

There are other ways around the problems associated with the production of human monoclonals which ex-

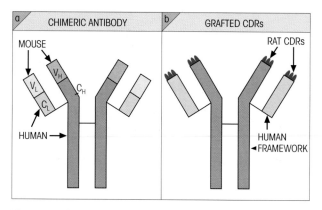

Figure 3.11 Genetically engineering rodent antibody specificities into the human. (a) Chimeric antibody with mouse variable regions fused to human immunoglobulin (Ig) constant region. (b) "Humanized" rat monoclonal in which gene segments coding for all six complementarity-determining regions (CDRs) are grafted onto a human Ig framework.

ploit the wiles of modern molecular biology. Reference has already been made to the "humanizing" of rodent antibodies (figure 3.11), but an important new strategy based upon bacteriophage expression and **selection** has achieved a prominent position. In essence, messenger RNA (mRNA) isolated from the B-cells of nonimmunized or preferably immunized donors is converted to complementary DNA (cDNA) and the antibody genes, or fragments therefrom, expanded by the polymerase chain reaction (PCR). Single constructs are then made in which the light- and heavy-chain genes are allowed to combine randomly in tandem with the bacteriophage *pIII* gene. This **combinatorial library** containing most random pairings of heavy- and light-chain genes encodes a huge repertoire of an-

tibodies (or their fragments) expressed as fusion proteins with the filamentous coat protein pIII on the bacteriophage surface. The extremely high number of phages can now be panned on solid-phase antigen to select those bearing the highest affinity antibodies attached to their surface. Because the genes that encode these antibodies are already present within the selected phage, they can readily be cloned and the antibody expressed in bulk. It should be recognized that this **selection** procedure has an enormous advantage over techniques which employ **screening** because the number of phages that can be examined is several logs higher.

Although a "test-tube" operation, this approach to the generation of specific antibodies does resemble the affinity maturation of the immune response *in vivo* in the sense that antigen is the determining factor in selecting out the highest affinity responders.

Fields of antibodies

Not only can the products of genes for a monoclonal antibody be obtained in bulk in the milk of lactating transgenic animals but plants can also be exploited for this purpose. So-called "**plantibodies**" have been expressed in bananas, potatoes and tobacco plants. One can imagine a high-tech farmer drawing the attention of a bemused visitor to one field growing anti-tetanus toxoid, another anti-meningococcal polysaccharide, and so on. Multifunctional plants might be quite profitable with, say, the root being harvested as a food crop and the leaves expressing some desirable gene product. At this rate there may not be much left for science fiction authors to write about!

REVISION

The basic immunoglobulin (Ig) structure is a four-peptide unit

• Immunoglobulins have a basic four-peptide structure of two identical heavy and two identical light chains joined by interchain disulfide links.

• Papain splits the molecule at the exposed flexible hinge region to give two identical univalent antigen-binding fragments (Fab) and a further fragment (Fc). Pepsin proteolysis gives a divalent antigen-binding fragment $F(ab')_2$ lacking the Fc.

Amino acid sequences reveal variations in Ig structure

• There are perhaps 10^8 or more different Ig molecules in normal serum.

• Analysis of myeloma proteins, which are homogeneous Ig produced by single clones of malignant plasma cells, has shown the N-terminal region of heavy and light chains to have a variable amino acid structure and the remainder to be relatively constant in structure.

Immunoglobulin genes

• Clusters of genes on three different chromosomes encode κ, λ and heavy Ig chains respectively. In each cluster there is a pool of 30–50 variable region (*V*) genes and around five small *J* minisegments. Heavy chain clusters in addition contain of the order of 25 *D* minigenes. There is a single gene encoding each constant region.

- A special splicing mechanism involving mutual recognition of 5' and 3' flanking sequences, catalysed by recombinase enzymes, effects the *VD*, *VJ* and *DJ* translocations.

Structural variants of the basic Ig molecule

- Isotypes are Ig variants based on different heavy chain constant structures, all of which are present in each individual; examples are the Ig classes, IgG, IgA, etc.
- Allotypes are heavy chain variants encoded by allelic (alternative) genes at single loci and are therefore genetically distributed; examples are Gm groups found on IgG molecules.
- An idiotype is the collection of antigenic determinants on an antibody, usually associated with the hypervariable regions, recognized by other antigen-specific receptors, either antibody (the anti-idiotype) or T-cell receptors.

Immunoglobulin domains serve different functions

- The variable region binds antigen, and three hypervariable loops on the heavy chain, termed complementarity-determining regions (CDRs), and three on the light chain, form the antigen-binding site.
- The constant region domains of the heavy chain (particularly the Fc) carry out secondary biological functions after the binding of antigen, e.g. complement fixation and binding to phagocytes.

Immunoglobulin classes and subclasses

- In the human there are five major types of heavy chain giving five classes of Ig. Immunoglobulin G is the most abundant Ig, particularly in the extravascular fluids where it neutralizes toxins and combats microorganisms by activating complement via the C1 pathway, and facilitating the binding to phagocytic cells by receptors for C3b and Fcγ. It crosses the placenta in late pregnancy and the intestine in the neonate.

Fcγ receptors

- There is an extensive family of receptors for IgG including FcγRI, FcγRII, FcγRIII and FcRn. By binding IgG, these receptors are crucial for many antibody functions such as phagocytosis, opsonization and antibody-dependent cellular cytotoxicity (ADCC). FcRn transfers circulating IgG across the placenta to the fetus.

Immunoglobulin A guards the mucosal surfaces

- Immunoglobulin A exists mainly as a monomer (basic four-peptide unit) in plasma. In the seromucous secretions, where it is the major Ig concerned in the defense of the external body surfaces, it is present as a dimer linked to a secretory component.
- Immunoglobulin A acts by inhibiting the adherence of coated organisms to mucosal cells.
- Phagocytic cells possess an FcαR and can be activated when the receptor is engaged by cross-linked IgA.

The other Igs have various functions in the immune response

- Immunoglobulin M is a pentameric molecule, essentially intravascular and produced early in the immune response. Because of its high valency it is a very effective bacterial agglutinator and mediator of complement-dependent cytolysis and is therefore a powerful first-line defense against bacteremia.
- Immunoglobulin D is largely present on the lymphocyte and functions as an antigen receptor.
- Immunoglobulin E binds firmly to mast cells and contact with antigen leads to local recruitment of antimicrobial agents through degranulation of the mast cells and release of inflammatory mediators. Immunoglobulin E is of importance in certain parasitic infections and is responsible for the symptoms of atopic allergy.
- Further diversity of function is possible through the subdivision of classes into subclasses based on structural differences in heavy chains all present in each normal individual.

Making antibodies to order

- Immortal hybridoma cell lines making monoclonal antibodies provide powerful immunologic reagents and insights into the immune response. Applications include enumeration of lymphocyte subpopulations, cell depletion, immunoassay, cancer diagnosis and imaging, and purification of antigen.
- Mouse monoclonal antibodies are immunogenic in humans. Chimeric constructs can be produced by splicing mouse *V* genes onto human *C* genes.
- Genetically engineered human antibody fragments can be derived by expanding the V_H and V_L genes from unimmunized or preferably immunized donors and expressing them as completely randomized combinatorial libraries on the surface of bacteriophage.

See the accompanying website (**www.roitt.com**) for multiple choice questions

FURTHER READING

Cedar, H. & Bergman, Y. (1999) Developmental regulation of immune system gene rearrangement. *Current Opinion in Immunology*, **11**, 64–9.

Delves, P.J. & Roitt, I.M. (eds) (1998) *Encyclopedia of Immunology*, 2nd edn. Academic Press, London. (Articles on IgG, IgA, IgM, IgD and IgE and immunoglobulin function and domains.)

Grawunder, U. & Harfst, E. (2001) How to make ends meet in V(D)J recombination. *Current Opinion in Immunology*, **13**, 186–94.

Grawunder, U., West, R.B. & Lieber, M.R. (1998) Antigen receptor gene rearrangement. *Current Opinion in Immunology*, **10**, 172–80.

Kinet, J-P. (1999) The high-affinity IgE receptor (FcεRI): from physiology to pathology. *Annual Review of Immunology*, **17**, 931–72.

Ravetch, J.V. & Bolland, S. (2001) IgG Fc receptors. *Annual Review of Immunology*, **19**, 275–90.

Membrane receptors for antigen

THE B-CELL SURFACE RECEPTOR FOR ANTIGEN

The B-cell inserts a transmembrane immunoglobulin (Ig) into its surface

In Chapter 2 we discussed the cunning system by which an antigen can be led inexorably to its doom by selecting the lymphocytes capable of making antibodies complementary in shape to itself through its ability to combine with a copy of the antibody molecule on the lymphocyte surface. It will be recalled that combination with the surface receptor activates the cell to proliferate and mature into a clone of plasma cells secreting antibody specific for the inciting antigen (cf. figure 2.6)

Immunofluorescent staining of live B-cells with labeled anti-Ig (e.g. figure 2.4c) reveals the earliest membrane Ig to be of the IgM class. The cell is committed to the production of just one antibody specificity and so transcribes its individual rearranged VJC_κ (or λ) and $VDJC\mu$ genes. The solution to the problem of secreting antibody with the same specificity as that present on the cell surface as a membrane Ig, is found in a **differential splicing** mechanism. The initial nuclear μ chain RNA transcript includes sequences coding for **hydrophobic transmembrane regions** which enable the IgM to sit in the membrane as the B-cell receptor (BCR) but, if these are spliced out, the antibody molecules can be secreted in a soluble form (figure 4.1).

As the B-cell matures, it co-expresses a BCR utilizing surface IgD of the same specificity. This surface combined IgM + IgD surface phenotype is abundant in the mantle zone lymphocytes of secondary lymphoid follicles (cf. figure 6.7c & d) and is achieved by differential splicing of a single transcript containing VDJ, Cμ and Cδ segments producing either membrane IgM or IgD. As the B-cell matures further, other isotypes such as IgG may be utilized in the BCR.

The surface immunoglobulin (sIg) is complexed with associated membrane proteins

The cytoplasmic tail of the surface IgM is only three amino acids long. In no way could this accommodate the structural motifs required for interaction with intracellular protein tyrosine kinases or G proteins which mediate the activation of signal transduction cascades. However, the sIg gets around this problem by transducing signals through a pair of associated membrane glycoproteins called Ig-α (CD79a) and Ig-β (CD79b) which become phosphorylated.

THE T-CELL SURFACE RECEPTOR FOR ANTIGEN

The receptor for antigen is a transmembrane heterodimer

The antigen-specific **T-cell receptor (TCR)** is a membrane-bound molecule composed of two disulfide-linked chains, α and β. Each chain folds into

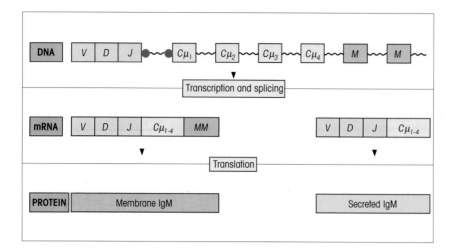

Figure 4.1 Splicing mechanism for the switch from the membrane to the secreted form of immunoglobulin M (IgM). The hydrophobic sequence encoded by the exons *M–M*, which anchors the receptor IgM to the membrane, is spliced out in the secreted form. For simplicity, the leader sequence has been omitted. ᨈ, introns.

two Ig-like domains, one having a relatively invariant structure, the other exhibiting a high degree of variability—rather like an Ig Fab fragment.

There are two classes of TCRs

Not long after the breakthrough in identifying the TCR αβ came reports of the existence of a second type of receptor composed of γ and δ chains. This TCR γδ appears earlier in thymic ontogeny than the TCR αβ.

In the human, γδ cells make up only 0.5–15.0% of the T-cells in peripheral blood, but they show greater dominance in the intestinal epithelium and in skin.

The encoding of TCRs is similar to that of Igs

The gene segments encoding the TCR β chains follow a similar arrangement of *V, D, J* and *C* segments to those described for the Igs (figure 4.2). As an immunocompetent T-cell is formed, rearrangement of *V, D* and *J* genes occurs to form a continuous *VDJ* sequence. The firmest evidence that B- and T-cells use similar recombination mechanisms comes from mice with severe combined immunodeficiency (SCID) due to a single autosomal recessive defect preventing successful linkage of *V, D* and *J* segments. Homozygous mutants fail to develop immunocompetent B- and T-cells and identical sequence defects in *VDJ* joint formation are seen in both pre-B- and pre-T-cell lines.

Looking first at the β-chain cluster, one of the two *Dβ* genes rearranges next to one of the *Jβ* genes. Note that the first *Dβ* gene, $D\beta_1$, can utilize any of the 13 *Jβ* genes, but $D\beta_2$ can only choose from the seven $J\beta_2$ genes. Next, one of the 50 or so *Vβ* genes is rearranged to the pre-

formed *DβJβ* segment. **Variability in junction formation** and the **random insertion of nucleotides** to create N-region diversity either side of the D segment, mirror the same phenomenon seen with Ig gene rearrangements. Sequence analysis emphasizes the analogy with the antibody molecule; each *V* segment contains two hypervariable regions, while the *DJ* sequence provides a **very hypervariable** CDR3 structure, making a total of six potential complementarity-determining regions for antigen binding in each TCR. As in the synthesis of antibody, the intron between *VDJ* and *C* is spliced out of the messenger RNA (mRNA) before translation with the restriction that rearrangements involving genes in the $D\beta_2 J\beta_2$ cluster can only link to $C\beta_2$.

All the other chains are encoded by genes formed through similar translocations. The α-chain gene pool lacks *D* segments but more than makes up for it with a prodigious number of *J* segments. The number of *Vγ* and *Vδ* genes is very small in comparison with *Vα* and *Vβ*. Like the α-chain pool, the γ chain cluster has no *D* segments.

The CD3 complex is an integral part of the TCR

The T-cell antigen recognition complex and its B-cell counterpart can be likened to specialized army platoons whose job is to send out a signal when the enemy has been sighted. When the TCR "sights the enemy," i.e. ligates antigen, it relays a signal through an associated complex of transmembrane polypeptides (**CD3**) to the interior of the T-lymphocyte, instructing it to awaken from its slumbering G0 state and do something useful —like becoming an effector cell. In all im-

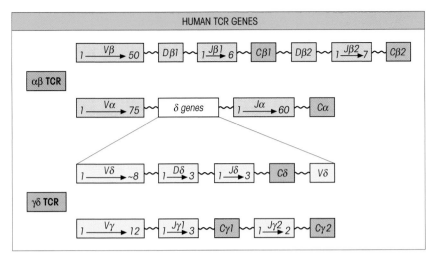
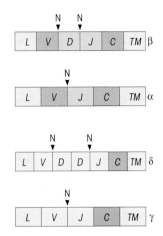

Figure 4.2 Genes encoding αβ and γδ T-cell receptors (TCRs). Genes encoding the δ chains lie between the $V\alpha$ and $J\alpha$ clusters and some V segments in this region can be used in either δ or α chains, i.e. as either $V\alpha$ or $V\delta$. T-cell receptor genes rearrange in a manner analogous to that seen with immunoglobulin genes.

munocompetent T-cells, the antigen receptor is noncovalently but still intimately linked with CD3 in a complex which contains two heterodimeric TCR αβ or γδ recognition units closely apposed to the invariant CD3 peptide chains γ and δ, two molecules of CD3ε plus the disulfide-linked ζ–ζ dimer. The total complex has the structure $TCR_2CD3\gamma\delta\epsilon_2\zeta_2$ (figure 4.3). The relationship of the CD3 molecules to the TCR heterodimer is therefore directly comparable to that of the Ig-α and Ig-β molecules to the sIg in the B-cell.

THE GENERATION OF DIVERSITY FOR ANTIGEN RECOGNITION

We know that the immune system has to be capable of recognizing virtually any pathogen that has arisen or might arise. The extravagant genetic solution to this problem of anticipating an unpredictable future involves the generation of millions of different specific antigen receptors, probably vastly more than the lifetime needs of the individual. Since this is likely to exceed the number of genes in the body, there must be some clever ways to generate all this diversity, particularly since the number of genes coding for antibodies and TCRs is only of the order of 400. We can now profitably examine the mechanisms which have evolved to generate tremendous diversity from such limited gene pools.

Intrachain amplification of diversity

Random VDJ combination increases diversity geometrically

Just as we can use a relatively small number of different building units in a child's construction set to create a rich variety of architectural masterpieces, so the individual receptor gene segments can be viewed as building blocks to fashion a multiplicity of antigen-specific receptors for both B- and T-cells.

Take, for example, the Ig heavy-chain genes (table 4.1). Although the precise number of gene segments varies from one individual to another, there are typically around 25 D and six J functional segments. If there were entirely **random joining** of any one D to any one J segment (cf. figure 3.5), we would have the possibility of generating 150 DJ combinations (25 × 6). Let us go to the next stage. Since each of these 150 DJ segments could join with any one of the approximately 50 V_H functional sequences, the net potential repertoire of VDJ genes encoding the heavy-chain variable region would be 50 × 150 = 7500. In other words, just taking our V, D and J genes, which in this example add up arithmetically to 81, we have produced a range of some 7500 different variable regions by **geometric recombination** of the basic elements. But that is only the beginning.

Playing with the junctions

Another ploy to squeeze more variation out of the germ line repertoire involves variable boundary re-

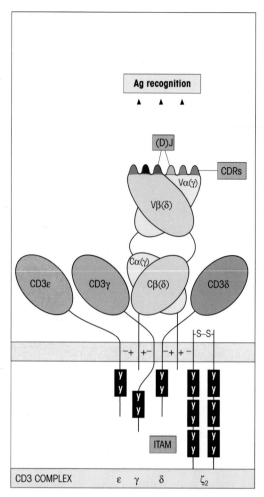

Figure 4.3 The T-cell receptor (TCR)/CD3 complex. The TCR resembles the immunoglobulin (Ig) Fab antigen-binding fragment in structure. The variable and constant segments of the TCR α and β chains (VαCα/VβCβ), and of the corresponding γ and δ chains of the $\gamma\delta$ TCR, belong structurally to the Ig-type domain family. The cytoplasmic domains of the CD3 peptide chains, shown in black, contact protein tyrosine kinases which activate cellular transcription factors.

combinations of *V*, *D* and *J* to produce different junctional sequences.

Further diversity arises from the insertion of nucleotides between the *V*, *D* and *J* segments, a process referred to as N-region diversity and associated with the expression of terminal deoxynucleotidyl transferase. This maneuver greatly increases the repertoire, especially for the TCR γ and δ genes which are otherwise rather limited in number.

Yet additional mechanisms relate specifically to the *D*-region sequence: particularly in the case of the TCR δ genes, where the *D* segment can be read in three different reading frames and two *D* segments can join together giving a *DD* combination.

Receptor editing

Recent observations have established that lymphocytes are not necessarily stuck with the antigen receptor they initially make; if they do not like it, they can change it. The replacement of an undesired receptor with one that has more acceptable characteristics is referred to as receptor editing. This process has been described for both Igs and for TCR, allowing the replacement of either nonfunctional or autoreactive rearrangements. Furthermore, receptor editing in the periphery may rescue low affinity B-cells from apoptotic cell death by replacing a low affinity receptor with a selectable one of higher affinity. The process involves reactivation of *RAG* genes followed by production of a new light or heavy chain which will change the Ig or TCR. Receptor editing occurs more readily in Ig light chains and TCR α chains than in Ig heavy chains and TCR β chains. Indeed, it has been suggested that the TCR α chain may undergo a series of rearrangements continuously deleting previously rearranged *VJ* segments until a selectable TCR is produced.

Interchain amplification

The immune system took an ingenious step forward when two different types of chain were utilized for the recognition molecules because the combination produces not only a larger combining site with potentially greater affinity but also new variability. Thus, when one heavy chain is paired with different light chains the specificity of the final antibody is altered.

This random association between TCR γ and δ chains, TCR α and β chains, and Ig heavy and light chains yields a further geometric increase in diversity. From table 4.1 it can be seen that approximately 230 functional TCR and 160 functional Ig germ line segments can give rise to 4.5 million and 2.4 million different combinations respectively, by straightforward associations *without* taking into account all of the fancy junctional mechanisms mechanisms described above.

Somatic hypermutation

There is inescapable evidence that Ig *V*-region genes can undergo significant somatic mutation.

A number of features of this somatic diversification phenomenon deserve mention. The mutations are the result of single nucleotide substitutions, they are restricted to the variable as distinct from the constant region, and occur in both framework and hypervariable regions. The mutation rate is remarkably high,

Table 4.1 Calculations of human *V* gene diversity. The minimum number of specificities generated by straightforward random combination of germ line segments are calculated. These will be increased by the further mechanisms listed.

	γδTCR (TCR1)		αβTCR (TCR2)		Ig		
	γ	δ	α	β	H	L (κ)	L (λ)
V gene segments	12	~8	75	50	50	40	30
D gene segments	-	3	-	1,1	25	-	-
J gene segments	3,2	3	60	6,7	6	5	4
Random combinatorial joining (without junctional diversity)	$V \times J$ 12 x5	$V \times D \times J$ 8 x 3 x3	$V \times J$ 75 x 60	$V \times D \times J$ 50(13+7)	$V \times D \times J$ 50 x 25 x 6	$V \times J$ 40 x 5	$V \times J$ 30 x 4
Total	60	72	4500	1000	7500	200	120
Combinatorial heterodimers	60 x 72		4500 x 1000		7500 x 200		7500 x 120
Total (rounded)	4.3×10^3		4.5×10^6		1.5×10^6		0.9×10^6
Other mechanisms: D's in 3 reading frames, junctional diversity, N region insertion; x10³	4.3×10^6		4.5×10^9		1.5×10^9		0.9×10^9
Somatic mutation	–		–		+++		+++

between 2 and 4% for V_H genes as compared with a value of < 0.0001% for a nonimmunologic lymphocyte gene. The mutational mechanism is bound up in some way with class switch since hypermutation is more frequent in IgG and IgA than in IgM antibodies. It is likely that somatic mutation does not add to the repertoire available in the early phases of the primary response, but occurs during the generation of memory and is probably responsible for tuning the response towards higher affinity.

T-cell receptor genes, on the other hand, **do not appear to undergo somatic mutation**. This is fortunate since, because TCRs already partly recognize self major histocompatibility complex (MHC) molecules, mutations could readily encourage the emergence of high affinity autoreactive receptors and resulting autoimmunity.

RECOGNITION OF ANTIGEN BY NATURAL KILLER (NK) CELLS

As was described in Chapter 1, one of the main functions of NK cells is to patrol the body looking for malignant or infected cells which have lost expression of the normally ubiquitously present MHC class I molecules. Activating receptors recognize molecules collectively present on all cell surfaces and inhibitory receptors recognize MHC class I molecules. Any nucleated cell lacking MHC class I will not engage the inhibitory receptors and will only trigger the activating receptors, resulting in its execution by the NK cell. Unlike the TCR on T-cells and the BCR on B-cells, this recognition system is not antigen specific. However, a second mode of killing which NK cells employ is antibody-dependent cellular cytotoxicity (ADCC, cf. p. 23) for which they are equipped with FcγRIII receptors in order to recognize antibody-coated target cells (figure 4.4). In this case the antibody alerts the NK cell to the presence of specific antigen.

THE MAJOR HISTOCOMPATIBILITY COMPLEX (MHC)

Molecules expressed by genes which constitute this complex chromosomal region were originally defined by their ability to provoke vigorous rejection of grafts exchanged between different members of a species. In Chapter 2, brief mention was made of the necessity for cell-surface antigens to be associated with class I or class II MHC molecules so that they can be recognized by T-lymphocytes. The intention now is to give more insight into the nature of these molecules.

Class I and class II molecules are membrane-bound heterodimers

Major histocompatibility complex class I

Class I molecules consist of a heavy polypeptide chain of 44 kDa noncovalently linked to a smaller 12 kDa peptide called β2-microglobulin. The largest part of the heavy chain is organized into three globular domains (α_1, α_2 and α_3; figure 4.5a) which protrude from the cell surface; a hydrophobic section anchors the molecule in the membrane and a short hydrophilic sequence carries the C-terminus into the cytoplasm.

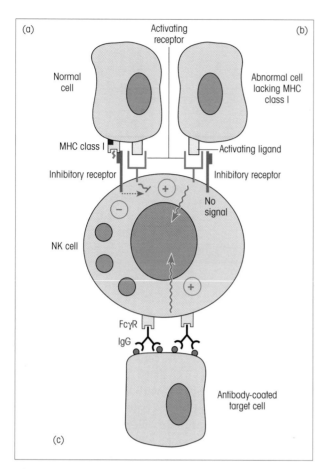

Figure 4.4 Natural killer (NK) cells. Natural killer cells possess both activating and inhibitory receptors. Engagement of an activating receptor by its ligand sends a stimulatory signal into the NK cell but this is normally subverted by a signal transmitted upon recognition of major histocompatibility complex (MHC) class I molecules by an inhibitory receptor (a). Any nucleated cell lacking class I is deemed abnormal and is killed following unimpeded transmission of the activation signal (b). Natural killer cells usually possess several different inhibitory and activating receptors and it is the balance of signals from these that determines whether the cell becomes activated. Like several other cell types, NK cells can utilize their Fcγ receptors to mediate antibody-dependent cellular cytotoxicity (ADCC) on target cells coated with antibody (c).

X-ray analysis of crystals of a human class I molecule provided an exciting leap forward in our understanding of MHC function. Both β_2-microglobulin and the α_3 region resemble classic Ig domains in their folding pattern. However, the α_1 and α_2 domains, which are most distal to the membrane, form two extended α-helices above a floor created by peptide strands held together in a β-pleated sheet, the whole forming an undeniable cavity (figure 4.5b,c). Another curious feature emerged. A linear molecule, now known to be a peptide, which had co-crystallized with the class I protein, occupied the cavity. The significance of these unique

findings for T-cell recognition of antigen will be revealed in Chapter 5.

Major histocompatibility complex class II

Class II MHC molecules are also transmembrane glycoproteins, in this case consisting of α and β polypeptide chains of molecular weight 34 kDa and 29 kDa respectively.

There is considerable sequence homology with class I. Structural studies have shown that the α_2 and β_2 domains, the ones nearest to the cell membrane, assume the characteristic Ig fold, while the α_1 and β_1 domains mimic the class I α_1 and α_2 in forming a groove bounded by two α-helices and a β-pleated sheet floor (figure 4.5a).

Several immune response related genes contribute to the class III region of the MHC

A variety of other genes that congregate within the MHC chromosome region are grouped under the heading of class III. Broadly, one could say that many are directly or indirectly related to immune defense functions. A notable cluster are the genes coding for complement components including C2, two C4 isotypes and factor B. The cytokines tumor necrosis factor (TNF) and lymphotoxin are also encoded under the class III umbrella.

Gene map of the MHC

The complete sequence of a human MHC was published at the very end of the last millennium. The sequence comprises 224 gene loci. An overall view of the main clusters of class I, II and III genes in the human MHC (human leukocyte antigen, HLA, system) may be gained from figure 4.6. A number of silent or pseudogenes have been omitted from this gene map in the interest of simplicity.

The genes of the MHC display remarkable polymorphism

Unlike the Ig and TCR systems where, as we have seen, variability is achieved in each individual by rearrangement of multiple gene segments, the MHC has evolved in terms of variability between individuals with a highly **polymorphic** (literally "many-shaped") system based on **multiple alleles** (i.e. alternative genes at each locus). A given MHC gene complex is referred to as a "haplotype" and is usually inherited *en bloc* as a single Mendelian trait. The class I and class II genes are

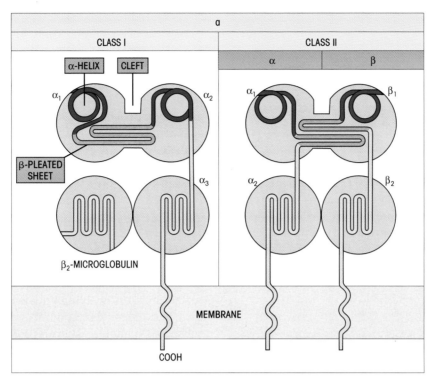

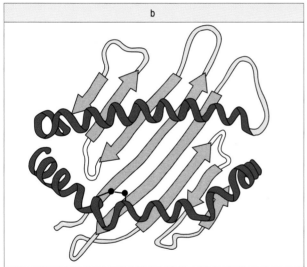

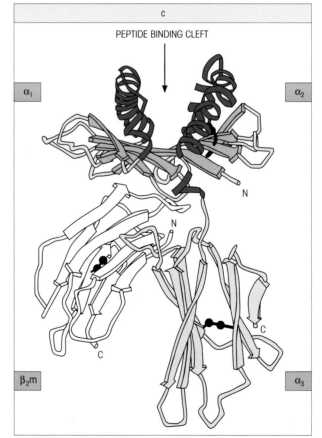

Figure 4.5 Class I and class II MHC molecules. (a) Diagram showing domains and transmembrane segments; the α-helices and β-sheets are viewed end on. (b) Schematic bird's eye representation of the top surface of a human class I molecule (HLA-A2) based on X-ray crystallographic structure. The strands making the β-pleated sheet are shown as thick gray arrows in the amino to carboxy direction; α-helices are represented as dark-red helical ribbons. The inside-facing surfaces of the two helices and the upper surface of the β-sheet form a cleft which binds and presents the peptide antigen to the T-cell. The two black spheres represent an intrachain disulfide bond. (c) Side view of the same molecule clearly showing the anatomy of the cleft and the typical immunoglobulin folding of the α_3- and β_2-microglobulin domains (four antiparallel β-strands on one face and three on the other). (Reproduced from P.J. Bjorkman *et al.* (1987) *Nature,* **329,** 506–12, with permission.)

The major histocompatibility complex														
MHC class	II				III						I			
HLA	DP	LMP &TAP	DQ	DR	C4	FB	C2	HSP70	TNF		B	C	E	A	G

Figure 4.6 Main genetic regions of the human major histocompatibility complex (MHC). HLA, human leukocyte antigen. Note that, although originally identified on leukocytes, HLA class I molecules are present on virtually all nucleated cells.

the most polymorphic genes in the human genome. For some of these genes, over 200 allelic variants have been identified. The amino acid changes responsible for these polymorphisms are restricted to the α_1 and α_2 domains of class I and to the α_1 and β_1 domains of class II. It is of enormous significance that they occur essentially in the β-sheet floor and the inner surfaces of the α-helices that line the central cavity (figure 4.5) and also on the upper surface of the helices.

The tissue distribution of MHC molecules

Essentially, all nucleated cells carry classical class I molecules. These are abundantly expressed on lymphoid cells, less so on liver, lung and kidney, and only sparsely on brain and skeletal muscle. In the human, the surface of the villous trophoblast lacks HLA-A and -B and bears HLA-G, which does not appear on any other body cell. Class II molecules are also restricted in their expression, being present only on antigen-presenting cells (APCs) such as B-cells, dendritic cells and macrophages and on thymic epithelium. When activated by agents such as interferon γ, capillary endothelia and many epithelial cells in tissues other than the thymus, they can develop surface class II and increased expression of class I.

Major histocompatibility complex functions

Although originally discovered through transplantation reactions, the MHC molecules are utilized for vital biological functions by the host. Their function as cell surface markers enabling infected cells to signal cytotoxic and helper T-cells will be explored in depth in subsequent chapters. There is no doubt that this role in immune responsiveness is immensely important, and in this respect the **rich polymorphism of the MHC** region would represent a species response to **maximize protection against diverse microorganisms**.

REVISION

The B-cell surface receptor for antigen
• The B-cell inserts its immunoglobulin (Ig) gene product containing a transmembrane segment into its surface where it acts as a specific receptor for antigen.
• The surface immunoglobulin (sIg) is complexed with the membrane proteins Ig-α and Ig-β which become phosphorylated on cell activation and transduce signals received through the Ig antigen receptor.

The T-cell surface receptor for antigen
• The receptor for antigen is a transmembrane dimer, each chain consisting of two Ig-like domains.
• The outer domains are variable in structure, the inner ones constant, rather like a membrane-bound Fab.
• Most T-cells express a receptor (T-cell receptor, TCR) with α and β chains. A separate lineage bearing γδ receptors is fairly abundant during early thymic ontogeny but is associated mainly with epithelial tissues in the adult.
• The encoding of the TCR is similar to that of Igs. The variable region coding sequence in the differentiating T-cell is formed by random rearrangement from clusters of

V, D (for β and δ chains) and J segments to form a single recombinant $V(D)J$ sequence for each chain.
• Like the Ig chains, each variable region has three hypervariable sequences which function in antigen recognition.
• The CD3 complex, composed of γ, δ, ε_2 and ζ_2, forms an intimate part of the receptor and has a signal transducing role following ligand binding by the TCR.

The generation of antibody diversity for antigen recognition
• The individual receptor gene segments can be viewed as building blocks to produce very large numbers of antigen-specific TCRs or B-cell receptors (BCRs).
• Further diversity is introduced at the junctions between V, D and J segments by variable recombination as they are spliced together by recombinase enzymes.
• In addition, after a primary response, B-cells, but not T-cells, undergo high rate somatic mutation affecting the V regions.

Major histocompatibility complex (MHC)
• Each vertebrate species has a MHC identified originally

through its ability to evoke very powerful transplantation rejection.

• Each contains three classes of genes. Class I encodes a polypeptide chain associated at the cell surface with β_2-microglobulin. Class II molecules are transmembrane heterodimers. Class III products are heterogeneous but include complement components and tumor necrosis factor (TNF).

• The genes display remarkable polymorphism. The particular set of MHC genes inherited by an individual is referred to as the haplotype.

• Classical class I molecules are present on virtually all nucleated cells in the body and signal cytotoxic T-cells.

• Class II molecules are particularly associated with B-cells, dendritic cells, macrophages and thymic epithelium, but can be induced on capillary endothelial cells and many epithelial cells by interferon γ. They signal T-helpers for B-cells and macrophages.

• Structural analysis indicates that the two domains distal to the cell membrane form a cavity bounded by two parallel α-helices sitting on a floor of β-sheet peptide strands; the walls and floor of the cavity and the upper surface of the helices are the sites of maximum polymorphic amino acid substitutions.

• Many class III gene products are associated with immune defense mechanisms, including complement proteins and TNF.

See the accompanying website (**www.roitt.com**) for multiple choice questions

---

FURTHER READING

Campbell, K.S. (1999) Signal transduction from the B-cell antigen-receptor. *Current Opinion in Immunology*, **11**, 256–64.

Campbell, R.D. & Trowsdale, J. (1997) Map of the human major histocompatibility complex. *Immunology Today*, **18** (1), pullout.

Campbell, R.D. & Trowsdale, J. (1993) Map of the human MHC. *Immunology Today*, **14**, 349–52.

Howard, J.C. (1991) Disease and evolution. *Nature*, **352**, 565–7.

Hughes, A.L., Yeager, M., Ten Elshof, A.E. & Chorney, M.J. (1999) A new taxonomy of mammalian MHC class I molecules. *Immunology Today*, **20**, 22–6.

CHAPTER 5

The primary interaction with antigen

WHAT IS AN ANTIGEN?

A man cannot be a husband without a wife and a molecule cannot be an antigen without a corresponding antiserum or antibody or T-cell receptor (TCR). The term **antigen** is used in two senses, the first to describe a molecule which generates an immune response (also called an **immunogen**), and the second a molecule which reacts with antibodies or primed T-cells. **Haptens** are small well-defined chemical groupings, such as dinitrophenyl (DNP) or *m*-aminobenzene sulfonate, which are not immunogenic on their own but will react with preformed antibodies induced by injection of the hapten linked to a "carrier" molecule which is itself an immunogen (figure 5.1).

The part of the hypervariable regions on the antibody which contacts the antigen is termed the **paratope**, and the part of the antigen which is in contact with the paratope is designated the **epitope** or **antigenic determinant**. It is important to be aware that each antigen usually bears several determinants on its surface, which may well be structurally distinct from each other; thus a monoclonal antibody reacting with one determinant will usually not react with any other determinants on the same antigen (figure 5.2). To get some idea of size, if the antigen is a linear peptide or carbohydrate, the combining site can usually accommodate up to five or six amino acid residues or hexose units. With a globular protein as many as 16 or so amino acid side-chains may be in contact with an antibody (figure 5.3).

The structure of antigens

In general, large proteins, because they have more potential determinants, are better antigens than small ones. Furthermore, the more foreign an antigen, that is the less similar to self configurations, the more effective it is in provoking an immune response. Although antibodies can be produced to almost any part of a foreign protein, certain areas of the antigen are more immunogenic and are called the immunodominant regions of the antigen. These sites of high epitope density are often those parts of the peptide chains that protrude significantly from the globular surface.

ANTIGEN AND ANTIBODY INTERACTIONS

Antigen and antibody interact due to complementarity in shape over a wide area of contact (figure 5.3), not so much as inflexible entities which fit together precisely in a "lock and key" manner but rather as mutually deformable surfaces—more like clouds than rocks. The interaction depends upon weak van der

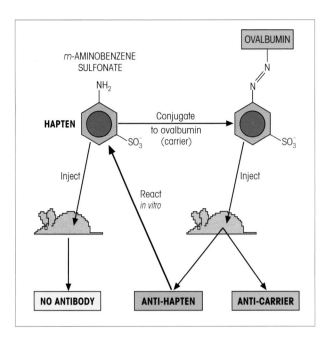

Figure 5.1 A hapten on its own will not induce antibodies. However, it will react *in vitro* with antibodies formed to a conjugate of the hapten with an immunogenic carrier.

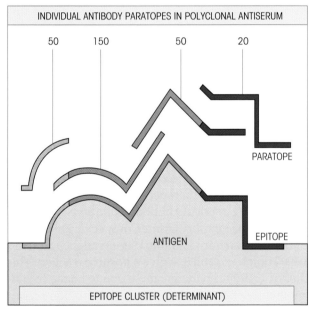

Figure 5.2 A globular protein antigen usually bears a mosaic of determinants (dominant epitope clusters) on its surface, defined by the heterogeneous population of antibody molecules in a given antiserum. This highly idealized diagram illustrates the idea that individual antibodies in a polyclonal antiserum with different combining sites (paratopes) can react with overlapping epitopes forming a determinant on the surface of the antigen. The numbers refer to the imagined relative frequency of each antibody specificity.

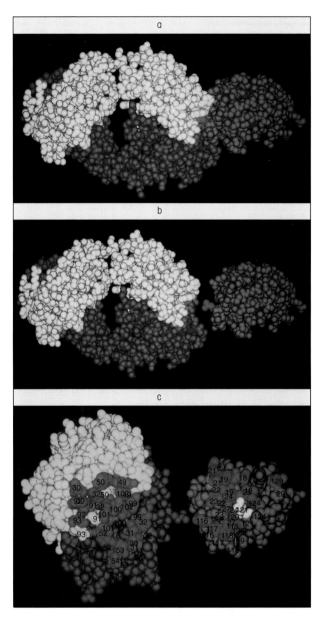

Figure 5.3 Structure of the contact regions between a monoclonal Fab antilysozyme and lysozyme. (a) Space-filling model showing Fab and lysozyme molecules fitting snugly together. Antibody heavy chain, blue; light chain, yellow; lysozyme, green with its glutamine-121 in red. (b) Fab and lysozyme models pulled apart to show how the protuberances and depressions of each are complementary to each other. (c) End-on views of antibody combining site (left) and the lysozyme epitope (right) obtained from (b) by rotating each molecule 90° about a vertical axis. (Reproduced with permission from A. Amit *et al.* (1986) *Science*, **233**, 747–53. Copyright 1986 by the AAAS.)

Waals, electrostatic, hydrophobic and hydrogen bonding forces which only become of significant magnitude when the interacting molecules are very close together. Thus, the more snugly the paratope and epitope fit together, the stronger the strength of binding, termed the **affinity**. This is defined as the equilibrium constant (K_a) of the reversible association of antibody with a single epitope (e.g. a hapten, figure 5.1), represented by the equation:

$$Ab + Hp \rightleftharpoons AbHp$$

Obviously a high affinity betokens strong binding. Usually, we are concerned with the interaction of an antiserum, i.e. the serum from an immunized individual with a multivalent antigen where the binding is geometrically increased relative to a monovalent hapten or single antigenic epitope. The term employed to express this binding is avidity, which being a measure of the functional affinity of an antiserum for the whole antigen is of obvious relevance to the reaction with antigen in the body. High avidity is superior to low for a wide variety of functions *in vivo*, including immune elimination of antigen, virus neutralization and the protective role against bacteria and other organisms.

THE SPECIFICITY OF ANTIGEN RECOGNITION BY ANTIBODY IS NOT ABSOLUTE

The strength of an antigen–antibody reaction can be quantified by the affinity or avidity of the antibody to that specific antigen. In so far as we recognize that an antiserum may have a relatively greater avidity for one antigen than another, by the same token we are saying that the antiserum is displaying relative rather than absolute specificity; in practice we speak of degrees of **cross-reactivity**. An antiserum raised against a given antigen can cross-react with a partially related antigen which bears one or more identical or similar determinants. In figure 5.4 it can be seen that an antiserum to antigen-1 (Ag_1) will react less strongly with Ag_2, which bears just one identical determinant, because only certain of the antibodies in the serum can bind. Antigen-3, which possesses a similar but not identical determinant, will not fit as well with the antibody, and hence the binding is even weaker. Antigen-4, which has no structural similarity at all, will not react significantly with the antibody. Thus, based upon stereochemical considerations, we can see why the avidity of the anti-

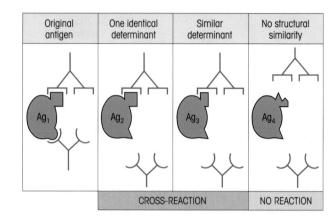

Figure 5.4 Specificity and cross-reaction. The avidity of the serum antibodies ⊣ and ⟩⟨ for antigen-1 (Ag_1) > Ag_2 > Ag_3 >> Ag_4.

serum for Ag_2 and Ag_3 is less than for the homologous antigen, while for the unrelated Ag_4 it is negligible. It would be customary to describe the antiserum as being highly specific for Ag_1 in relation to Ag_4 but cross-reacting with Ag_2 and Ag_3 to different extents. These principles have significance in human autoimmune diseases since an antibody may react not only with the antigen which stimulated its production but also with some quite unrelated molecules.

IN VITRO ANTIGEN–ANTIBODY REACTIONS

The specificity of antigen–antibody reactions enables us to detect the presence of specific antibody in serum or other fluid by combining it with the known antigen under strict laboratory conditions. Not only will positive reactions tell us that specific antibodies are present but by testing a series of antibody dilutions we can get an idea of the quantity, or titer, of specific antibody in the fluid. To take an example, a serum might be diluted 10 000 times and still just give a positive reaction. This titer of 1 : 10 000 enables comparison to be made with another much weaker serum which has a titer of, say, 1 : 100, i.e. it can only be diluted out 100 times before the test becomes negative. The titer is of crucial importance in interpreting the significance of antibodies in patients with clinical disease. Many normal individuals, for example, may have low titer antibodies to cytomegalovirus resulting from previous, perhaps subclinical, infection. In active infection titers may be high and increasing.

Numerous techniques are available to detect the presence and the titer of an antibody

Precipitation

When an antigen solution is added progressively to a potent antiserum, antigen–antibody precipitates are formed which can be detected by a variety of laboratory techniques. This precipitation can be enhanced by countercurrent immunoelectrophoresis. For example, antigen and antiserum can be placed in wells punched in an agar gel and a current applied to the system. The antigen migrates steadily into the antibody zone and forms a precipitin line where the complex forms. This provides a fairly sensitive and rapid test that has been applied to the detection of many clinically significant antibodies and, by the same means, antigen.

Nonprecipitating antibodies can be detected by nephelometry

The small aggregates formed when dilute solutions of antigen and antibody are mixed create a cloudiness or turbidity that can be measured by forward angle scattering of an incident light source (nephelometry). Greater sensitivity can be obtained by using monochromatic light from a laser.

Agglutination of antigen-coated particles

Whereas the cross-linking of multivalent protein antigens by antibody leads to precipitation, cross-linking of cells or large particles by antibody directed against surface antigens leads to agglutination.

Agglutination reactions are used to identify bacteria and to type red cells. They have been observed with leukocytes and platelets and even with spermatozoa in cases of male infertility due to sperm antibodies.

Immunoassay for antibody using solid-phase antigen

The antibody content of a serum can be assessed by its ability to bind to antigen that has been attached to a plastic tube or micro-agglutination tray with multiple wells. Immunoglobulin (Ig) binding to the antigen may then be detected by addition of a labeled secondary antibody, i.e. an anti-Ig raised in another species (figure 5.5). Consider, for example, the determination of DNA autoantibodies in systemic lupus erythematosus (SLE). When a patient's serum is added to a microwell coated with antigen (in this case DNA), the autoantibodies will bind to the immobilized DNA and remaining serum proteins can be readily washed away. Bound antibody can now be estimated by addition of enzyme-labeled rabbit anti-human IgG. After rinsing out excess unbound reagent, the enzyme activity of the tube will clearly be a measure of the autoantibody content of the patient's serum. The distribution of antibody in different classes can be determined by using specific antisera. For example, to detect IgE antibodies in allergic individuals the allergen such as pollen extract is covalently coupled to a paper disc or plastic well to which is added patient serum. The amount of specific IgE bound to antigen can be estimated by the addition of enzyme-labeled anti-IgE. Enzymes such as horseradish peroxidase and alkaline phosphatase, which give a colored soluble reaction product, are widely employed in these enzyme-linked immunosorbent assays (ELISAs).

Identification and measurement of antigen

Antigens can be readily identified and quantitated *in vitro*, provided that specific antibody is available in the reaction mixture. Laboratory techniques similar to those employed to detect antibodies can be used to

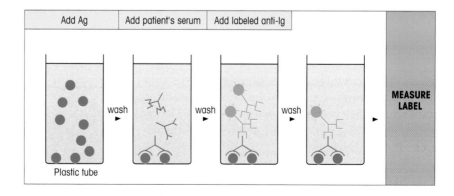

Figure 5.5 Solid-phase immunoassay for antibody. The anti-immunoglobulin (anti-Ig) may be labeled by radioactive iodine or, more usually, by an enzyme which gives a soluble colored or chemiluminescent reaction product. Ag, antigen.

detect antigens. For example, precipitation reactions can be carried out in gels to detect an abnormal protein in serum or urine secreted by a B-cell or plasma-cell tumor. The monoclonal paraprotein localizes as a dense compact "M" band of defined electrophoretic mobility, and its antigenic identity is then revealed by immunofixation with specific precipitating anti-serums applied in paper strips overlying parallel lanes in the electrophoresis gel.

The nephelometric assay for antigen

If antigen is added to a solution of excess antibody, the amount of complex assessed by forward light scatter in a nephelometer is linearly related to the concentration of antigen. With the ready availability of a huge range of monoclonal antibodies which facilitate the standardization of the method, nephelometry is commonly used to detect a wide array of serum proteins including Igs, C3, C4, haptoglobin, ceruloplasmin and C-reactive protein (CRP).

Immunoassay on multiple microspots

The field of DNA microarray technology has led to the area of miniaturization of immunoassays. This depends on spotting multiple antigens, or when necessary antibodies, in an ordered dense array on a solid support such as a glass slide. Patient serum or other bodily fluid is layered over the slide and the presence of binding is detected with chemiluminescent or enzyme-labeled secondary antibodies. Expression is recorded by sophisticated analytical apparatus and stored in a database. Sensitivities compare very favorably with the best immunoassays and, with such miniaturization, arrays of microspots which capture antibodies of different specificities can be placed on a single chip. This opens the door to multiple analyte screening in a single test, with each analyte being identified by its grid coordinates in the array.

WHAT THE T-CELL SEES

We have on several occasions alluded to the fact that the TCR sees antigen on the surface of cells associated with a major histocompatibility complex (MHC) class I or II molecule. Now is the time for us to go into the nuts and bolts of this relationship.

Haplotype restriction reveals the need for MHC participation

It has been established that T-cells bearing $\alpha\beta$ recep-

tors, with some exceptions, only respond when the antigen-presenting cells (APCs) express the same MHC haplotype as the host from which the T-cells were derived. This **haplotype restriction** on T-cell recognition tells us unequivocally that MHC molecules are intimately and necessarily involved in the interaction of the antigen-bearing cell with its corresponding antigen-specific T-lymphocyte. We also learn that cytotoxic T-cells recognize antigen in the context of class I MHC, and helper T-cells respond when the antigen is associated with class II molecules on APCs.

One of the seminal observations which helped to elucidate the role of the MHC was the dramatic Nobel Prize-winning revelation by Peter Doherty and Rolf Zinkernagel that cytotoxic T-cells taken from an individual recovering from a viral infection will only kill virally infected cells which share an MHC haplotype with the host. For example, on recovery from influenza, individuals bearing the MHC haplotype HLA-A2 have $CD8^+$ T-cells which kill HLA-A2 target cells infected with influenza virus but not cells of a different HLA-A tissue-type specificity.

T-cells recognize a linear peptide sequence from the antigen

With any complex antigen only certain linear peptides can be recognized by a specific T-cell. When clones of identical specificity are derived from these T-cells, each clone reacts with only one of the peptides; in other words, like B-cell clones, each clone is specific for one corresponding epitope. Therefore, when either cytotoxic or helper T-cell clones are stimulated by APCs to which certain peptides derived from the original antigen had been added, the clones can be activated. By synthesizing a series of such peptides, the T-cell epitope can be mapped with some precision.

The conclusion is that the **T-cell recognizes both MHC and peptide**, and we now know that the peptide which acts as a T-cell epitope lies along the groove formed by the α-helices and the β-sheet floor of the class I and class II outermost domains. Just how does it get there?

PROCESSING OF INTRACELLULAR ANTIGEN FOR PRESENTATION BY CLASS I MHC

Within the cytosol lurk proteolytic structures, the **proteasomes**, involved in the routine turnover and cellular degradation of proteins. Cytosolic proteins destined for antigen presentation, including viral pro-

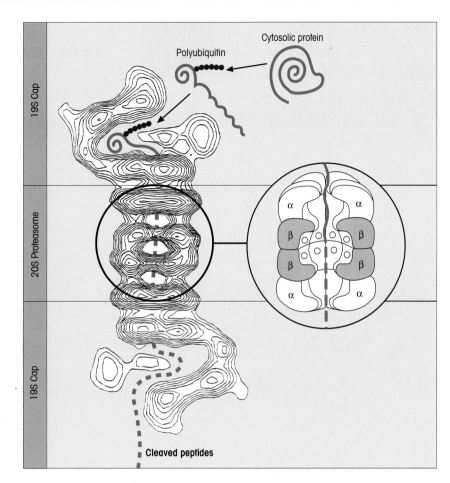

Figure 5.6 Cleavage of cytosolic proteins by the proteasome. The whole 26S protease complex consisting of the 20S proteasome with twin 19S caps is displayed as a contour plot derived from electron microscopy and image analysis. The cross-section of the proteasome reveals the sites of peptidase activity (o) within the inner core of the seven-membered rings of β-subunits. (Based on J.-M. Peters *et al.* (1993) *Journal of Molecular Biology*, **234**, 932–7 and D.M. Rubin & D. Finley (1995) *Current Biology*, **5**, 854–8.)

teins, link to a small polypeptide called ubiquitin and are fed into a specialized proteasome, the immunoproteasome, where they are degraded (figure 5.6). The degraded peptides now attach to transporter proteins called TAP1/TAP2 (transporters associated with antigen processing) which moves them into the endoplasmic reticulum (ER). The immunoproteasome contains the nonpolymorphic MECL-1 molecule together with two MHC-linked low molecular weight proteins, LMP2 and LMP7, which are polymorphic and may serve to optimize delivery of the peptides to the TAP1/TAP2 (figure 5.7). Now within the lumen of the ER, the peptides complex with the membrane-bound class I MHC molecules thereby releasing peptide from their association with the TAP transporter. Thence, the complex traverses the Golgi stack, presumably picking up carbohydrate side-chains en route, and reaches the surface where it is a sitting target for the cytotoxic T-cell. It is worth pointing out at this stage that the cytokine interferon γ (IFNγ), which is actively produced by T-cells during cell-mediated immune responses, increases the production of the proteasomal subunits

LMP2 and LMP7 and thereby amplifies antigen processing.

PROCESSING OF ANTIGEN FOR CLASS II MHC PRESENTATION FOLLOWS A DIFFERENT PATHWAY

Class II MHC complexes with antigenic peptide are generated by a fundamentally different intracellular mechanism, since the APCs which interact with T-helper cells need to sample the antigen from both the *extra*cellular and *intra*cellular compartments. In essence, a trans-Golgi vesicle containing class II has to intersect with a late endosome containing exogenous protein antigen taken into the cell by an endocytic mechanism.

First let us consider the class II molecules themselves. These are assembled from α and β chains in the ER in association with the transmembrane **invariant chain** (figure 5.8), which has several functions. It acts as a dedicated chaperone to ensure correct folding of the nascent class II molecule and it inhibits the

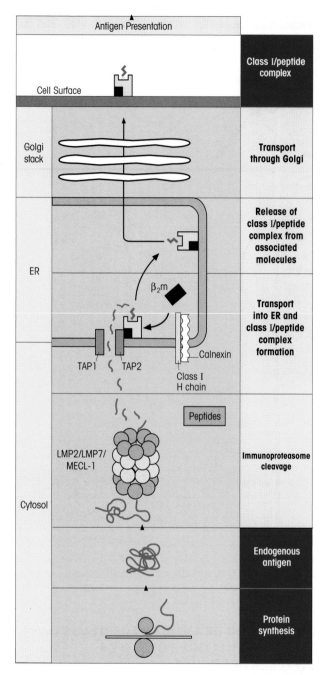

Figure 5.7 Processing and presentation of endogenous antigen by class I major histocompatibility complex (MHC). Cytosolic proteins are degraded by the proteasome complex into peptides which are transported into the endoplasmic reticulum (ER). There, they bind to membrane-bound class I MHC formed by β₂-microglobulin (β₂m)-induced dissociation of nascent class I heavy chains from their calnexin chaperone. The peptide/MHC complex is now released from its association with the TAP transporter, traverses the Golgi system, and appears on the cell surface ready for presentation to the T-cell receptor.

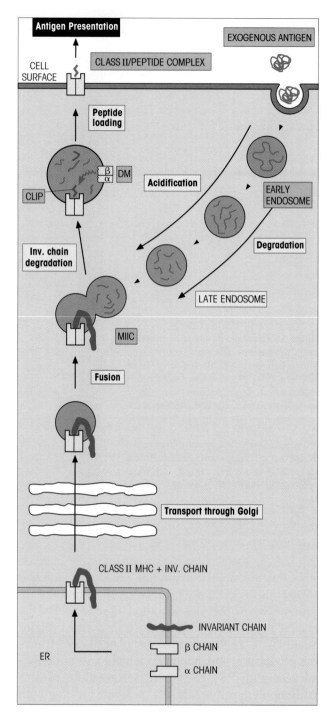

Figure 5.8 Processing and presentation of exogenous antigen by class II major histocompatibility complex (MHC). Class II molecules with invariant chain are assembled in the endoplasmic reticulum (ER) and transported through the Golgi to the trans-Golgi reticulum. There they are sorted to a late endosomal vesicle with lysosomal characteristics known as MIIC (meaning MHC class II enriched compartment) containing partially degraded protein derived from the endocytic uptake of exogenous antigen. Degradation of invariant chains leaves the CLIP (class II-associated invariant chain peptide) peptides lying in the groove but, under the influence of the MHC-related dimeric molecule (DM), they are replaced by other peptides in the vesicle including those derived from exogenous antigen, and the complexes are transported to the cell surface for presentation to T-helper cells.

precocious binding of peptides in the ER before the class II reaches the endocytic compartment containing antigen. Additionally, combination of the invariant chain with the αβ class II heterodimer inactivates a retention signal and allows transport to the Golgi.

Meanwhile, exogenous protein is taken up by endocytosis and is subjected to partial degradation as the early endosome undergoes progressive acidification. The late endosome having many of the characteristics of a lysosomal granule now fuses with the vacuole containing the class II-invariant chain complex. Under the acidic conditions within this MHC class II-enriched compartment the invariant chain is degraded and replaced with other vesicular peptides, after which the complexes are transported to the membrane for presentation to T-helper cells.

Processing of antigens for class II presentation is not confined to soluble proteins taken up from the exterior but can also encompass proteins and peptides within the ER, and microorganisms whose antigens reach the lysosomal structures, either after direct phagocytosis or prolonged intracellular cohabitation. Conversely, class I-restricted responses can be generated against exogenous antigens. This may occur either by a TAP-dependent pathway in phagocytic cells where proteins are transferred from the phagosome to the cytosol, or by endocytosis of cell surface MHC class I molecules which then arrive in the class II-enriched compartments where peptide exchange occurs with sequences derived from the endocytic processing pathway.

Binding to MHC class I

The peptides binding along the length of the groove are predominantly 8–9 residues long. Except in the case of viral infection, the natural class I ligands will be self peptides derived from proteins endogenously synthesized by the cell, histones, heat-shock proteins, enzymes, leader signal sequences and so on. It turns out that 75% or so of these peptides originate in the cytosol.

Binding to MHC class II

The open nature of the class II groove places no constraint on the length of the peptide, which can dangle nonchalantly from each end of the groove, quite unlike the straitjacket of the class I ligand site (figure 5.9). Thus, each class II molecule binds a collection of peptides with a spectrum of lengths ranging from 8 to 30 mers.

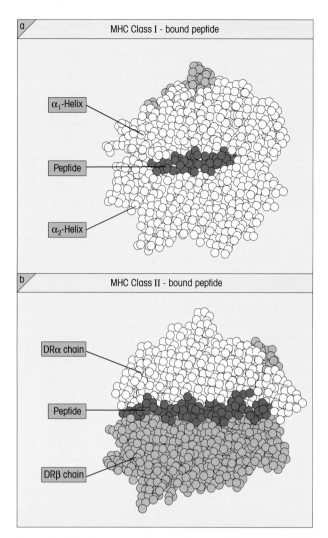

Figure 5.9 Binding of peptides to the major histocompatibility complex (MHC) cleft. T-cell receptor "view" looking down on the α-helices lining the cleft represented in space-filling models. (a) Peptide 309–317 from HIV-1 reverse transcriptase bound tightly within the class I HLA-A2 cleft. (b) Influenza hemagglutinin 306–318 lying in the class II HLA-DR1 cleft. In contrast with class I, the peptide extends out of both ends of the binding groove. (Based on D.A.A. Vignali & J.L. Strominger (1994) *The Immunologist*, **2**, 112, with permission of the authors and publisher.)

T-CELLS WITH A DIFFERENT OUTLOOK

The family of CD1 non-MHC class I-like molecules can present exotic antigens

After MHC class I and class II, the CD1 family represents a third lineage of antigen-presenting molecules recognized by T-lymphocytes. The CD1 polypeptide chain also associates with β$_2$-microglobulin and the overall structure is similar to that of classical class I molecules. CD1 molecules present lipid and glycolipid microbial antigens, especially those derived from *Mycobacterium tuberculosis* to T-cells. Because antigen recognition by CD1-restricted T-cells involves clonally diverse αβ and γδ TCRs, it is likely that CD1 can present a broad range of such antigens. Just like their proteinaceous colleagues, exogenously derived lipid and glycolipid antigens are delivered to the acidic endosomal compartment. Antigens derived from endogenous pathogens can also be presented by the CD1 pathway, but in a process that, unlike class I-mediated presentation, is independent of TAP.

Some T-cells have natural killer (NK) markers

A group of T-cells which possess various markers characteristic of NK cells, together with a TCR, are called NK-T-cells or NK1.1$^+$ T-cells. These cells are a major component of the T-cell compartment, accounting for 20–30% of T-cells in bone marrow and liver, and up to 1% of spleen cells. They are most abundant in the liver, and unique molecular and cellular mechanisms control their migration and/or retention in this organ.

The NK-T-cells rapidly secrete high levels of interleukin-4 (IL-4) and IFNγ following stimulation and therefore have important regulatory functions. Although substantial numbers of NK-T-cells are CD1-restricted, others are restricted by classical MHC molecules indicating that there are subsets within this group.

γδ T-cell receptors have some features of antibody

Unlike αβ T-cells, γδ T-cells recognize antigens directly without a requirement for antigen processing. Whilst some T-cells bearing a γδ receptor are capable of recognizing MHC molecules, neither the polymorphic residues associated with peptide binding nor the peptide itself are involved. Thus, a γδ T-cell clone specific for the herpes simplex virus glycoprotein-1 can be stimulated by the native protein bound to plastic, suggesting that the cells are triggered by cross-linking of their receptors by antigen, which they recognize in the intact native state just as antibodies do. The X-ray crystallographic structure of a TCR variable domain highlights that the γδ TCR indeed incorporates key structural elements of both Ig and TCR V regions.

γδ T-cells can be stimulated by a variety of antigens including heat-killed bacteria, bacterial extracts and both peptide and non-peptide components of *Mycobacterium tuberculosis*. Stressed or damaged cells appear to be powerful activators of γδ cells, and there is evidence that molecules such as heat-shock proteins can stimulate γδ T-cells. Low molecular weight non-proteinaceous antigens, such as isopentenyl pyrophosphate and ethyl phosphate, which occur in a range of microbial and mammalian cells, have been identified as potent stimulators. In fact, responses of γδ T-cells are evident in almost every infectious disease. There is now extensive evidence that these cells are important in terminating host immune responses. This is mediated by activated γδ T-cells which acquire cytotoxic activity and kill stimulatory macrophages, leading to resolution of inflammatory immune responses and prevention of chronic inflammatory disease.

The above characteristics provide the γδ cells with a distinctive role complementary to that of the αβ population and enable them to function in the recognition of microbial pathogens and damaged or stressed host cells as well as regulating immune responses.

SUPERANTIGENS STIMULATE WHOLE FAMILIES OF LYMPHOCYTE RECEPTORS

Bacterial toxins represent one major group of T-cell superantigens

Individual peptides complexed to MHC will react only with antigen-specific T-cells, which represent a relatively small percentage of the T-cell pool. Molecules called superantigens stimulate the 5–20% of the total T-cell population, which express the same TCR Vβ family structure irrespective of their antigen specificity. Superantigens include *Staphylococcus aureus* enterotoxins (staphylococcal enterotoxin A, SEA; staphylococcal enterotoxin B, SEB; and several others), which are single-chain proteins responsible for food poisoning. They are strongly mitogenic for T-cells expressing particular Vβ families in the presence of MHC class II accessory cells. Superantigens are not processed by the APC, but cross-link the class II and Vβ independently of direct interaction between MHC and TCR molecules (figure 5.10). Staphylococcal enterotoxin A is one of the most potent T-cell mitogens known, causing marked T-cell proliferation with release of copious amounts of cytokines, including IL-2 and lymphotoxin. Superantigens can also cause the release of mast cell leukotrienes, and this probably forms the basis of toxic shock syndrome. This is a multisystem febrile illness caused by staphylococci or Group A streptococci seen more often in menstruating women using tampons. It is due to bacterial toxins acting as superantigens, inducing sustained release of inflammatory mediators from T-cells, macrophages and mast cells.

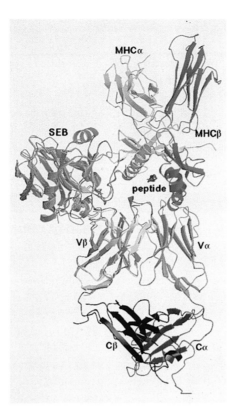

Figure 5.10 Interaction of superantigen with major histocompatibility complex (MHC) and T-cell receptor (TCR). In this composite model, the interaction with the superantigen staphylococcal enterotoxin B (SEB) involves SEB wedging itself between the TCR Vβ chain and the MHC, effectively preventing interaction between the TCR and the peptide in the groove, and between the TCR β chain and the MHC. Thus, direct contact between the TCR and the MHC is limited to Vα amino acid residues. (Reproduced from H. Li *et al.* (1999) *Annual Review of Immunology* **17**, 435–66, with permission.)

REVISION

The nature of antigens
- An antigen is defined by its antibody. The contact area with an antibody is called an **epitope** and the corresponding area on an antibody is a **paratope**.
- Antisera recognize a series of dominant epitope clusters on the surface of an antigen; each cluster is called a determinant.

Antigens and antibodies interact by spatial complementarity, not by covalent binding
- The forces of interaction include electrostatic, hydrogen-bonding, hydrophobic and van der Waals.
- Antigen–antibody bonds are readily **reversible**.
- Antigens and antibodies are mutually deformable.
- The strength of binding to a single antibody combining site is measured by the **affinity**.
- The reaction of multivalent antigens with the heterogeneous mixture of antibodies in an antiserum is defined by **avidity (functional affinity)**.
- **Specificity** of antibodies is not absolute and they may cross-react with other antigens to different extents measured by their relative avidities.

In vitro antigen–antibody reactions
- Antibody can be detected in serum or other fluids by its ability to bind to specific antigens.
- The level of antibodies in a solution is called the antibody titer.

Numerous techniques are available for the estimation of antibody
- Antibody in solution can be assayed by the formation of frank precipitates which can be enhanced by countercurrent electrophoresis in gels.

(*continued*)

- Nonprecipitating antibodies can be measured by laser nephelometry.
- Antibodies can also be detected by macroscopic agglutination of antigen-coated particles, and by enzyme-linked immunosorbent assays (ELISA), a two-stage procedure in which antibody bound to solid-phase antigen is detected by an enzyme-linked anti-immunoglobulin (anti-Ig).

Identification and measurement of antigen

- Antigens can be quantified by their reaction in gels with antibody using single radial immunodiffusion.
- Higher concentrations of antigens are frequently estimated by nephelometry.
- Spotting multiple antigens or antibodies onto glass slides or chips can miniaturize immunoassays. This will allow multiple analyte screening in a single test.

T-cell recognition

- $\alpha\beta$ T-cells see antigen in association with major histocompatibility complex (MHC) molecules.
- They are restricted to the haplotype of the cell that first primed the T-cell.
- Protein antigens are processed by antigen-presenting cells (APCs) to form small linear peptides which associate with the MHC molecules, binding to the central groove formed by the α-helices and the β-sheet floor.

Processing of antigen for presentation by class I MHC

- Endogenous cytosolic antigens such as viral proteins link to ubiquitin and are cleaved by proteasomes. The peptides so-formed are transported to the endoplasmic reticulum (ER) by the TAP1/TAP2 system.
- The peptide then dissociates and forms a stable heterotrimer with newly synthesized class I MHC heavy chain and β_2-microglobulin.
- This peptide–MHC complex is then transported to the surface for presentation to cytotoxic T-cells.

Processing of antigen for presentation by class II MHC

- The $\alpha\beta$ **class II molecule** is synthesized in the ER and complexes with membrane-bound **invariant chain**.
- This facilitates transport of the vesicles containing class II across the Golgi and directs it to the late endosomal compartment.

- The antigen is degraded to peptides which bind to class II now free of invariant chain.
- The **class II-peptide** complex now appears on the cell surface for presentation to T-helper cells.

The nature of the peptide

- Class I peptides are held in extended conformation within the MHC groove.
- They are usually 8–9 residues in length.
- Class II peptides are between 8 and 30 residues long and extend beyond the groove.

T-cells with a different outlook

- CD1 molecules present lipid and glycolipid antigens to T-cells.
- Both exogenous and endogenous lipids can be presented by CD1.
- A group of T-cells, which in addition to a T-cell receptor (TCR) also have natural killer (NK) cell markers, are called NK-T-cells.
- NK-T-cells produce cytokines such as interleukin-4 (IL-4) and interferon γ (IFNγ) which are important in regulating immune responses.

$\gamma\delta$ T-cells

- This subpopulation of T-cells can recognize antigen in its native, unprocessed state.
- These cells are activated by stressed or damaged cells and by numerous bacteria
- $\gamma\delta$ T-cells play an important regulatory role in terminating immune responses by killing activated macrophages.

Superantigens

- These are potent mitogens that stimulate whole T-cell subpopulations sharing the same TCR Vβ family independently of antigen specificity.
- *Staphylococcus aureus* enterotoxins are powerful human superantigens that cause food poisoning and toxic shock syndrome.
- They are not processed but cross-link MHC class II and TCR Vβ independently of their direct interaction.

See the accompanying website (**www.roitt.com**) for multiple choice questions

FURTHER READING

Carding, S.R., & Egan, P.J. (2000) The importance of γδ T cells in the resolution of pathogen-induced inflammatory immune response. *Immunological Reviews*, **173**, 98–108.

Eisen, H.N. (2001) Specificity and degeneracy in antigen recognition: Yin and yang in the immune system. *Annual Review of Immunology*, **19**, 1–21.

van den Elsen, P.J. & Rudensky, A. (eds) (2004) Section on antigen processing and recognition. *Current Opinion in Immunology*, **16**, 63–125.

Hennecke, J. & Wiley, D.C. (2001) T cell receptor–MHC interactions up close. *Cell*, **104**, 1–4.

Moss, D.J. & Khanna, R. (1999) Major histocompatibility complex: From genes to function. *Immunology Today*, **20**, 165–7.

Van den Eynde, B.J. & Morel, S. (2001) Differential processing of class I-restricted epitopes by the standard proteasome and the immunoproteasome. *Current Opinion in Immunology*, **13**, 147–53.

CHAPTER 6

The anatomy of the immune response

THE SURFACE MARKERS OF CELLS IN THE IMMUNE SYSTEM

In order to discuss the events that occur in the operation of the immune system as a whole, it is imperative to establish a nomenclature which identifies the surface markers on the cells involved. These are usually functional molecules reflecting the state of cellular differentiation. The nomenclature system is established as follows. Immunologists from the far corners of the world who have produced monoclonal antibodies directed to surface molecules on cells involved in the immune response get together every so often to compare the specificities of their reagents in international workshops. Where a cluster of monoclonals are found to react with the same polypeptide, they clearly represent a series of reagents defining a given marker and we label it with a CD (**cluster of differentiation**) number. There are now over 250 CD specificities assigned and some of them are shown in table 6.1.

Detection of surface markers

Because fluorescent dyes such as fluorescein and rhodamine can be coupled to antibodies without destroying their specificity, the conjugates can combine with antigen present in a tissue section and be visualized in the fluorescence microscope (figure 6.1a). In this way the distribution of antigen throughout a tissue and within cells can be demonstrated.

In place of fluorescent markers, other workers have evolved methods in which enzymes such as alkaline phosphatase or horseradish peroxidase are coupled to antibodies and these can be visualized by conventional histochemical methods at the level of both the light microscope (figure 6.1b) and the electron microscope.

When enumerating cells in suspensions such as in blood or other fluids, surface antigens can be detected by the use of labeled antibodies. It is possible to stain single cells with several different fluorochromes and analyse the cells in individual droplets as they flow past a laser beam in a flow cytometer. The laser light excites the fluorochrome and the intensity of the fluorescence is measured by detectors (fig 6.2). With the impressive number of monoclonal antibodies to hand, highly detailed phenotypic analysis of single-cell populations is now a practical proposition. Of the ever-growing number of applications, the contribution to diagnosis and classification of leukemia and lymphoma is quite notable.

THE NEED FOR ORGANIZED LYMPHOID TISSUE

For an effective immune response an intricate series of cellular events must occur. Antigen must bind and if necessary be processed by antigen-presenting cells (APCs), which must then make contact with and activate T- and B-cells. In addition T-helper cells must assist certain B-cells and cytotoxic T-cell precursors to perform their functions, which include amplification of the numbers of potential effector cells by proliferation and the generation of the mediators of humoral and cellular immunity. In addition, memory cells for secondary responses must be formed and the whole

Table 6.1 Some of the major clusters of differentiation (CD) markers on human cells.

CD	Expression	Functions
CD1	IDC, B subset	Presents glycolipid and other non-peptide antigens to T-cells
CD2	T, NK	Receptor for CD58 (LFA-3) costimulator. Binds sheep rbc
CD3	T	Transducing elements of T-cell receptor
CD4	T-helper, Mo, Mφ	MHC class II. HIV receptor
CD5	T, B subset	Involved in antigen receptor signaling
CD8	T-cytotoxic	MHC class I receptor
CD14	G, Mo, Mφ	LPS/LBP complex receptor
CD16	G, NK, B, Mφ, IDC	FcγRIII (medium affinity IgG receptor)
CD19	B, FDC	Part of B-cell antigen receptor complex
CD20	B	Unknown, but able to provide intracellular signals
CD21	B, FDC	CR2. Receptor for C3d and Epstein–Barr virus. Part of B-cell antigen receptor complex
CD23	B, Mo, FDC	FcεRII (low affinity IgE receptor)
CD25	*T, *B, *Mo, *Mφ	IL-2 receptor α chain
CD28	T, *B	Receptor for CD80/CD86 (B7.1 and B7.2) costimulators
CD32	Mo, Mφ, IDC, FDC, G, NK, B,	FcγRII (low affinity IgG receptor)
CD34	Progenitors	Adhesion molecule. Stem cell marker
CD40	B, Mφ, IDC, FDC	Receptor for CD40L costimulator
CD45RA	Resting/Naive T-cells, B, G, Mo, NK	Phosphatase, cell activation
CD45RO	Activated/Memory T-cells, Mo, DC	Phosphatase, cell activation
CD64	Mo, Mφ, DC	FcγRI (high affinity IgG receptor)
CD79a/CD79b	B	Transducing elements of B-cell receptor
CD80	*B, *T, Mφ, DC	B7.1 receptor for CD28 costimulator and for CTLA4 inhibitory signal
CD86	B, IDC, Mo	B7.2 receptor for CD28 costimulator and for CTLA4 inhibitory signal
CD95	Widespread	Fas. Receptor for FasL. Transmits apoptotic signals

*, activated; B, B-lymphocytes; FDC, follicular dendritic cells; G, granulocytes; IDC, interdigitating dendritic cells; Mφ, macrophages; Mo, monocytes; NK, natural killer cells; T, T-lymphocytes.

response controlled so that it is adequate but not excessive and is appropriate to the type of infection being dealt with. The integration of the complex cellular interactions which form the basis of the immune response takes place within the organized architecture of peripheral, or secondary, lymphoid tissue, which includes the lymph nodes, spleen and unencapsulated tissue lining the respiratory, gastrointestinal and genitourinary tracts.

These tissues become populated by cells of reticular origin and by macrophages and lymphocytes derived from bone marrow stem cells; the T-cells first differentiating into immunocompetent cells by a high-intensity training period in the thymus, the B-cells undergoing their education in the bone marrow itself (figure 6.3). In essence, the lymph nodes filter off and, if necessary, respond to foreign material draining body tissues, the spleen monitors the blood, and the unencapsulated lymphoid tissue is strategically integrated into mucosal surfaces of the body as a forward defensive system based on immunoglobulin A (IgA) secretion. The bone marrow also contributes substantially to antibody production.

Communication between these tissues and the rest of the body is maintained by a pool of recirculating lymphocytes which pass from the blood into the lymph nodes, spleen and other tissues and back to the blood by the major lymphatic channels such as the thoracic duct (figure 6.4).

LYMPHOCYTES TRAFFIC BETWEEN LYMPHOID TISSUES

This traffic of lymphocytes between the tissues, the bloodstream and the lymph nodes enables antigen-sensitive cells to seek the antigen and to be recruited to sites at which a response is occurring, while the dissemination of memory cells enables a more widespread response to be organized throughout the lymphoid system. Thus, antigen-reactive cells are depleted from the circulating pool of lymphocytes within 24h of antigen first localizing in the lymph nodes or spleen; several days later, after proliferation at the site of antigen localization, a peak of activated cells appears in the thoracic duct.

Lymphocytes home to their specific tissues

Naive lymphocytes enter a lymph node through the afferent lymphatics and by guided passage across the specialized **high-walled endothelium of the postcapillary venules (HEVs)** (figure 6.5). Comparable HEVs offer the transit of cells concerned with mucosal immu-

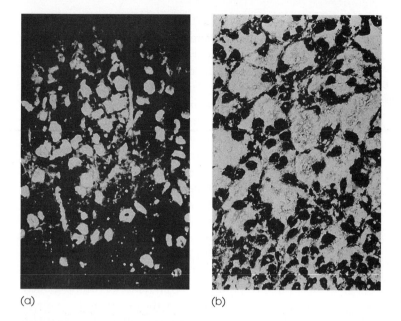

(a)   (b)

Figure 6.1 Staining of gastric parietal cells by (a) fluorescein (white cells) and (b) peroxidase-linked antibody (black cells). The sections were sequentially treated with human parietal cell autoantibodies and then with the conjugated rabbit anti-human immunoglobulin G (IgG). The enzyme was visualized by the peroxidase reaction. (Courtesy of Miss V. Petts.)

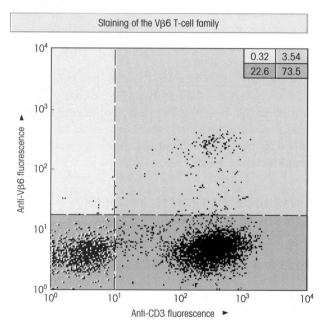

Figure 6.2 Cytofluorometric analysis of human peripheral blood lymphocytes. Cells stained with fluoresceinated anti-T-cell receptor (TCR) Vβ6 and phycoerythrin conjugated anti-CD3. Each dot represents an individual lymphocyte and the numbers refer to the percentage of lymphocytes lying within the four quadrants formed by the two gating levels arbitrarily used to segregate positive from negative values. Virtually no lymphocytes bearing the TCRs belonging to the Vβ6 family lack CD3, while 4.6% (3.5 out of 77.0) of the mature T-cells express Vβ6. (Data kindly provided by D. Morrison.)

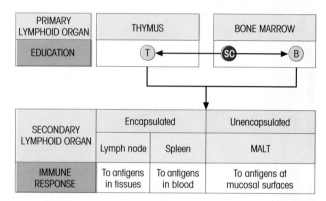

Figure 6.3 The functional organization of lymphoid tissue. Stem cells (SC) arising in the bone marrow differentiate into immunocompetent T- and B-cells in the primary lymphoid organs and then colonize the secondary lymphoid tissues where immune responses are organized. The mucosa-associated lymphoid tissue (MALT) produces the antibodies for mucosal secretions.

nity to Peyer's patches. In other cases involving migration into normal and inflamed tissues, the lymphocytes bind to and cross nonspecialized flatter endothelia in response to locally produced mediators.

This highly organized traffic is orchestrated by directing the relevant lymphocytes to different parts of the lymphoid system and the various other tissues by a series of **homing receptors**. These include members of the integrin superfamily and also a member of the selectin family, L-selectin. These homing receptors recognize their complementary ligands, termed **vascular addressins**, on the surface of the appropriate endothelial cells of the blood vessels. Endothelium expressing these addressins acts as a selective gateway which allows lymphocytes access to the appropriate tissue. Chemokines presented by vascular endothelium play a key role in triggering lymphocyte arrest, the chemokine receptors on the lymphocyte being involved in the functional upregulation of integrin-homing receptors.

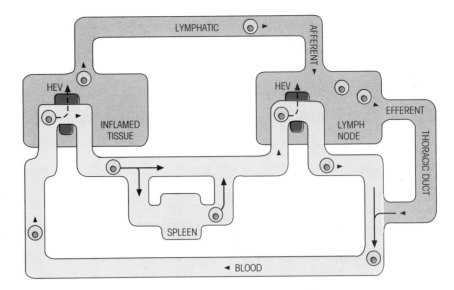

Figure 6.4 Traffic and recirculation of lymphocytes through encapsulated lymphoid tissue and sites of inflammation. Blood-borne lymphocytes enter the tissues and lymph nodes passing through the high-walled endothelium of the postcapillary venules (HEV) and leave via the draining lymphatics. The efferent lymphatics, finally emerging from the last node in each chain, join to form the thoracic duct, which returns the lymphocytes to the bloodstream. In the spleen, lymphocytes enter the lymphoid area (white pulp) from the arterioles, pass to the sinusoids of the erythroid area (red pulp) and leave by the splenic vein. Traffic through the mucosal immune system is elaborated in figure 6.10.

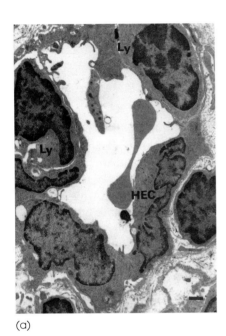

(a)

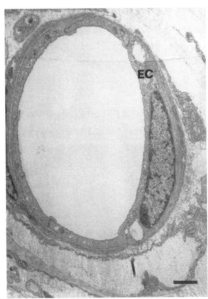

(b)

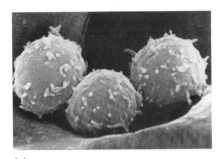

(c)

Figure 6.5 Lymphocyte association with postcapillary venules. (a) High-walled endothelial cells (HEC) of postcapillary venules in rat cervical lymph nodes showing intimate association with lymphocytes (Ly). (b) Flattened capillary endothelial cell (EC) for comparison. (c) Lymphocytes adhering to HEC (scanning electron micrograph). ((a) and (b) kindly provided by Professor Ann Ager and (c) by Dr W. van Ewijk.)

Transmigration

Lymphocytes normally travel in the fast lane down the centre of the blood vessels. However, for the lymphocyte to become attached to the endothelial cell it has to overcome the shear forces that this creates. This is effected by a force of attraction between homing receptors on the lymphocytes and their ligands on the vessel wall. After this tethering process, the lymphocyte rolls along the endothelial cell, partly through the **selectin** interactions but now increasingly through the binding of various **integrins** to their respective ligands.

This process leads to activation and recruitment of members of the β_2-integrin family to the surface of the lymphocyte. In particular, molecules such as LFA-1 (lymphocyte function-associated antigen-1) will become activated and will bind very strongly to ICAM-1 and 2 (intercellular adhesion molecule-1 and 2) on the

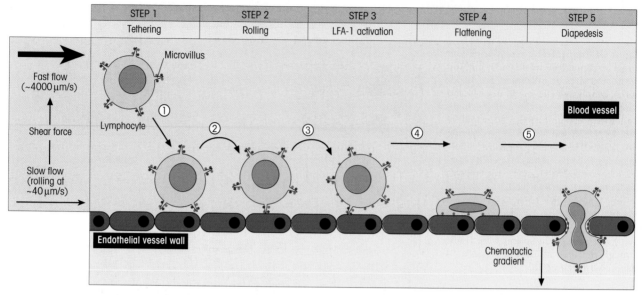

STEP 1	STEP 2	STEP 3	STEP 4	STEP 5
Tethering	Rolling	LFA-1 activation	Flattening	Diapedesis

Figure 6.6 Homing and transmigration of lymphocytes. Fast-moving lymphocytes are tethered (Step 1) to the vessel walls of the tissue they are being guided to enter through an interaction between specific homing receptors and their ligands. After rolling along the surface of the endothelial cells making up the vessel wall, activation of β_2 integrins occurs (Step 3), which leads to firm binding, cell flattening and (Step 5) migration of the lymphocyte between adjacent endothelial cells.

endothelial cell. This intimate contact will cause the lymphocyte to flatten (figure 6.6, step 4) and it may now elbow its way between the endothelial cells and into the tissue (figure 6.6, step 5). Similar homing mechanisms enable lymphocytes bearing receptors for mucosa-associated lymphoid tissue (MALT) to circulate within and between the collections of lymphoid tissue guarding the external body surfaces (see figure 6.10).

ENCAPSULATED LYMPH NODES

The encapsulated tissue of the lymph node contains a meshwork of reticular cells and their fibers organized into sinuses. These act as a filter for lymph draining the body tissues and possibly bearing foreign antigens; this lymph enters the subcapsular sinus by the afferent vessels and diffuses past the lymphocytes in the cortex to reach the macrophages of the medullary sinuses (figure 6.7a,c) and thence the efferent lymphatics. What is so striking about the organization of the lymph node is that the T- and B-lymphocytes are very largely separated into different anatomical compartments.

B-cell areas

The follicular aggregations of B-lymphocytes are a prominent feature of the outer cortex. In unstimulated nodes they are present as spherical collections of cells termed **primary follicles** (figure 6.7f), which are composed of a mesh of follicular dendritic cells (FDCs). Spaces within this meshwork are filled with recirculating but resting small B-lymphocytes. After antigenic challenge they form **secondary follicles** which consist of a corona or mantle of concentrically packed, resting, small B-lymphocytes possessing both IgM and IgD on their surface surrounding a pale-staining **germinal center** (figure 6.7b,c). This contains large, usually proliferating, B-blasts and a tight network of specialized FDCs. Germinal centers are greatly enlarged in secondary antibody responses (figure 6.7d), and they are regarded as important sites of B-cell maturation and the generation of B-cell memory.

A proportion of the B-cells that are shunted down the **memory** cell pathway take up residence in the mantle zone population, the remainder joining the recirculating B-cell pool. Other cells differentiate into plasmablasts, with a well-defined endoplasmic reticulum, prominent Golgi apparatus and cytoplasmic Ig; these migrate to become plasma cells in the medullary cords of lymphoid cells which project between the medullary sinuses. This maturation of antibody-forming cells at a site distant from that at which antigen triggering has occurred is also seen in the spleen, where plasma cells are found predominantly in the marginal zone. The remainder of the outer cortex is also essentially a B-cell area with scattered T-cells.

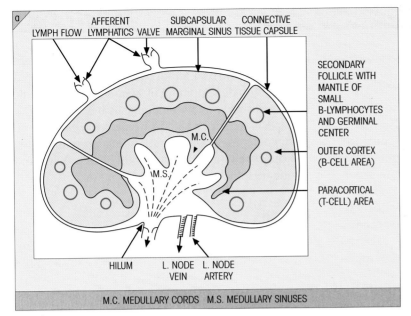

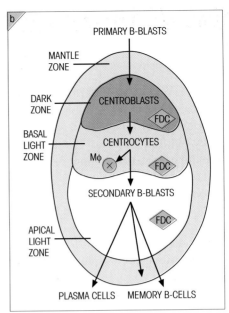

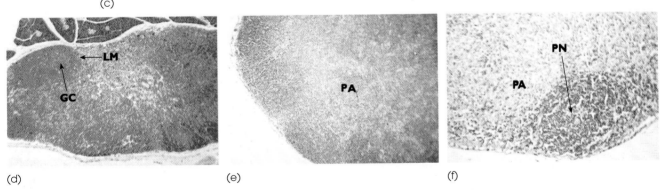

(c)

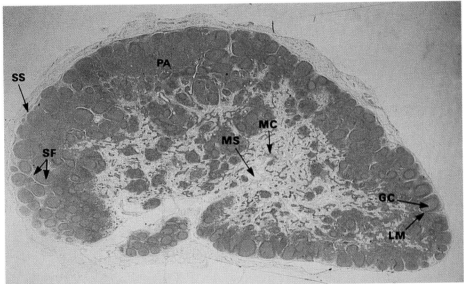

(d)   (e)   (f)

Figure 6.7 Lymph node. (a) Diagrammatic representation of section through a whole node. (b) Diagram showing differentiation of B-cells during passage through different regions of an active germinal center. ×, apoptotic B-cell; FDC, follicular dendritic cell; Mφ, macrophage. (c) Human lymph node, low-power view. GC, germinal center; LM, lymphocyte mantle of SF; MC, medullary cords; MS, medullary sinus; PA, paracortical area; SF, secondary follicle; SS, subcapsular sinus. (d) Secondary lymphoid follicle showing germinal center in a mouse immunized with the thymus-independent antigen, pneumococcus polysaccharide SIII, revealing prominent stimulation of secondary follicles with germinal centers. GC, germi-

nal center; LM, lymphocyte mantle of secondary follicle. (e) Methyl Green/Pyronin stain of lymph node draining site of skin painted with the contact sensitizer oxazolone, highlighting the generalized expansion and activation of the paracortical T-cells, the T-blasts being strongly basophilic. PA, paracortical area. (f) The same study in a neonatally thymectomized mouse shows a lonely primary nodule (follicle) with complete lack of cellular response in the paracortical area. PA, paracortical area; PN, primary nodule. ((c) Courtesy of Professor P.M. Lydyard and (d–f) courtesy of Dr M. de Sousa and Professor D.M.V. Parrott.)

T-cell areas

T-cells are mainly confined to a region referred to as the paracortical (or thymus-dependent) area (figure 6.7a); in nodes taken from children with selective T-cell deficiency (cf. figure 13.4) or neonatally thymectomized mice the paracortical region is seen to be virtually devoid of lymphocytes (figure 6.7f). Furthermore, when a T-cell-mediated response is elicited, say by a skin graft or by exposure to poison ivy which induces contact hypersensitivity, there is a marked proliferation of cells in the thymus-dependent area and typical lymphoblasts are evident (figure 6.7e). In contrast, stimulation of antibody formation by thymus-independent antigens leads to proliferation in the cortical lymphoid follicles with development of germinal centers, while the paracortical region remains inactive (figure 6.7d). As expected, nodes taken from children with congenital hypogammaglobulinemia associated with failure of B-cell development conspicuously lack primary and secondary follicles.

SPLEEN

On a fresh section of spleen, the lymphoid tissue forming the white pulp is seen as circular or elongated gray

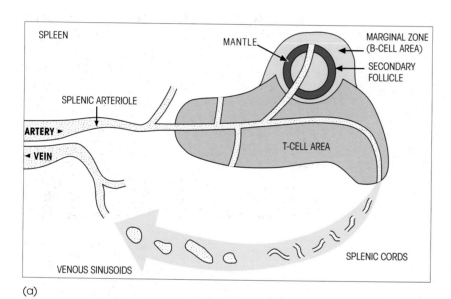

(a)

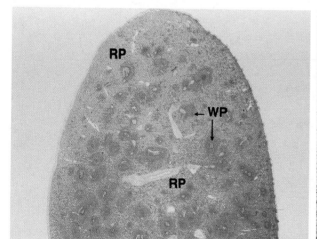

(b)

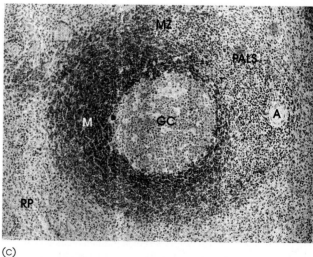

(c)

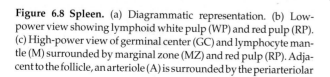

Figure 6.8 Spleen. (a) Diagrammatic representation. (b) Low-power view showing lymphoid white pulp (WP) and red pulp (RP). (c) High-power view of germinal center (GC) and lymphocyte mantle (M) surrounded by marginal zone (MZ) and red pulp (RP). Adjacent to the follicle, an arteriole (A) is surrounded by the periarteriolar lymphoid sheath (PALS) predominantly consisting of T-cells. Note that the marginal zone is only present above the secondary follicle. ((b) Photographs by Professor P.M. Lydyard and (c) by Professor N. Milicevic.)

areas (figure 6.8b,c) within the erythrocyte-filled red pulp, which consists of splenic cords lined with macrophages and venous sinusoids. As in the lymph node, T- and B-cell areas are segregated (figure 6.8a). The spleen is a very effective blood filter, removing effete red and white cells and responding actively to blood-borne antigens, the more so if they are particulate. Plasmablasts and mature plasma cells are present in the marginal zone extending into the red pulp (figure 6.8c).

MUCOSA-ASSOCIATED LYMPHOID TISSUE (MALT)

The respiratory, gastrointestinal and genitourinary tracts are guarded immunologically by subepithelial accumulations of lymphoid tissue which are not constrained by a connective tissue capsule (figure 6.9). These may occur as diffuse collections of lymphocytes, plasma cells and phagocytes throughout the lung and the lamina propria of the intestinal wall (figure 6.9a,b)

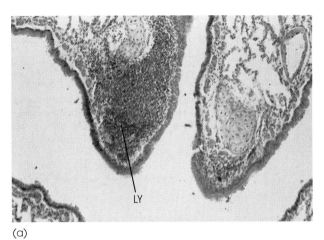

(a)

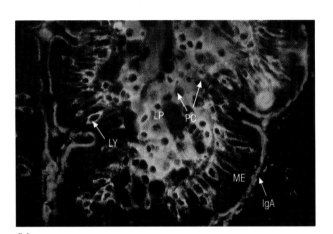

(b)

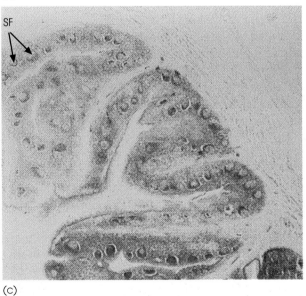

(c)

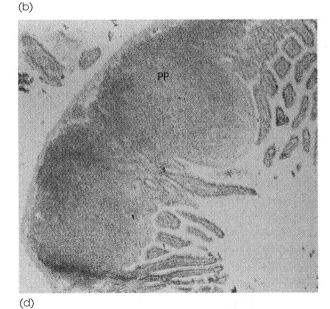

(d)

Figure 6.9 The immunoglobulin A (IgA) secretory immune system (mucosa-associated lymphoid tissue, MALT). (a) Section of lung showing a diffuse accumulation of lymphocytes (LY) in the bronchial wall. (b) Section of human jejunum showing lymphoid cells (LY) stained green by a fluorescent anti-leukocyte monoclonal antibody, in the mucosal epithelium (ME) and in the lamina propria (LP). A red fluorescent anti-IgA conjugate stains the cytoplasm of plasma cells (PC) in the lamina propria and detects IgA in the surface mucus, altogether a super picture! (c) Low-power view of human tonsil showing the MALT with numerous secondary follicles (SF) containing germinal centers. (d) Peyer's patches (PP) in mouse ileum. The T-cell areas are stained brown by a peroxidase-labeled monoclonal antibody to Thy 1. ((a) Kindly provided by Professor P.M. Lydyard, (b) by Professor G. Jannosy, (c) by Mr C. Symes and (d) by Dr E. Andrew.)

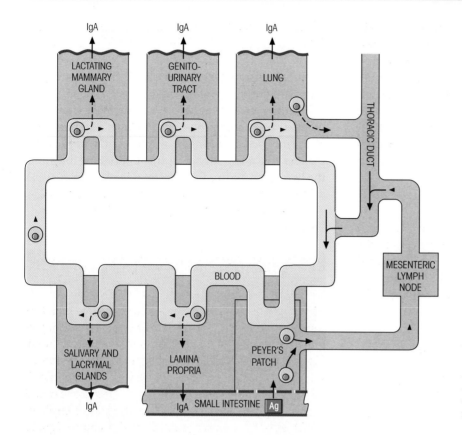

Figure 6.10 Circulation of lymphocytes within the mucosal-associated lymphoid system. Antigen-stimulated cells move from Peyer's patches (and probably lung and maybe all the mucosal member sites) to colonize the lamina propria and the other mucosal surfaces ( ).

or as more clearly organized tissue with well-formed follicles. The latter includes tonsils (figure 6.9c), the small intestinal Peyer's patches (figure 6.9d) and the appendix. Mucosa-associated lymphoid tissue forms a separate interconnected secretory system within which cells committed to IgA or IgE synthesis may circulate.

In the gut, antigen enters the Peyer's patches (figure 6.9d) across specialized epithelial cells called M-cells (cf. figure 6.12) and stimulates the antigen-sensitive lymphocytes. After activation these drain into the lymph and, after a journey through the mesenteric lymph nodes and the thoracic duct, pass from the bloodstream into the lamina propria (figure 6.10). Here they become IgA-forming cells which protect a wide area of the bowel with protective antibody. The cells also appear in the lymphoid tissue of the lung and in other mucosal sites guided by the interactions of specific homing receptors with appropriate HEV addressins as discussed earlier.

Intestinal lymphocytes

The intestinal lamina propria is home to a predominantly activated T-cell population. These T-cells bear a phenotype comparable to that of peripheral blood lymphocytes: viz., > 95% T-cell receptor (TCR) $\alpha\beta$ and a CD4 : CD8 ratio of 7 : 3. There is also a generous sprinkling of activated B-blasts and plasma cells secreting IgA for transport by the poly-Ig receptor to the **intestinal lumen. Intestinal intraepithelial lymphocytes**, however, are different. They are also mostly T-cells but 10–40% are TCR $\gamma\delta^+$ cells. This relatively high proportion of TCR $\gamma\delta$ cells is unusual.

THE ENJOYMENT OF PRIVILEGED SITES

Certain selected parts of the body, brain, anterior chamber of the eye and testis have been designated **privileged immunologic sites**, in the sense that antigens located within them do not provoke reactions against themselves. It has long been known, for example, that foreign corneal grafts are not usually rejected even without immunosuppressive therapy.

Generally speaking, privileged sites are protected by rather strong blood–tissue barriers and low permeability to hydrophilic compounds. Functionally insignificant levels of complement reduce the threat of acute inflammatory reactions and unusually high concentrations of immunomodulators, such as interleukin-10 (IL-10) and transforming growth factor-β (TGFβ) endow macrophages with an immunosuppressive capacity. It has also been shown that tissues in immune privileged sites may constitutively express FasL (Fas-ligand), which by attaching to Fas on infiltrating leukocytes could result in their death by apoptosis. However, inflammatory reactions at the blood–tissue barrier can open the gates to invasion by immunologic marauders—witness the inability of corneal grafts to take in the face of a local pre-existing inflammation.

THE HANDLING OF ANTIGEN

Where does antigen go when it enters the body? If it penetrates the tissues, it will tend to finish up in the draining lymph nodes. Antigens that are encountered in the upper respiratory tract or intestine are trapped by local MALT, whereas antigens in the blood provoke a reaction in the spleen.

Macrophages are general APCs

Antigens draining into lymphoid tissue are taken up by macrophages. They are then partially, if not completely, broken down in the lysosomes; some may escape from the cell in a soluble form to be taken up by other APCs and a fraction may reappear at the surface, as a processed peptide associated with class II major histocompatibility molecules. Some antigens, such as polymeric carbohydrates, cannot be degraded because the macrophages lack the enzymes required; in these instances specialized macrophages in the marginal zone of the spleen or the lymph node subcapsular sinus trap and present the antigen to B-cells directly, apparently without any processing or intervention from T-cells.

Dendritic cells (DCs) are professional APCs

Although macrophages are important APCs there is one function where they are seemingly deficient, namely the priming of naive lymphocytes. This function is performed by DCs of which there are at least two populations. The first is derived from myeloid cells and includes Langerhans' cells in the skin and interdigitating DCs (IDCs) found in all other tissues. The second consist of plasmacytoid DCs that, on exposure to viruses, secrete large amounts of type 1 interferon, a cytokine with potent antiviral activity. In peripheral tissues DCs are in an immature form and express a variety of **pattern recognition receptors** (PRRs), including **Toll-like receptors** (TLRs), that can recognize molecular patterns expressed by pathogens. Once activated by contact with microbial products or by proin-

flammatory cytokines such as tumor necrosis factor (TNF), interferon γ (IFNγ) or IL-1 they undergo maturation into competent APCs, bearing high levels of major histocompatibility complex (MHC), costimulatory and adhesion molecules.

In addition to their antigen-presenting function, DCs are important producers of chemokines, especially T-cell attracting chemokines. Once these cells get together, there are a number of receptor-ligand interactions involved in DC activation of T-cells aside from MHC–peptide recognition by the TCR. These include B7–CD28 and CD40–CD40L (CD40-ligand).

Interdigitating DCs present antigen to T-lymphocytes

The scenario for T-cell priming appears to be as follows. Peripheral immature DCs such as the Langerhans' cells can pick up and process antigen. As their maturation proceeds, they upregulate expression of the chemokine receptor CCR7 and travel as "veiled" cells in the lymph to the paracortical T-cell zone of the draining lymph node. There, its maturation complete, the DC delivers the antigen with costimulatory signals to naive specific T-cells which take advantage of the large surface area to bind to the MHC–peptide complex on the membrane of the DC (figure 6.11). Sites of chronic T-cell inflammation seem to attract these cells, since abnormally high numbers are found closely adhering to activated T-lymphocytes in synovial tissue from patients with ongoing rheumatoid arthritis and in the glands of subjects with chronic autoimmune thyroiditis lesions.

Follicular dendritic cells (FDCs) stimulate B-cells in germinal centers

Another type of cell with dendritic morphology, but this time of mesenchymal origin, is the **FDC**. These are nonphagocytic and lack lysosomes but have very elongated processes which can make contact with numerous lymphocytes present in the germinal centers of secondary follicles. Their surface receptors for IgG Fc and for C3b enable them to trap complexed antigen very efficiently and hold the antigen on their surface for extended periods, in keeping with the memory function of secondary follicles. This would explain how secondary antibody responses can be boosted by quite small amounts of immunogen. These complex with circulating antibody and fix C3 so that they localize very effectively on the surface of the FDCs within the germinal centers of secondary follicles.

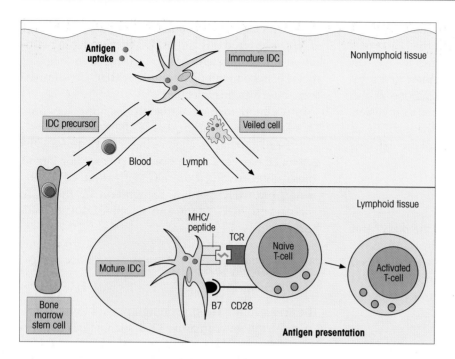

Figure 6.11 Migration and maturation of interdigitating dendritic cells (IDCs). The precursors of the IDCs are derived from bone marrow stem cells. They travel via the blood to nonlymphoid tissues. These immature IDCs, e.g. Langerhans' cells in skin, are specialized for antigen uptake. Subsequently they travel via the afferent lymphatics as veiled cells to take up residence within secondary lymphoid tissues where they express high levels of major histocompatibility complex (MHC) class II and costimulatory molecules such as B7. These cells are highly specialized for the activation of naive T-cells.

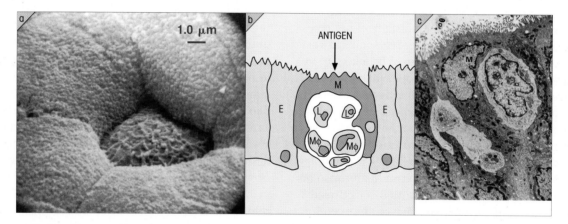

Figure 6.12 M-cell within Peyer's patch epithelium. (a) Scanning electron micrograph of the surface of the Peyer's patch epithelium. The antigen-sampling M-cell in the center is surrounded by absorptive enterocytes covered by closely packed, regular microvilli. Note the irregular and short microfolds of the M-cell. (b) After uptake and transcellular transport by the M-cell (M), antigen is processed by macrophages and thence by dendritic cells, which present antigen to T-cells in Peyer's patches and mesenteric lymph nodes. E, enterocyte; L, lymphocyte; Mφ, macrophage. (c) Electron photomicro-graph of an M-cell (M in nucleus) with adjacent lymphocyte (L in nucleus). Note the flanking epithelial cells are both absorptive enterocytes with a typical brush border. (Lead citrate and uranyl acetate, × 1600.) ((a) Reproduced with permission of the authors and publishers from T. Kato & R.L. Owen (1999) in R. Ogra *et al.* (eds) *Mucosal Immunology*, 2nd edn. Academic Press, San Diego, pp. 115–32; (b) Based on T. Sminia & G. Kraal (1998) in P.J. Delves & I.M. Roitt (eds) *Encyclopedia of Immunology*, 2nd edn. Academic Press, London, p. 188.)

M-cells provide the gateway to the mucosal lymphoid system

The mucosal surface is in the front line facing a very unfriendly sea of microbes and, for the most part, antigens are excluded by the epithelium with its tight junctions and mucous layer. Gut lymphoid tissue, such as Peyer's patches, is separated from the lumen by a single layer of columnar epithelium interspersed with M-cells; these are specialized antigen-transporting cells. They overlay intraepithelial cells and macrophages (figure 6.12). A diverse array of foreign material including bacteria is taken up by M-cells (figure 6.12) and passed on to the underlying APCs which, in turn, migrate to the local lymphoid tissue to stir the appropriate lymphocytes into action.

REVISION

The surface markers of cells in the immune system

• Individual surface molecules are assigned a cluster of differentiation (CD) number defined by a cluster of monoclonal antibodies reacting with that molecule.

• Antigens can be localized if stained by fluorescent antibodies and viewed in an appropriate microscope.

• Antibodies can be labeled by enzymes for histochemical definition of antigens.

• Cells in suspension can be labeled with fluorescent antibodies and analysed in a flow cytometer.

Organized lymphoid tissue

• The complexity of immune responses is catered for by a sophisticated structural organization.

• Lymph nodes filter and screen lymph flowing from the body tissues while spleen filters the blood.

• B- and T-cell areas are separated. B-cell structures appear in the lymph node cortex as primary follicles which become secondary follicles with germinal centers after antigen stimulation.

• Germinal centers with their meshwork of follicular dendritic cells (FDCs) expand B-cell blasts produced by secondary antigen challenge and direct their differentiation into memory cells and antibody-forming plasma cells.

• A pool of recirculating lymphocytes moves from the blood into lymphoid tissue and back again via the major lymphatic channels.

Lymphocyte traffic

• Lymphocyte recirculation between the blood and lymphoid tissues is guided by specialized homing receptors on the surface of the high-walled endothelium of the postcapillary venules (HEV).

• Lymphocytes are tethered and then roll along the surface of the selected endothelial cells through interactions between selectins and integrins and their respective ligands. Flattening of the lymphocyte and transmigration across the endothelial cell follow LFA-1 activation.

• Entry of memory T-cells into sites of inflammation is facilitated by upregulation of integrin molecules on the lymphocyte and corresponding binding ligands on the vascular endothelium.

Lymph nodes and spleen

• Lymphoid follicles consist predominantly of B-cells and FDCs. B-cells may mature into plasma cells.

• T-cells reside in the paracortical areas of the lymph nodes.

Mucosal-associated lymphoid tissue

• Lymphoid tissue guarding the gastrointestinal tract is unencapsulated and somewhat structured (tonsils, Peyer's patches, appendix) or present as diffuse cellular collections in the lamina propria.

• Together with the subepithelial accumulations of cells lining the mucosal surfaces of the respiratory and genitourinary tracts, this lymphoid tissue forms the "secretory immune system" which bathes the surface with protective immunoglobulin A (IgA) antibodies.

Other sites

• Bone marrow is a major site of antibody production.

• The brain, anterior chamber of the eye and testis are privileged sites in which antigens can be safely sequestered.

The handling of antigen

• Macrophages are general antigen-presenting cells (APCs) for primed lymphocytes but cannot stimulate naive T-cells.

• Immature dendritic cells (DCs) are situated in peripheral tissues and recognize and respond to antigen. Once activated they mature, upregulate chemokine receptor CCR7 and migrate to draining lymph nodes where they settle down as interdigitating dendritic cells (IDCs) which powerfully initiate primary T-cell responses.

• Follicular DCs in germinal centers bind immune complexes to their surface through Ig and C3b receptors. The complexes are long-lived and provide a sustained source of antigenic stimulation for B-cells.

• Specialized antigen-transporting M-cells in the gut provide the gateway for antigens to the mucosal lymphoid tissue.

See the accompanying website (**www.roitt.com**) for multiple choice questions

FURTHER READING

Bradley, L.M. & Watson, S.R. (1996) Lymphocyte migration into tissue: The paradigm derived from CD4 subsets. *Current Opinion in Immunology*, **8**, 312–20.

Brandtzaaeg, P., Farstad, I.N. & Haraldsen, G. (1999) Regional specialization in the mucosal immune system: Primed cells do not always home along the same track. *Immunology Today*, **20**, 267–77.

Cavanagh, L.L. & Von Andrian, U.H. (2002) Travellers in many guises: The origins and destinations of dendritic cells. *Immunology and Cell Biology*, **80**, 448–62

Lane, P.J.L. & Brocker, T. (1999) Developmental regulation of dendritic cell function. *Current Opinion in Immunology*, **11**, 308–13.

Peters, J.H., Gieseler, R., Thiele, B. & Steinbach, F. (1996) Dendritic cells: From ontogenetic orphans to myelomonocytic descendants. *Immunology Today* **17**, 273–8.

Lymphocyte activation

IMMUNOCOMPETENT T- AND B-CELLS DIFFER IN MANY RESPECTS

The differences between immunocompetent T- and B-cells are sharply demarcated at the cell surface (table 7.1). The most clear-cut discrimination is established by reagents which recognize anti-CD3 for T-cells and anti-CD19 or anti-CD20 for B-cells. In laboratory practice these are the markers most often used to enumerate the two lymphocyte populations. B-cells also possess surface membrane immunoglobulin (Ig) whilst T-cells bear the T-cell receptor (TCR).

Differences in the cluster of differentiation (CD) markers determined by monoclonal antibodies reflect disparate functional properties and in particular define specialized T-cell subsets. CD4 is, generally speaking, a marker of T-helper cell populations, which promote activation and maturation of B-cells and cytotoxic T-cells, and control antigen-specific chronic inflammatory reactions through stimulation of macrophages. CD4 forms subsidiary links with class II major histocompatibility complex (MHC) molecules on antigen-presenting cells (APCs). Similarly, the CD8 molecules on cytotoxic T-cells associate with MHC class I (figure 7.1).

T-LYMPHOCYTES AND APCs INTERACT THROUGH SEVERAL PAIRS OF ACCESSORY MOLECULES

The affinity of an individual TCR for its specific MHC–antigen peptide complex is relatively low and a sufficiently stable association with the APC can only be achieved by the interaction of complementary pairs of accessory molecules such as LFA-1/ICAM-1 (lymphocyte function-associated antigen-1/intercellular adhesion molecule-1) and CD2/LFA-3 (figure 7.2). However, these molecular couplings are not necessarily concerned just with intercellular adhesion.

THE ACTIVATION OF T-CELLS REQUIRES TWO SIGNALS

It has been known for some time that two signals are required to induce RNA and protein synthesis in a resting T-cell (figure 7.2) and to move it from G0 into the G1 phase of the mitotic cycle. Antigen in association with MHC class II on the surface of APCs is clearly capable of providing one of these signals for the CD4$^+$ T-cell population. Complex formation between the TCR, antigen and MHC thus provides signal 1 through the receptor–CD3 complex, and this is greatly enhanced by the coupling of CD4 with the MHC. The T-cell is now exposed to a costimulatory signal 2 from the APC in the form of two related molecules called B7.1 (CD80) and B7.2 (CD86). These bind to CD28 on the T-helper cell, and also to a receptor called CTLA-4 (cytotoxic T-lymphocyte antigen-4) on activated T-cells. Thus, antibodies to the B7 molecules can block activation of resting T-cells. Surprisingly, this renders the T-cell **anergic**, i.e. unresponsive to any further stimulation by antigen. As we shall see in later chapters, the principle that two signals activate but one may induce anergy in an antigen-specific cell provides a potential for targeted immunosuppressive therapy. A further costimulatory interaction is between CD40 on the APC and

Table 7.1 Comparison of human T- and B-cells.

	T-cells	B-cells
% in peripheral blood	65–80	8–15
ANTIGEN RECOGNITION	Processed	Native
CELL SURFACE MOLECULES		
Antigen receptor	TCR/CD3	Surface Ig
MHC class I	+	+
MHC class II	only after activation	+
CD2	+	–
CD4	MHC class II-restricted (helper)	–
CD5	+	only on B1a minor subset
CD8	MHC class I-restricted (cytotoxic)	–
CD19	–	+
CD20	–	+
CD21 (CR2: C3d and EBV receptor	–	+
CD23 (FcεRII)	–	+
CD32 (FcγRII)	–	+
POLYCLONAL ACTIVATION	Anti-CD3 Phytohemagglutinin	Anti-Ig Epstein-Barr virus

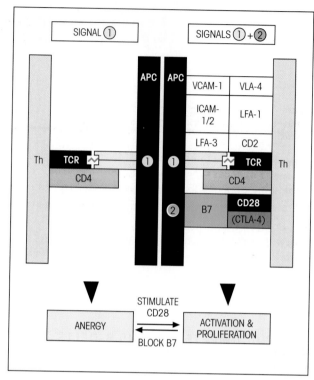

Figure 7.2 Activation of resting T-cells. Interaction of costimulatory molecules leads to activation of resting T-lymphocyte by antigen-presenting cell (APC) on engagement of the T-cell receptor (TCR) with its antigen–major histocompatibility complex (MHC). Engagement of the TCR signal 1 without accompanying costimulatory signal 2 leads to anergy. Note, a cytotoxic rather than a helper T-cell would, of course, involve coupling CD8 to MHC class I. Engagement of the CTLA-4 (cytotoxic T-lymphocyte antigen-4) molecule (CD152) with B7 downregulates signal 1. ICAM-1/2, intercellular adhesion molecule-1/2; LFA-1/2, intercellular adhesion molecule-1/2; VCAM-1, vascular cell adhesion molecule-1; VLA-4, very late integrin antigen-4. (Based on Y. Liu & P.S. Linsley (1992) *Current Opinion in Immunology*, **4**, 265–70.)

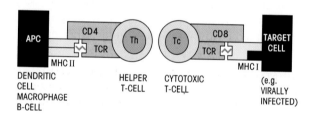

Figure 7.1 Helper and cytotoxic T-cell subsets are restricted by major histocompatibility complex (MHC) class. CD4 on helpers contacts MHC class II; CD8 on cytotoxic cells associates with class I.

PROTEIN TYROSINE PHOSPHORYLATION IS AN EARLY EVENT IN T-CELL SIGNALING

The major docking forces that conjugate the APC and its T-lymphocyte counterpart come from the complementary accessory molecules such as ICAM-1/LFA-1 and LFA-3/CD2, rather than through the relatively low-affinity TCR–MHC/peptide links. Nonetheless, cognate antigen recognition by the TCR remains a *sine qua non* for T-cell activation. Interaction of the TCR with peptide bound to MHC molecules triggers a remarkable cascade of signaling events that culminates in cell cycle progression and cytokine production.

The initial signal for T-cell activation through the TCR is greatly enhanced by bringing the CD4-associated protein tyrosine kinase (PTK), Lck, close to the CD3-

CD40L (CD40-ligand) on the T-cell. Although this interaction does not activate the T-cells directly, it increases the production of the B7 molecules by the APCs and also stimulates these cells to release cytokines that enhance T-cell activity.

Adhesion molecules such as ICAM-1, VCAM-1 (vascular cell adhesion molecule-1) and LFA-3 are not themselves costimulatory but augment the effect of other signals—an important distinction.

Activation of CD8⁺ T-cells requires an interaction of the TCR with peptides within the groove of class I MHC molecules, and costimulatory adhesion molecules also strengthen this interaction. The CD4 and CD8 responses, however, are not separate entities and a variety of cytokines produced by CD4⁺ cells can activate CD8⁺ cells, almost acting as a second signal.

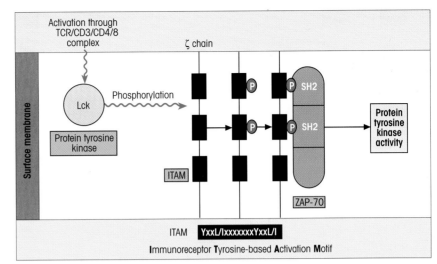

Figure 7.3 Signals through the T-cell receptor (TCR)/CD3/CD4/8 complex initiate a tyrosine protein kinase (TPK) cascade. The TPK Lck phosphorylates the tyrosine within the immunoreceptor tyrosine-based activation motif (ITAM) sequences of CD3 ζ-chains. These bind the ζ-associated protein (ZAP-70) through its SH2 domains and this in turn acquires TPK activity for downstream phosphorylation of later components in the chain. The other CD3 chains each bear a single ITAM.

associated ζ-chains. Immunoreceptor tyrosine-based activation motifs (ITAMs) on the ζ-chains become phosphorylated and bind to ZAP-70, which now becomes an active PTK (figure 7.3) capable of initiating a series of downstream biochemical events. It is now becoming clear that very large numbers of TCRs interact with only a few peptide–MHC complexes, and it has been suggested that each MHC–peptide complex can serially engage up to 200 TCRs. This they do for a prolonged period of time during which the TCRs move across the surface of the APC. The T-cells thereby undergo a sustained increase in intracellular calcium levels which is required for the induction of proliferation and cytokine production.

DOWNSTREAM EVENTS FOLLOWING TCR SIGNALING

Following TCR signaling, there is an early increase in the level of active Ras–GTP (guanosine triphosphate) complexes, which regulate pivotal mitogen-activated protein kinases (MAPKs) through sequential kinase cascades. As illustrated in figure 7.4, there are a number of different pathways involved in T-cell activation.

Within 15 s of TCR stimulation, phospholipase C activates the phosphatidylinositol pathway, is phosphorylated and its catalytic activity increased. This ultimately triggers the release of Ca^{2+} into the cytosol. The raised Ca^{2+} level synergizes with diacylglycerol to activate protein kinase C (PKC) and to act together with calmodulin to increase the activity of calcineurin.

Control of interleukin-2 (IL-2) gene transcription

Transcription of IL-2 is one of the key elements in preventing the signaled T-cell from lapsing into anergy and is controlled by multiple receptors for transcriptional factors in the promoter region (figure 7.4)

Under the influence of calcineurin, NFκB (nuclear factor-kappa B) and $NFAT_c$ (cytoplasmic component of the nuclear factor of activated T-cells) become activated. The NFκB is released from its inhibitor in the cytoplasm, IκB, and then both NFκB and $NFAT_c$ translocates to the nucleus. Here $NFAT_c$ forms a binary complex with $NFAT_n$, its partner which is constitutively expressed in the nucleus, and the NFAT complex together with NFκB bind to IL-2 regulatory sites resulting in cytokine production (figure 7.4). Note here that the calcineurin effect is blocked by the anti-T-cell drugs cyclosporin and FK506 (see Chapter 15).

We have concentrated on IL-2 transcription as an early and central consequence of T-cell activation, but more than 70 genes are newly expressed within 4 h of T-cell activation, leading to proliferation and the synthesis of several cytokines and their receptors.

Damping T-cell enthusiasm

We have frequently reiterated the premise that no self-respecting organism would permit the operation of an expanding enterprise such as a proliferating T-cell population without some sensible controlling mechanisms. Control of T-cell function will be described in Chapter 9, but it is worth pointing out that whereas

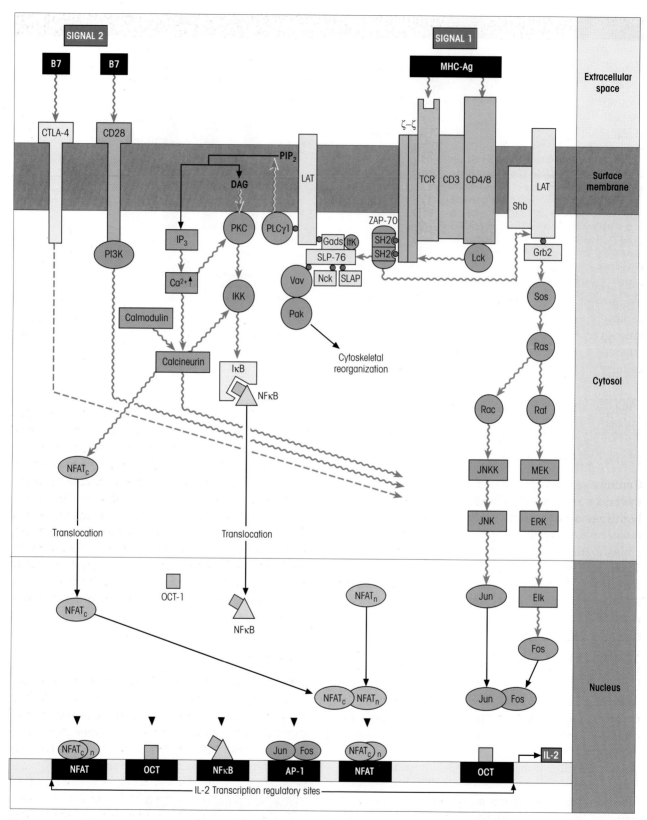

Figure 7.4 T-cell signaling leads to activation. The signals through the MHC (major histocompatibility complex)–antigen complex (signal 1) and costimulator B7 (signal 2) initiate a protein kinase cascade and a rise in intracellular calcium, thereby activating transcription factors which control entry in the cell cycle from G0 and regulate the expression of interleukin-2 (IL-2) and many other cytokines. The scheme presented omits several molecules which are thought to play important additional roles in signal transduction. DAG, diacylglycerol; ERK, extracellular signal regulated kinase; IP$_3$, inositol triphosphate; JNK, Jun N-terminal kinase; LAT, linker for activated T-cells; NFκB, nuclear factor-kappa B; NFAT, nuclear factor of activated T-cell; OCT-1, octamer-binding factor; Pak, p21-activated kinase; PI3K, phosphatidylinositol 3-kinase; PIP$_2$, phosphatidylinositol diphosphate; PKC, protein kinase C; PLC, phospholipase C; SH2, Src-homology domain 2; SLAP, SLP-76-associated phosphoprotein; SLP-76, SH2-domain containing leukocyte-specific 76kDa phosphoprotein; ZAP-70, ζ-chain-associated protein kinase; ⌇⌇⌇➤, positive signal transduction; – – ➤, negative signal transduction; ▢, adapter proteins; ▨, guanine nucleotide exchange factors; ▨, kinases; ▨, transcription factors; ▨, other molecules.

CD28 is constitutively expressed on T-cells, CTLA-4 is not found on the resting cell but is rapidly upregulated following activation. It has a 10–20-fold higher affinity for both B7.1 and B7.2 and, in contrast to costimulatory signals generated through CD28, B7 engagement of CTLA-4 downregulates T-cell activation (figure 7.4).

THE NATURE OF B-CELL ACTIVATION

B-cells are stimulated by cross-linking surface immunoglobulin (sIg)

Cross-linking of B-cell surface receptors, e.g. by thymus independent antigens, induces early activation events. Within 1 min of sIg ligation, Src family kinases rapidly phosphorylate the Syk kinase, Bruton's tyrosine kinase (Btk) and the ITAMs on the sIg receptor chains Ig-α and Ig-β. This is followed by a rise in intracellular calcium and activation of phosphokinase C.

B-cells respond to T-independent and T-dependent antigens

Thymus-independent antigens

Certain linear antigens that are not readily degraded in the body and which have an appropriately spaced, highly repeating determinants such as the *Pneumococcus* polysaccharide, are thymus-independent in their ability to stimulate B-cells directly without the need for T-cell involvement. They persist for long periods on the surface of specialized macrophages located at the subcapsular sinus of the lymph nodes and the splenic marginal zone. This type of antigen binds to antigen-specific B-cells with great avidity through their multivalent attachment to the complementary Ig receptors which they cross-link (figure 7.5). This cross-linking induces early B-cell activation events. In general, the thymus-independent antigens give rise to predominantly low-affinity IgM responses, and relatively poor, if any, memory.

Thymus-dependent antigens

Many antigens are thymus-dependent in that they provoke little or no antibody response in animals which have been thymectomized at birth. Such antigens cannot fulfill the molecular requirements for direct stimulation, and if they bind to B-cell receptors, they will sit on the surface just like a hapten and do nothing to trigger the B-cell (figure 7.6). Cast your mind back to the definition of a hapten—a small molecule that binds to preformed antibody (e.g. the surface receptor of a specific B-cell) but fails to stimulate anti-

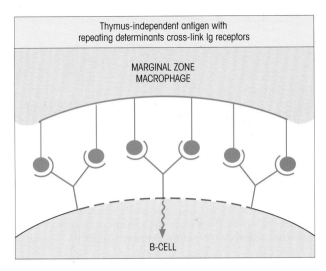

Figure 7.5 B-cell recognition of thymus-independent antigens. The complex gives a sustained signal to the B-cell because of the long half-life of this type of molecule. ⟿, activation signal; ⊥, surface immunoglobulin (sIg) receptor; — — —, cross-linking of receptors.

body production (i.e. stimulate the B-cell). Remember also that haptens become immunogenic when coupled to an appropriate carrier protein. Building on the knowledge that both T- and B-cells are necessary for antibody responses to thymus-dependent antigens, we now know that the carrier functions to stimulate T-helper cells, which cooperate with B-cells to enable them to respond to the hapten by providing accessory signals (figure 7.6). It should also be evident from figure 7.6 that while one determinant on a typical protein antigen is behaving as a hapten in binding to the B-cell, the other determinants subserve a carrier function in recruiting T-helper cells.

Antigen processing by B-cells

Although we think of B-cells primarily as antibody-producing cells, they in fact play an important role in antigen processing and presentation to T-cells. Primed B-cells, in fact, work at much lower antigen concentrations than conventional APCs because they can focus antigen through their surface receptors. Antigen bound to sIg is internalized in endosomes which then fuse with vesicles containing MHC class II molecules with their invariant chain. Processing of the protein antigen then occurs as described in Chapter 5 and the resulting antigenic peptide is recycled to the surface in association with the class II molecules. There it is available for recognition by the TCR on a carrier-specific T-helper cell (figure 7.7). With the assistance of costimulatory signals arising from the interaction of **CD40 with its ligand CD40L**, B-cell activation is ensured.

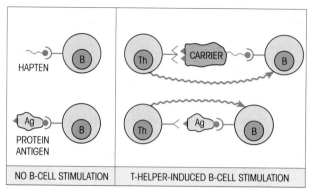

Figure 7.6 T-helper cells cooperate through protein carrier determinants to help B-cells respond to hapten or equivalent determinants on antigens by providing accessory signals. (For simplicity we are ignoring the major histocompatibility complex (MHC) component and epitope processing in T-cell recognition, but we won't forget it.)

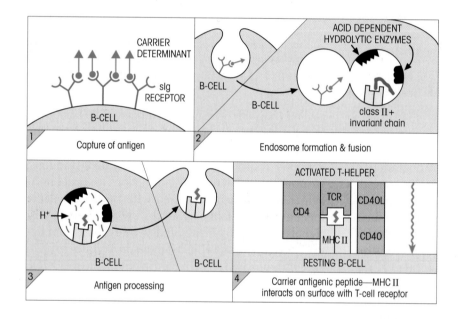

Figure 7.7 B-cell handling of a thymus-dependent antigen. Antigen captured by the surface immunoglobulin (sIg) receptor is internalized within an endosome, processed and expressed on the surface with major histocompatibility complex (MHC) class II (cf. figure 5.8). Costimulatory signals through the CD40–CD40L interaction are required for activation of the resting B-cell by the T-helper. ⟿, activation signal.

REVISION

Immunocompetent T- and B-cells differ in many respects

• The CD3 cell surface antigen can be used to identify T-cells, whilst CD19 and CD20 are characteristic of B-cells.

• The antigen-specific TCR on T-cells and surface immunoglobulin (sIg) on B-cells also provide a clear distinction between these two cell types.

• Differences in CD markers define specialized T-cell subsets.

T-lymphocytes and antigen-presenting cells (APCs) interact through pairs of accessory molecules

• The docking of T-cells and APCs depends upon strong mutual interactions between complementary molecular pairs on their surfaces: major histocompatibility complex (MHC) II/CD4; MHC I/CD8; ICAM-1/LFA-1; LFA-3/CD2; B7/CD28 (and CTLA-4).

Activation of T-cells requires two signals

• Two signals activate T-cells, but one alone produces unresponsiveness (anergy).

• One signal is provided by the low-affinity cognate T-cell receptor (TCR)/MHC–peptide interaction.

• The second costimulatory signal is mediated through ligation of CD28 by B7.1 or B7.2.

Protein tyrosine phosphorylation is an early event in T-cell signaling

- The TCR signal is transduced and amplified through a protein tyrosine kinase (PTK) enzymic cascade. This culminates in cell division and cytokine production.
- Large numbers of TCRs interact with only a few peptide–MHC complexes.
- As activation proceeds, intracellular calcium levels increase, and protein kinase C (PKC) and calcineurin are activated.
- Under the influence of calcineurin the transcription factors NFAT and NFκB are activated, resulting in transcription of genes for cytokines such as interleukin-2 (IL-2).
- There are a number of mechanisms that control T-cell activity including the association of B7 with CTLA-4.

B-cells respond to two different types of antigen

- Thymus-independent antigens are polymeric molecules which cross-link many sIg receptors and, because of their long half-lives, provide a persistent signal to the B-cell.
- Thymus-dependent antigens require the cooperation of helper T-cells to stimulate antibody production by B-cells.
- Antigen captured by specific sIg receptors is taken into the B-cell, processed, and expressed on the surface as a peptide in association with MHC II.
- This complex is recognized by the T-helper cell, which activates the resting B-cell.

The nature of B-cell activation

- Cross-linking of sIg receptors (e.g. thymus-independent antigens) activates B-cells.
- T-helper cells activate resting B-cells through TCR recognition of MHC II–carrier peptide complexes and co-stimulation through CD40L/CD40 interactions (analogous to the B7/CD28 second signal for T-cell activation).

See the accompanying website (**www.roitt.com**) for multiple choice questions

FURTHER READING

Acuto, O. & Cantrell, D. (2000) T cell activation and the cytoskeleton. *Annual Reviews in Immunology*, **18**, 165–84.

Borst, J. & Cope, A. (1999) Turning the immune system on. *Immunology Today*, **20**, 156–8.

Jenkins, M.K., Khoruts, A., Ingulli, E. *et al.* (2001) *In vivo* activation of antigen-specific CD4 T cells. *Annual Review of Immunology* **19**, 23–45.

Myung, P.S., Boerthe, N.J. & Koretzky, G.A. (2000) Adaptor proteins in lymphocyte antigen-receptor signaling. *Current Opinion in Immunology*, **12**, 256–66.

CHAPTER 8

The production of effectors

A SUCCESSION OF GENES ARE UPREGULATED BY T-CELL ACTIVATION

We have dwelt upon the early events in lymphocyte activation consequent upon the engagement of the T-cell receptor (TCR) and the provision of an appropriate costimulatory signal. A complex series of tyrosine and serine/threonine phosphorylation reactions produces the factors which push the cell into the mitotic cycle and drive clonal proliferation and differentiation to effector cells. Within the first half hour, nuclear transcription factors which regulate interleukin-2 (IL-2) expression and the cellular proto-oncogene c-*myc* are expressed, but the next few hours see the synthesis of a range of **soluble cytokines and their receptors** (figure 8.1). Much later we see molecules like the transferrin receptor related to cell division and very late antigens such as the adhesion molecule VLA-1.

CYTOKINES ACT AS INTERCELLULAR MESSENGERS

In contrast to the initial activation of T-cells and T-dependent B-cells, which involves intimate contact with the antigen-presenting cells (APCs), subsequent proliferation and maturation of the response is orchestrated by soluble mediators generically termed cytokines. These relay information between cells as soluble messengers. A list of some of these protein mediators is shown in table 8.1.

Cytokine action is transient and usually short range

These low molecular weight secreted proteins mediate cell growth, inflammation, immunity, differentiation, migration and repair. They are highly potent, often acting at femtomolar (10^{-15} M) concentrations, combining with small numbers of high-affinity cell surface receptors to produce changes in the pattern of RNA and protein synthesis. Unlike endocrine hormones, the majority of cytokines normally act locally in a paracrine or even autocrine fashion. Thus, cytokines derived from lymphocytes rarely persist in the circulation. Nonlymphoid cells such as macrophages can however be triggered by bacterial products to release cytokines, which may be detected in the bloodstream, often to the detriment of the host. Certain cytokines, including IL-1 and tumor necrosis factor (TNF), also exist in membrane forms which could exert their stimulatory effects without becoming soluble.

Cytokines act through cell surface receptors

There are six major cytokine receptor structural families of which the largest is the family of hematopoietin receptors. These generally consist of one or two polypeptide chains responsible for cytokine binding and an additional shared (common or "c") chain involved in signal transduction. The γc-chain is used by the IL-2, IL-4, IL-7, IL-9, IL-15 and IL-21 receptors,

ACTIVATION	0 min		
EARLY	15 min	cfos/cjun	Nuclear binding transcription factor; binds to AP-1
		c-*myc*	Cellular oncogene; controls GO → G1
		Nur77	Function in TCR-mediated apoptosis in immature T-cells
	30 min	NFAT	Nuclear transcription factor of activated-T; regulates IL-2 gene
		NFκB	Nuclear binding protein; regulates expression of many genes
		IκB-α	Inhibitor of NFκB
		PAC-1	Nuclear phosphatase which inactivates ERKs
MEDIUM TERM	Several hours	IL-2/3/4/5/6	Cytokines and their receptors influencing growth and differentiation of myeloid and lymphoid cells, controlling viral growth and mediating chronic inflammatory processes
		IL-9/10/13	
		GM-CSF	
		IFNγ TGFβ	
LATE	14h	Transferrin receptor	Related to cell division
	16h	c-*myb*	Cellular oncogene
	3-5 days	Class II MHC	Antigen presentation
	7-14 days	VLA-1	Very late "antigen"; adhesion molecule

Figure 8.1 Sequential gene activation on T-cell stimulation, appearance of messenger RNA (mRNA). AP-1, activator protein-1; ERKs, extracellular signal-regulated kinases; GM-CSF, granulocyte-macrophage colony-stimulating factor; IL, interleukin; IFNγ, interferon γ; MHC, major histocompatibility complex; NFκB, nuclear factor-kappa B; NFAT, nuclear factor of activated T-cell; TCR, T-cell receptor; TGFβ, transforming growth factor-β.

and the βc-chain by IL-3, IL-5 and granulocyte-macrophage colony-stimulating factor (GM-CSF) receptors. Other families include the interferon (IFN) receptors, the TNF receptors, the immunoglobulin superfamily (IgSF) receptors (including the IL-1 receptor), the large family of chemokine receptors and the receptors for transforming growth factors (TGFs) such as TGFβ. The interaction of cytokine with its receptor initiates cell signalling which generally utilizes either the Janus kinase (JAK)-STAT or the Ras-MAP kinase pathways.

Cytokines often have multiple effects

In general, cytokines are pleiotropic, i.e. exhibit multiple effects on growth and differentiation of a variety of cell types (table 8.1). There is considerable overlapping and redundancy between them with respect to individual functions, partially accounted for by the sharing of receptor components and the utilization of common transcription factors. For example many of the biological activities of IL-4 overlap with those of IL-13.

Their roles in the generation of T- and B-cell effec-tors, and in the regulation of chronic inflammatory reactions (figure 8.2a,b) will be discussed later in this chapter. We should note here the important role of cytokines in the control of hematopoiesis (figure 8.2c). The differentiation of stem cells to become the formed elements of blood within the environment of the bone marrow is carefully nurtured through the production of cytokines such as GM-CSF by the stromal cells and by T-cells and macrophages. It is not surprising, therefore, that during a period of inflammation the cytokines produced recruit new precursors into the hematopoietic differentiation pathway, giving rise to the leukocytosis so often seen in patients with active infection.

Network interactions

The complex and integrated relationships between the different cytokines are mediated through cellular events. For example, the genes for IL-3, IL-4, IL-5 and GM-CSF are all tightly linked on chromosome 5 in a region containing genes for macrophage colony-stimulating factor (M-CSF) and its receptor and several other growth factors and receptors. Interaction may

Table 8.1 Cytokines: their origin and function. Note that there is not an interleukin-14 (IL-14). This designation was given to an activity that, upon further investigation, could not be unambiguously assigned to a single cytokine. Interleukin-8 is a member of the chemokine family. These cytokines are listed separately in table 8.2.

CYTOKINE	SOURCE	EFFECTOR FUNCTION
INTERLEUKINS		
IL-1α, IL-1β	Mono, Mφ, DC, NK, B, Endo, Eosino	Costimulates T activation by enhancing production of cytokines including IL-2 and its receptor; enhances B proliferation and maturation; NK cytotoxicity; induces IL-1,-6,-8, TNF, GM-CSF and PGE$_2$ by Mφ; proinflammatory by inducing chemokines and ICAM-1 and VCAM-1 on endothelium; induces fever, APP, bone resorption by osteoclasts
IL-2	Th1, Eosino	Induces proliferation of activated T- and B-cells; enhances NK cytotoxicity and killing of tumor cells and bacteria by monocytes and Mφ
IL-3	T, NK, MC, Eosino	Growth and differentiation of hematopoietic precursors; MC growth
IL-4	Th2, Tc2, NK, NK-T, γδ T, MC, Eosino	Induces Th2 cells; stimulates proliferation of activated B, T, MC; upregulates MHC class II on B and Mφ, and CD23 on B; downregulates IL-12 production and thereby inhibits Th1 differentiation; increases Mφ phagocytosis; induces switch to IgG1 and IgE
IL-5	Th2, MC, Eosino	Induces proliferation of eosino and activated B; induces switch to IgA
IL-6	Th2, Mono, Mφ, DC, BM stroma, Eosino	Differentiation of myeloid stem cells and of B into plasma cells; induces APP; enhances T proliferation
IL-7	BM and thymic stroma	Induces differentiation of lymphoid stem cells into progenitor T and B; activates mature T
IL-8	Mono, Mφ, Endo, Eosino	Mediates chemotaxis and activation of neutrophils
IL-9	Th	Induces proliferation of thymocytes; enhances MC growth; synergizes with IL-4 in switch to IgG1 and IgE
IL-10	Th (Th2 in mouse), Tc, B, Mono, Mφ, Eosino	Inhibits IFNγ secretion by mouse, and IL-2 by human, Th1 cells; downregulates MHC class II and cytokine (including IL-12) production by mono, Mφ and DC, thereby inhibiting Th1 differentiation; inhibits T proliferation; enhances B differentiation
IL-11	BM stroma	Promotes differentiation of pro-B and megakaryocytes; induces APP
IL-12	Mono, Mφ, DC, B	Critical cytokine for Th1 differentiation; induces proliferation and IFNγ production by Th1, CD8$^+$ T and γδ T and NK; enhances NK and CD8$^+$ T cytotoxicity
IL-13	Th2, MC, Eosino	Inhibits activation and cytokine secretion by Mφ; co-activates B proliferation; upregulates MHC class II and CD23 on B and mono; induces switch to IgG1 and IgE; induces VCAM-1 on endo
IL-15	T, NK, Mono, Mφ, DC, B	Induces proliferation of T, NK and activated B and cytokine production and cytotoxicity in NK and CD8$^+$ T; chemotactic for T; stimulates growth of intestinal epithelium
IL-16	Th, Tc, Eosino	Chemoattractant for CD4 T, mono and eosino; induces MHC class II
IL-17	T	Proinflammatory; stimulates production of cytokines including TNF, IL-1β,-6,-8, G-CSF
IL-18	Mφ, DC	Induces IFNγ production by T; enhances NK cytotoxicity
IL-19	Mono	Modulation of Th1 activity
IL-20	Keratinocytes?	Regulation of inflammatory responses to skin?
IL-21	Th	Regulation of hematopoiesis; NK differentiation; B activation; T costimulation
IL-22	T	Inhibits IL-4 production by Th2
IL-23	DC	Induces proliferation and IFNγ production by Th1; induces proliferation of memory cells
COLONY STIMULATING FACTORS		
GM-CSF	Th, Mφ, Fibro, MC, Endo, Eosino	Stimulates growth of progenitors of mono, neutro, eosino and baso; activates Mφ
G-CSF	Fibro, Endo	Stimulates growth of neutro progenitors
M-CSF	Fibro, Endo, Epith	Stimulates growth of mono progenitors
SLF	BM stroma	Stimulates stem cell division (c-*kit* ligand)
TUMOR NECROSIS FACTORS		
TNF (TNFα)	Th, Mono, Mφ, DC, MC, NK, B, Eosino	Tumor cytotoxicity; cachexia (weight loss); induces cytokine secretion; induces E-selectin on endo; activates Mφ; antiviral
Lymphotoxin (TNFβ)	Th1, Tc	Tumor cytotoxicity; enhances phagocytosis by neutro and Mφ; involved in lymphoid organ development; antiviral
INTERFERONS		
IFNα	Leukocytes	Inhibits viral replication; enhances MHC class I
IFNβ	Fibroblasts	Inhibits viral replication; enhances MHC class I
IFNγ	Th1, Tc1, NK	Inhibits viral replication; Enhances MHC class I and II; activates Mφ; induces switch to IgG2a; antagonizes several IL-4 actions; inhibits proliferation of Th2
OTHERS		
TGFβ	Th3, B, Mφ, MC, Eosino	Proinflammatory by, e.g., chemoattraction of mono and Mφ but also anti-inflammatory by, e.g. inhibiting lymphocyte proliferation; induces switch to IgA; promotes tissue repair
LIF	Thymic epith, BM stroma	Induces APP
Eta-1	T	Stimulates IL-12 production and inhibits IL-10 production by Mφ
Oncostatin M	T, Mφ	Induces APP

APP, acute phase proteins; B, B-cell; baso, basophil; BM, bone marrow; Endo, endothelium; eosino, eosinophil; Epith, epithelium; Fibro, fibroblast; GM-CSF, granulocyte-macrophage colony-stimulating factor; IL, interleukin; LIF, leukemia inhibitory factor; Mφ, macrophage; MC, mast cell; Mono, monocyte; neutro, neutrophil; NK, natural killer; SLF, steel locus factor; T, T-cell; TGFβ, transforming growth factor-β.

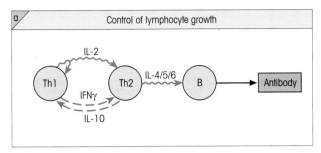

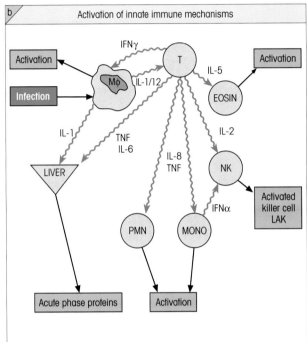

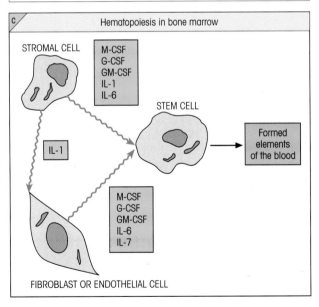

Figure 8.2 Cytokine action. A general but not entirely comprehensive guide to indicate the scope of cytokine interactions. EOSIN, eosinophil; G-CSF, granulocyte colony-stimulating factor; GM-CSF, granulocyte-macrophage colony-stimulating factor; IFN, interferon; IL, interleukin; LAK, lymphokine activated killer; Mφ, macrophage; M-CSF, macrophage colony-stimulating factor; MONO, monocyte; NK, natural killer cell; PMN, polymorphonuclear neutrophil; TNF, tumor necrosis factor.

occur through a cascade in which one cytokine induces the production of another, through transmodulation of the receptor for another cytokine and through synergism or antagonism of two cytokines acting on the same cell (figure 8.3). Furthermore, as mentioned above, many cytokines share the same signaling pathways and this too may contribute to the redundancy in their effect.

DIFFERENT CD4 T-CELL SUBSETS CAN MAKE DIFFERENT CYTOKINE PATTERNS

The bipolar Th1/Th2 concept

T-helper cells (Th) can be classified into various subsets depending on the cytokines they secrete. Th0 cells secrete IL-2, IL-3, IL-4, IL-5, IFNγ and GM-CSF. These cells can develop into Th1 cells which characteristically secrete IL-2, IFNγ and lymphotoxin and promote cell-mediated immunity, especially cytotoxic and delayed hypersensitivity reactions and macrophage activation. Alternatively the Th0 cells can differentiate into Th2 cells, which secrete IL-4, IL-5, IL-6, IL-10 and IL-13, and activate B-lymphocytes resulting in upregulation of antibody production. The characteristic cytokines produced by Th1 and Th2 cells have mutually inhibitory effects on the reciprocal phenotype. Interferon γ will inhibit the proliferation of Th2 cells and IL-10 will downregulate Th1 cells. Although the factors involved in directing immune responses to these two subpopulations are not fully elucidated, it appears that APCs and, in particular, dendritic cells (DCs) appear to be pivotal in driving differentiation towards a Th1 or Th2 phenotype. Also the cytokine environment in which these cells develop may influence their ultimate phenotype. Therefore IL-12 produced by APCs will stimulate IFNγ production from natural killer (NK) cells, and both these cytokines will drive differentiation of Th1 cells and inhibit Th2 responses. On the other side of the coin, when Th are activated by antigen in the presence of IL-4 they develop into Th2 cells (figure 8.4).

The different patterns of cytokine production by these T-cell subtypes are of importance in protection against different classes of microorganisms. Th1 cells producing cytokines such as IFNγ would be especially effective against viruses and intracellular organisms that grow in macrophages. Th2 cells are very good helpers for B-cells and seem to be adapted for defence against parasites that are vulnerable to IL-4-switched IgE and IL-5-induced eosinophilia, and against pathogens that are removed primarily through humoral mechanisms.

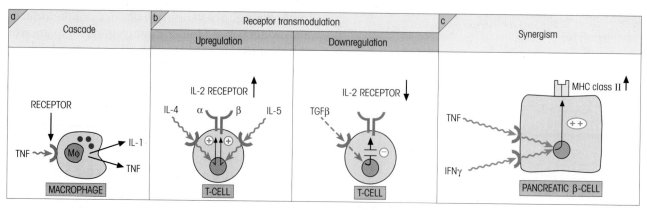

Figure 8.3 Network interactions of cytokines. (a) Cascade: in this example tumor necrosis factor (TNF) induces secretion of interleukin-1 (IL-1) and of itself (autocrine) in the macrophage. (Note all diagrams in this figure are simplified in that the effects on the nucleus are due to messengers resulting from combination of cytokine with its surface receptor.) (b) Receptor transmodulation showing upregulation of each chain forming the high-affinity IL-2 receptor in an activated T-cell by individual cytokines and downregulation by transforming growth factor-β (TGFβ). (c) Synergy of TNF and interferon γ (IFNγ) in upregulation of surface major histocompatibility complex (MHC) class II molecules on cultured pancreatic insulin-secreting cells. Mφ, macrophage.

Infections with *Mycobacterium tuberculosis*, the etiologic agent of tuberculosis, demonstrate well the clinical significance of these Th subsets. Successful control of infection is dependent upon an adequate Th1 response. These cells, by promoting IFNγ production, activate macrophages to reduce bacterial load and to release TNF, which is essential for granuloma production.

Infections with *Leishmania* organisms are also influenced by the pattern of cytokines produced by Th1 and Th2 cells. In the localized cutaneous form of the disease, IL-2 and IFNγ predominate in the lesions, indicating that Th1 cells are limiting the infection. In the more severe chronic mucocutaneous disease, however, the lesions have an abundance of IL-4, suggesting a predominantly Th2 response with inadequate cellular control. In the most severe visceral form of the disease, circulating lymphocytes are unable to produce IFNγ or IL-12 in response to the etiologic agent, *Leishmania donovani*, but addition of anti-IL-10 antibody results in an augmented IFNγ response. These findings may have significant therapeutic possibilities as therapies that increase activity of Th1 cytokines or decrease Th2 cytokines may enhance resolution of *Leishmania* lesions. Interferon γ in particular, since it enhances macrophage killing of parasites, has been shown to have some beneficial effect in treating severely ill patients and those with refractory disease.

Interactions with cells of the innate immune system biases the Th1/Th2 response

Antigen-presenting cells and, in particular, DCs appear to be pivotal in driving differentiation towards a Th1 or Th2 phenotype. Whilst there is some evidence indicating the existence of subpopulations of DCs specialized for the stimulation of either Th1 or Th2 populations, this is an area that is still under intensive investigation. Interleukin-12 seems to be particularly important for the production of Th1 cells and IL-4 for the production of Th2 cells. Invasion of phagocytic cells by intracellular pathogens induces copious secretion of IL-12, which in turn stimulates IFNγ production by NK cells. These two cytokines selectively drive differentiation of Th1 development and inhibit Th2 responses (figure 8.4). However, IL-4 effects appear to be dominant over IL-12 and, therefore, the amounts of IL-4 relative to the amounts of IL-12 and IFNγ will be of paramount importance in determining the differentiation of Th0 cells into Th1 or Th2.

ACTIVATED T-CELLS PROLIFERATE IN RESPONSE TO CYTOKINES

Amplification of T-cells following activation is critically dependent upon IL-2 (figure 8.5). This cytokine acts only on cells which express high-affinity IL-2 receptors. These receptors are not present on resting cells, but are synthesized within a few hours after activation (figure 8.1). The number of these receptors on the cell increases under the action of antigen and IL-2,

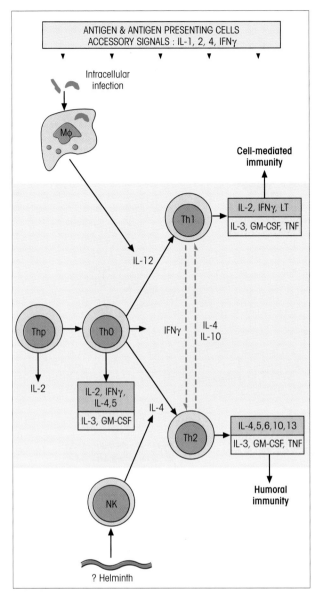

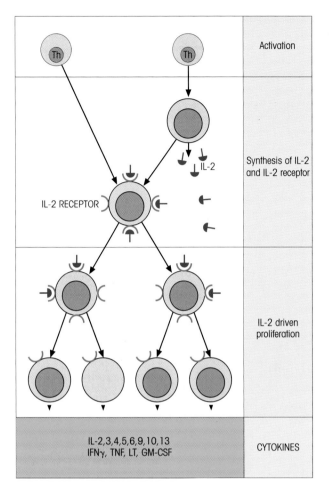

Figure 8.4 The generation of Th1 and Th2 CD4 subsets. Following initial stimulation of T-cells, a range of cells producing a spectrum of cytokine patterns emerges. Under different conditions, the resulting population can be biased towards two extremes. Interleukin-12 (IL-12), possibly produced through an "innate" type effect of an intracellular infection on macrophages, encourages the development of Th1 cells which produce the cytokines characteristic of cell-mediated immunity. In contrast IL-4, possibly produced by interaction of infectious agents with natural killer (NK) cells, skews the development to production of Th2 cells whose cytokines assist the progression of B-cells to antibody secretion and the provision of humoral immunity. Cytokines produced by polarized Th1 and Th2 subpopulations are mutually inhibitory. LT, lymphotoxin; Th0, early helper cell producing a spectrum of cytokines; Thp, T-helper precursor; other abbreviations as in table 8.1.

Figure 8.5 Activated T-blasts expressing surface receptors for interleukin-2 (IL-2) proliferate in response to IL-2 produced by itself or by another T-cell subset. The expanded population secretes a wide variety of biologically active cytokines of which IL-4 also enhances T-cell proliferation. GM-CSF, granulocyte-macrophage colony-stimulating factor; IFNγ, interferon γ; LT, lymphotoxin; Th, T-helper cell; TNF, tumor necrosis factor.

and as antigen is cleared, so the receptor numbers decline and, with that, the responsiveness to IL-2.

The T-cell blasts also produce an impressive array of other cytokines and the proliferative effect of IL-2 is reinforced by the action of IL-4 and IL-15 which react with corresponding receptors on the dividing T-cells. We must not lose sight of the importance of control mechanisms such as TGFβ, which blocks IL-2-induced proliferation (figure 8.3b) and the cytokines IFNγ, IL-4 and IL-12, which mediate the mutual antagonism of Th1 and Th2 subsets. Should the T-cells be repeatedly activated, IL-2 will be responsible for activation-induced cell death of the T-cells, thereby further controlling the extent of the immune response.

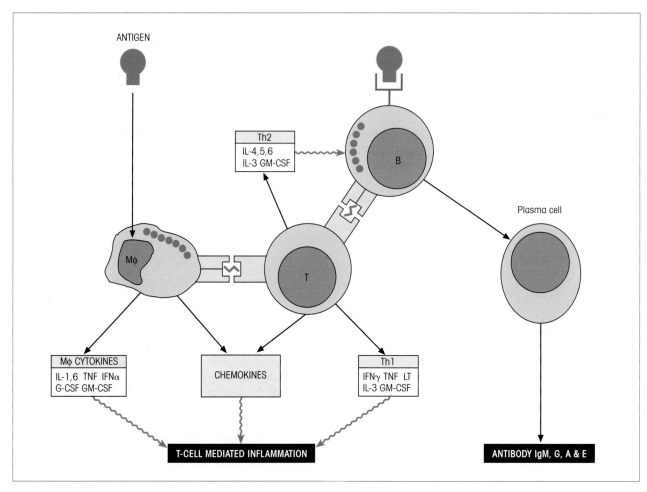

Figure 8.6 Cytokines controlling the antibody and T-cell-mediated inflammatory responses. Abbreviations as in table 8.1.

T-CELL EFFECTORS IN CELL-MEDIATED IMMUNITY

Cytokines mediate chronic inflammatory responses

In addition to their role in the adaptive response, the T-cell cytokines are responsible for generating antigen-specific chronic inflammatory reactions which deal with intracellular microorganisms (figure 8.6).

Early events

The initiating event is probably a local inflammatory response to tissue injury caused by the infectious agent that would upregulate the synthesis of adhesion molecules such as VCAM-1 (vascular cell adhesion molecule-1) and ICAM-1 (intercellular adhesion molecule-1) on adjacent vascular endothelial cells.

These would permit entry of memory T-cells to the infected site through their VLA-4 (very late antigen-4) and LFA-1 (lymphocyte function-associated antigen-1) homing receptors. Contact with processed antigen derived from the intracellular organism will activate the specific T-cell and induce the release of secreted cytokines. Tumor necrosis factor will further enhance the expression of endothelial accessory molecules and increase the chances of other memory cells in the circulation homing in to meet the antigen provoking the inflammation.

Chemotaxis

The recruitment of T-cells and macrophages to the inflammatory site is greatly enhanced by the action of chemotactic cytokines termed **chemokines** (chemoattractant cytokine). The main stimuli to the production of chemokines are the proinflammatory cytokines such as IL-1 and TNF, but bacterial and viral products

Table 8.2 Chemokines and their receptors. The chemokines are grouped according to the arrangement of their cysteines. The letter L designates ligand (i.e. the individual chemokine), whereas the letter R designates receptors. Names in parentheses refer to the murine homologs of the human chemokine where the names of these differ, or the murine chemokine alone if no human equivalent has been described.

FAMILY	CHEMOKINE	ALTERNATIVE NAMES	CHEMOTAXIS	RECEPTORS
CXC	CXCL1	GROα/MGSAα	Neutro	CXCR2>CXCR1
	CXCL2	GROβ/MGSAβ	Neutro	CXCR2
	CXCL3	GROγ/MGSAγ	Neutro	CXCR2
	CXCL4	PF4	Eosino, Baso	CXCR3
	CXCL5	ENA-78	Neutro	CXCR2
	CXCL6	GCP-2/(CKα-3)	Neutro	CXCR1, CXCR2
	CXCL7	NAP-2	Neutro	CXCR2
	CXCL8	IL-8	Neutro	CXCR1, CXCR2
	CXCL9	Mig	T, NK	CXCR3
	CXCL10	IP-10	T, NK	CXCR3
	CXCL11	I-TAC	T, NK	CXCR3
	CXCL12	SDF-1α/β	T, B, DC, Mono	CXCR4
	CXCL13	BLC/BCA-1	B	CXCR5
	CXCL14	BRAK/Bolekine	?	?
	CXCL15	Lungkine	Neutro	?
C	XCL1	Lymphotactin/SCM-1α/ATAC	T	XCR1
	XCL2	SCM-1β	T	XCR1
CX3C	CX3CL1	Fractalkine/Neurotactin	T, NK, Mono	CX3CR1
CC	CCL1	I-309/(TCA-3/P500)	Mono	CCR8
	CCL2	MCP-1/MCAF	T, NK, DC, Mono, Baso	CCR2
	CCL3	MIP-1α/LD78 α	T, NK, DC, Mono, Eosino	CCR1, CCR5
	CCL4	MIP-1β	T, NK, DC, Mono	CCR5
	CCL5	RANTES	T, NK, DC, Mono, Eosino, Baso	CCR1, CCR3, CCR5
	(CCL6)	(C10/MRP-1)	Mono	?
	CCL7	MCP-3	T, NK, DC, Mono, Eosino, Baso	CCR1,CCR2, CCR3
	CCL8	MCP-2	T, NK, DC, Mono, Baso	CCR3
	(CCL9/10)	(MRP-2/CCF18/MIP-1γ)	?	?
	CCL11	Eotaxin-1	T, DC, Eosino, Baso	CCR3
	(CCL12)	(MCP-5)	T, NK, DC, Mono, Baso	CCR2
	CCL13	MCP-4	T, NK, DC, Mono, Eosino, Baso	CCR2, CCR3
	CCL14	HCC-1/HCC-3	T, Mono, Eosino	CCR1
	CCL15	HCC-2/Leukotactin-1/MIP-1δ	T	CCR1, CCR3
	CCL16	HCC-4/LEC/(LCC-1)	T	CCR1
	CCL17	TARC	T, DC, Mono	CCR4
	CCL18	DCCK1/PARC/AMAC-1	T	?
	CCL19	MIP-3β/ELC/Exodus-3	T, B, DC	CCR7
	CCL20	MIP-3α/LARC/Exodus-1	DC	CCR6
	CCL21	6Ckine/SLC/Exodus-2/(TCA-4)	T, DC	CCR7
	CCL22	MDC/STCP-1/ABCD-1	T, DC, Mono	CCR4
	CCL23	MPIF-1	T	CCR1
	CCL24	MPIF-2/Eotaxin-2	T, DC, Eosino, Baso	CCR3
	CCL25	TECK	T, DC, Mono	CCR9
	CCL26	SCYA26/Eotaxin-3	T	CCR3
	CCL27	CTACK/ALP/ESkine	T	CCR10

B, B-cell; Baso, basophil; DC, dendritic cell; Eosino, eosinophil; Mono, monocyte; Neutro, neutrophil; NK, natural killer; T, T-cell.

may also do this. There are now more than 50 chemokines described and they bind to at least 19 functional receptors, predominantly on leukocytes. There are four chemokine families termed the CC and CXC chemokines, which are the predominant ones, and the CX3C and the C chemokines, which are smaller families (table 8.2). Receptor activation leads to a cascade of cellular events that ultimately results in activation of the cellular machinery necessary to direct the cell to a particular location. Despite the fact that a single chemokine can sometimes bind to more than one receptor, and a single receptor can bind several chemokines, many chemokines exhibit a strong tissue and receptor specificity. They play important roles in inflammation, lymphoid organ development, cell trafficking, cell compartmentalization within lymphoid tissues, Th1/Th2 development, angiogenesis and wound healing. Although the receptors are specific for chemokines, the CCR5 and CXCR4 receptors are now known to also act as co-receptors for the human immunodeficiency virus (HIV), allowing the virus that has attached to the CD4 molecule to gain entrance to the T-cell or the monocyte.

Macrophage activation

Macrophages with intracellular organisms are activated by agents such as IFNγ, GM-CSF, IL-2 and TNF and become endowed with microbicidal powers. During this process, some macrophages may die (perhaps helped along by cytotoxic T-cells (Tc)) and release living organisms, but these will be dealt with by fresh macrophages brought to the site by chemotaxis and activated by local cytokines.

Combating viral infection

Virally-infected cells require a different strategy, and one strand of that strategy exploits the innate IFN mechanism to deny the virus access to the cell's replicative machinery. Tumor necrosis factor has cytotoxic potential against virally infected cells, which is particularly useful since death of an infected cell before viral replication has occurred is obviously beneficial to the host. The cytotoxic potential of TNF was first recognized using tumor cells as targets (hence the name), and IFNγ and lymphotoxin can act synergistically with TNF setting up the cell for destruction by inducing the formation of TNF receptors.

Killer T-cells

The generation of cytotoxic T-cells

Cytotoxic T-cells (Tc), also referred to as cytotoxic T-lymphocytes (CTLs), represent the other major arm of the cell-mediated immune response, and are of strategic importance in the killing of virally infected cells and possibly in contributing to the postulated surveillance mechanisms against cancer cells.

The cytotoxic cell precursors (Tcp) recognize antigen on the surface of cells in association with class I major histocompatibility complex (MHC) molecules, and like B-cells they usually, but not always, require help from other T-cells. The mechanism by which help is proffered may, however, be quite different. Effective

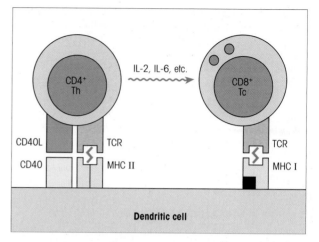

Figure 8.7 T-helper cell (Th) activation of cytotoxic T-cells (Tc). Activation of the CD4$^+$ Th by the dendritic cell (DC) involves a CD40–CD40L (CD40 ligand) (CD154) costimulatory signal and recognition of peptide presented to the T-cell receptor (TCR) by major histocompatibility complex (MHC) class II. The release of cytokines from the activated Th cells stimulates the differentiation of the CD8$^+$ precursor into an activated, MHC class I-restricted Tc.

T–B collaboration involves capture of the native antigen by the surface Ig receptors on the B-cells, which process it internally and present it to the Th as a peptide in association with MHC class II. With Th and Tcp interactions, it seems most likely that both cells bind to the same APC which has processed viral antigen and displays processed viral peptides in association with both MHC class II (for the Th cell) and class I (for the Tcp) on its surface. It is possible that the APC could be the virally infected cell itself. Cytokines from the triggered Th and from DCs will be released in close proximity to the Tcp, which is engaging the antigen–MHC signal, and these cells will be stimulated to proliferate and differentiate into a CTL under the influence of IL-2, IL-6, IL-12 and IL-15 (Figure 8.7).

The lethal process

Most Tc are of the CD8 subset and their binding to the target cell through TCR recognition of antigen plus class I MHC is assisted by association between CD8 and MHC class I and by other accessory molecules such as LFA-1 and CD2 (see figure 7.2). In some circumstances CD4$^+$ T-cells may also mediate cytotoxicity through the Fas–FasL (Fas ligand) pathway.

Cytotoxic T-cells are **unusual secretory cells** which use a modified lysosome to secrete their lytic proteins. Following delivery of the TCR/CD3 signal, the **lytic granules** are driven along the microtubule system and

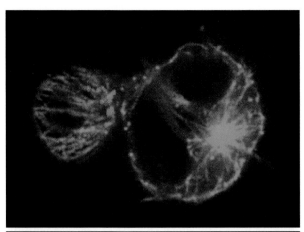

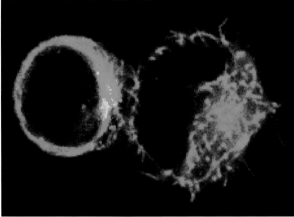

Figure 8.8 Conjugation of a cytotoxic T-cell (on left) to its target, here a mouse mastocytoma, showing polarization of the granules towards the target at the point of contact. The cytoskeletons of both cells are revealed by immunofluorescent staining with an antibody to tubulin (green) and the lytic granules with an antibody to granzyme A (red). Twenty minutes after conjugation the target cell cytoskeleton may still be intact (above), but this rapidly becomes disrupted (below). (Photographs kindly provided by Dr Gillian Griffiths.)

delivered to the point of contact between the Tc and its target (figure 8.8). This guarantees the specificity of killing dictated by TCR recognition of the target and limits any damage to bystander cells. As with NK cells which have comparable granules, exocytosis of the granule contents, including perforins, granzymes and TNF, produces lesions in the target cell membrane and death by inducing apoptosis. Cytotoxic T-cells are endowed with a second killing mechanism involving Fas and its ligand (cf. pp. 13 and 179).

Video microscopy shows that the Tc are serial killers. After the "kiss of death," the T-cell can disengage and seek a further victim, there being rapid synthesis of new granules. At some stage the expansion of the CD8 cells will need to be contracted and this occurs when the newly activated CD8 cells kill the activating APCs. One should also not lose sight of the fact that CD8 cells synthesize other cytokines such as IFNγ which also have antiviral potential.

Inflammation must be regulated

Once the inflammatory process has cleared the inciting agent, the body needs to switch off the response to that antigen. A variety of anti-inflammatory cytokines are produced during humoral and cell-mediated immune responses. Interleukin-10 has profound anti-inflammatory and immunoregulatory effects, acting on macrophages and Th1 cells to inhibit release of proinflammatory factors such as IL-1 and TNF. Furthermore IL-10 downregulates surface TNF receptor and induces the release of soluble TNF receptors which are endogenous inhibitors of TNF. Interleukin-1, a potent proinflammatory cytokine, can be regulated by soluble IL-1 receptors released during inflammation which act to decoy IL-1, and by the IL-1 receptor antagonist (IL-1Ra). This latter cytokine, which is structurally similar to IL-1, is produced by monocytes and macrophages during inflammation and competes with IL-1 for IL-1 receptors thereby antagonizing IL-1 activity. Production of IL-1Ra is stimulated by IL-4, which also inhibits IL-1 production and, as we have indicated previously, also acts to constrain Th1 cells. The role of TGFβ is more difficult to tease out because it has some pro and other anti-inflammatory effects, although it undoubtedly promotes tissue repair after resolution of the inflammation.

These anti-inflammatory cytokines have considerable potential for the treatment of those human diseases where proinflammatory cytokines are responsible for clinical manifestations. Such a situation exists in septic shock, where many of the clinical features are due to the massive production of IL-1, TNF and IL-6. Studies in rabbits showed that pre-treatment with IL-1Ra blocked endotoxin-induced septic shock and death. In studies in humans, however, treatment with IL-1Ra has not been shown to reduce mortality in patients with sepsis, and further trials on this and other anti-inflammatory cytokines are in progress.

PROLIFERATION AND MATURATION OF B-CELL RESPONSES ARE MEDIATED BY CYTOKINES

The activation of B-cells by Th through the TCR recognition of MHC-linked antigenic peptide plus the costimulatory **CD40L–CD40 interaction** leads to upregulation of the surface receptors for IL-4. Copious

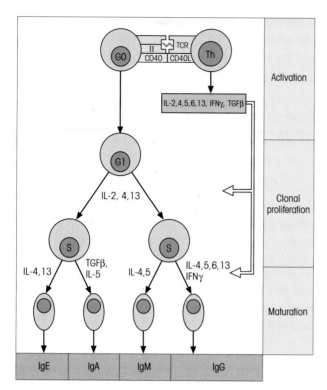

Figure 8.9 B-cell response to thymus-dependent (TD) antigen: clonal expansion and maturation of activated B-cells under the influence of T-cell-derived soluble factors. Costimulation through the CD40 ligand (CD40L)–CD40 interaction is essential for primary and secondary immune responses to TD antigens and for the formation of germinal centers and memory. IFNγ, interferon γ; IL, interleukin; Ig, immunoglobulin; TCR, T-cell receptor; TGFβ, transforming growth factor-β; Th, T-helper cell.

local release of this cytokine from the Th then drives powerful clonal proliferation and expansion of the activated B-cell population (figure 8.9). Interleukin-2 and IL-13 also contribute to this process.

Immunoglobulin M plasma cells emerge under the tutelage of IL-4 plus IL-5, and IgG producers result from the combined influence of IL-4, IL-5, IL-6, IL-13 and IFNγ. Under the influence of IL-4 and IL-13, the expanded clones can differentiate and mature into IgE-synthesizing cells. Transforming growth factor-β and IL-5 encourage cells to switch their Ig class to IgA (figure 8.9).

Thymus-independent antigens can activate B-cells directly but nonetheless still need cytokines for efficient proliferation and Ig production.

WHAT IS GOING ON IN THE GERMINAL CENTER?

Secondary challenge with antigen or immune com-

plexes induces enlargement of germinal centers, formation of new ones, appearance of B-memory cells and development of Ig-producing cells of higher affinity. B-cells entering the germinal center become **centroblasts**, which divide with a very short cycle time of 6 h, and then become nondividing centrocytes in the basal light zone, many of which die from apoptosis (figure 8.10). As the surviving centrocytes mature, they differentiate either into **immunoblast plasma cell precursors**, which secrete Ig in the absence of antigen, or **memory B-cells**.

What then is the underlying scenario? Following secondary antigen challenge, primed B-cells may be activated by paracortical Th cells in association with interdigitating DCs or macrophages, and migrate to the germinal center. There they divide in response to powerful stimuli from complexes on follicular dendritic cells (FDCs) and from cytokines released by T-cells in response to antigen-presenting B-cells. **Somatic hypermutation** of B-cell Ig genes occurs with high frequency during this stage of cell division. Mutated cells with surface antibody of higher affinity will be positively selected, so leading to **maturation of antibody affinity** during the immune response. The cells also undergo **Ig class switching** and further differentiation will now occur. The cells either migrate to the sites of plasma cell activity (e.g. lymph node medulla) or go to expand the memory B-cell pool.

IMMUNOGLOBULIN CLASS-SWITCHING OCCURS IN INDIVIDUAL B-CELLS

The synthesis of antibodies belonging to the various Ig classes proceeds at different rates. Usually there is an early IgM response which tends to fall off rapidly. Immunoglobulin G antibody synthesis builds up to its maximum over a longer time period. On secondary challenge with antigen, the synthesis of IgG antibodies rapidly accelerates to a much higher titer and there is a relatively slow fall-off in serum antibody levels (figure 8.11). The same probably holds for IgA, and in a sense both these Ig classes provide the main immediate defense against future penetration by foreign antigens.

Antibody synthesis in most classes shows considerable dependence upon T-cooperation in that the responses in T-deprived animals are strikingly deficient. Similarly, the switch from IgM to IgG and other classes is largely under T-cell control critically mediated by CD40 and by cytokines as described earlier. In addition to being brisker, the secondary responses tend to be of higher affinity because once the primary response gets under way and the antigen concentration declines to

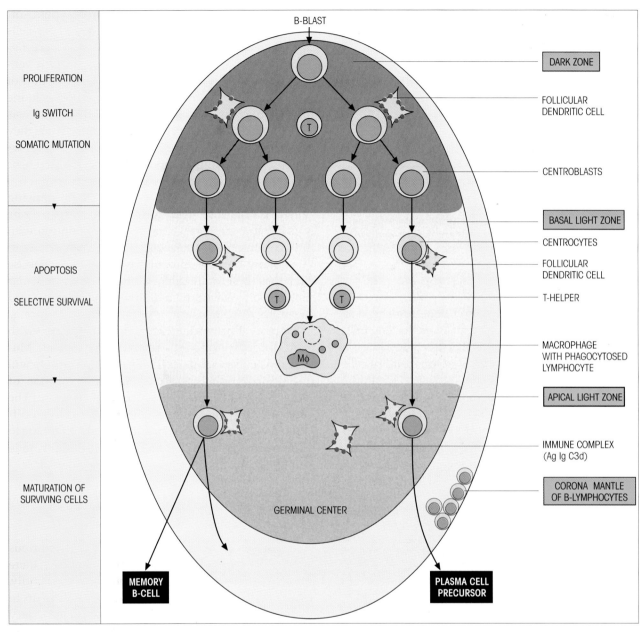

Figure 8.10 The events occurring in lymphoid germinal centers. Germinal center B-cells show numerous mutations in antibody genes. Expression of LFA-1 (lymphocyte function-associated antigen-1) and ICAM-1 (intercellular adhesion molecule-1) on B-cells and follicular dendritic cells (FDCs) in the germinal center makes them "sticky." Through their surface receptors, FDCs bind immune complexes containing antigen and C3 which, in turn, are very effective B-cell stimulators since coligation of the surface receptors for antigen and C3 lowers their threshold for activation. The costimulatory molecules CD40 and B7 play pivotal roles, and antibodies to CD40 or B7 prevent formation of germinal centers. Ag, antigen; Ig, immunoglobulin; Mφ, macrophage.

low levels, only successively higher-affinity cells will bind sufficient antigen to maintain proliferation.

MEMORY CELLS

Memory of early infections such as measles is long-lived and the question arises as to whether the memory cells are long-lived or are subject to repeated antigen stimulation from persisting antigen or subclinical reinfection. Fanum in 1847 described a measles epidemic on the Faroe Islands in the previous year in which almost the entire population suffered from infection

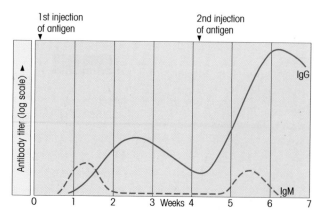

Figure 8.11 Synthesis of immunoglobulin M (IgM) and IgG antibody classes in the primary and secondary responses to antigen.

in the germinal center to capture and process this complexed antigen and then present it to memory T-cells.

The memory population is not simply an expansion of corresponding naive cells

In general, memory cells are more readily stimulated by a given dose of antigen because they have a higher affinity. In the case of B-cells, we have been satisfied by the evidence linking mutation and antigen selection to the creation of high-affinity memory cells within the germinal center of secondary lymph node follicles. Virgin B-cells lose their surface IgM and IgD and switch receptor isotype on becoming memory cells. The costimulatory molecules B7.1 (CD80) and B7.2 (CD86) are rapidly upregulated on memory B-cells, and their potent antigen-presenting capacity for T-cells could well account for the brisk and robust nature of secondary responses.

Memory T-cells augment their binding avidity for APCs through increased expression of accessory adhesion molecules such as CD2, LFA-1, LFA-3 and ICAM-1. Since several of these molecules also function to enhance signal transduction, the memory T-cell is more readily triggered than its naive counterpart. Indeed, memory cells enter cell division and secrete cytokines more rapidly than naive cells, and there is some evidence that they may secrete a broader range of cytokines than naive cells.

except for a few old people who had been infected 65 years earlier. While this evidence favors the long half-life hypothesis, it is envisaged that B-cell memory is a dynamic state in which survival of the memory cells is maintained by recurrent signals from FDCs in the germinal centers, the only long-term repository of antigen.

T-cell memory exists for both CD4 and CD8 cells and may be maintained even in the absence of the antigen. Usually, however, antigen persists as complexes on FDCs. There is, therefore, the potential for APCs with-

- Early interaction of antigen with macrophages producing IL-12 or with a T-cell subset secreting IL-4 will skew the responses to Th1 or Th2 respectively.
- Different patterns of cytokine production influence the severity and clinical manifestations of various infectious diseases.

Activated T-cells proliferate in response to cytokines

- Interleukin-2 acts as an autocrine growth factor for Th1 and paracrine for Th2 cells that have upregulated their IL-2 receptors.
- Cytokines act on cells which express receptors.

T-cell effectors in cell-mediated immunity

- Cytokines mediate chronic inflammatory responses.
- α-Chemokines are cytokines which chemoattract neutrophils, and β-chemokines attract T-cells, macrophages and other inflammatory cells.
- CCR5 and CXCR4 chemokine receptors act as co-receptors for the human immunodeficiency virus (HIV).
- Tumor necrosis factor synergizes with IFNγ in killing cells.

Killer T-cells

- Cytotoxic T-cells (Tc) are generated against cells (e.g. virally infected) that have intracellularly-derived peptide associated with surface major histocompatibility complex (MHC) class I.
- Cytotoxic T-cells proliferate under the influence of IL-2 released by Th in close proximity.
- Cytotoxic T-cells are CD8 cells that secrete lytic proteins to the point of contact between the Tc and its target.
- The granules contain perforins and TNF, which produce lesions in the target cell membrane, and granzymes, which cause death by apoptosis.

Control of inflammation

- Various anti-inflammatory cytokines are produced during the immune response.
- T-cell-mediated inflammation is strongly downregulated by IL-10.

- Interleukin-1 is inhibited by the IL-1 receptor antagonist (IL-1Ra) and by IL-4.

Proliferation of B-cell responses is mediated by cytokines

- Early proliferation is mediated by IL-4, which also aids immunoglobulin E (IgE) synthesis.
- Immunoglobulin A producers are driven by transforming growth factor-β (TGFβ) and IL-5.
- Interleukin-4 plus IL-5 promotes IgM, and IL-4, IL-5, IL-6 and IL-13 plus IFNγ stimulate IgG synthesis.

Events in the germinal center

- There is clonal expansion, isotype switch and mutation in the centroblasts.
- The B-cell centroblasts become nondividing centrocytes which differentiate into plasma cell precursors or into memory cells.

Immunoglobulin class-switching occurs in individual B-cells

- Immunoglobulin M produced early in the response switches to IgG, particularly with thymus-dependent antigens. The switch is under T-cell control.
- Immunoglobulin G, but not IgM, responses improve on secondary challenge.
- Secondary responses show increased affinity for antigen.

Memory cells

- It has been suggested that activated memory cells are sustained by recurrent stimulation with antigen.
- This must occur largely in the germinal centers since the complexes on the surface of follicular dendritic cells (FDCs) are the only long-term source of antigen.
- Memory cells have higher affinity than naive cells.

See the accompanying website (**www.roitt.com**) for multiple choice questions

FURTHER READING

Borish, L. & Steinke, J.W. (2003) Cytokines and chemokines. *Journal of Allergy and Clinical Immunology*, **111** (Suppl.), S460–75.

Camacho, S.A., Kosco-Vilbois, M.H. & Berek, C. (1998) The dynamic structure of the germinal center. *Immunology Today*, **19**, 511–14.

Kelsoe, G. (1999) VDJ hypermutation and receptor revision. *Current Opinion in Immunology*, **11**, 70–5.

Sprent, J & Surh, C.D. (2001) Generation and maintenance of memory T cells. *Current Opinion in Immunology*, **13**, 248–54.

Weiss, A. & Cambier, J.C. (eds) (2004) Section on lymphocyte activation. *Current Opinion in Immunology*, **16**, 285–387.

Control mechanisms

ANTIGEN IS A MAJOR FACTOR IN CONTROL

The acquired immune response evolved so that it would come into play when contact with an infectious agent was first made. The appropriate antigen-specific cells expand, the effectors eliminate the antigen, and then the response quietens down and leaves room for reaction to other infections. Feedback mechanisms must operate to limit antibody production; otherwise, after antigenic stimulation, we would become overwhelmed by the responding clones of antibody-forming cells and their products. There is abundant evidence to support the view that antigen is a major regulatory factor and that antibody production is driven by the presence of antigen, falling off in intensity as the antigen concentration drops (figure 9.1). Furthermore, clearance of antigen by injection of excess antibody during the course of an immune response leads to a dramatic decrease in antibody synthesis and in the number of antibody-secreting cells.

ANTIBODY EXERTS FEEDBACK CONTROL

A useful control mechanism is to arrange for the product of a reaction to be an inhibitor, and this type of negative feedback is seen with antibody. Thus, removal of circulating antibody by plasmapheresis during an ongoing response leads to an increase in synthesis, whereas injection of preformed immunoglobulin G (IgG) antibody markedly hastens the fall in the number of antibody-forming cells consistent with feedback control on overall synthesis probably mediated through the B-cell Fcγ receptor.

IDIOTYPE NETWORK

Jerne's network hypothesis

The hypervariable loops on the Ig molecule which form the antigen-combining site have individual characteristic shapes that can be recognized by the appropriate antibodies as idiotypic determinants. There are hundreds of thousands of different idiotypes in one individual.

Jerne reasoned that the great diversity of idiotypes would, to a considerable extent, mirror the diversity of antigenic shapes in the external world. Thus, Jerne stated that if lymphocytes can recognize a whole range of foreign antigenic determinants, then they should be able to recognize the idiotypes on other lymphocytes. They would therefore form a large network or series of networks depending upon idiotype–anti-idiotype recognition between lymphocytes of the various T- and B-subsets (figure 9.2). The response to an external antigen would be proliferation of the specific clone of lymphocytes with expansion of the particular idiotype and then subsequent triggering of anti-idiotype responses to downregulate the specific lymphocyte population. There is no doubt that the elements which can form an idiotypic network are present in the body. Individuals can be immunized against idiotypes on their own antibodies, and such autoanti-idiotypes have been identified during the course of responses induced by antigens. It seems likely that similar interactions will be established for newly expanding T-cell clones, possibly linking with the B-cell network. Certainly, anti-idiotypic reactivity can be demonstrated

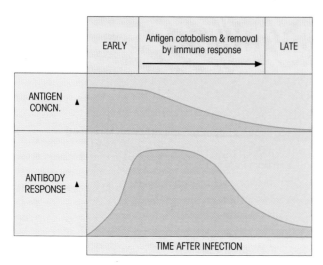

Figure 9.1 Antigen drives the immune response. As the antigen concentration falls due to catabolism and elimination by antibody, the intensity of the immune response declines but is maintained for some time at a lower level by antigen trapped on the follicular dendritic cells of the germinal centers.

in T-cell populations, and it is likely that relatively closed idiotype–anti-idiotype circuits contribute to a regulatory system.

T-CELL REGULATION

Activation-induced cell death

Termination of T-cell responses may result from ultraviolet or gamma-irradiation, hypoxia, high-dose corticosteroids, or various cytotoxic cytokines. It may also follow a decline in activating stimuli or growth factors, or be due to programmed cell death (apoptosis). Activation of T-cells by antigen does not continually produce proliferation but eventually sets off a train of events that culminate in activation-induced cell death by apoptosis. There are two main pathways of apoptosis, the CD95–CD95L (CD95 ligand) (Fas) death system and the mitochondrial pathway. Both pathways depend on the activation of a group of proteases belonging to the caspase family and result in T-cell numbers declining to pre-immunization levels.

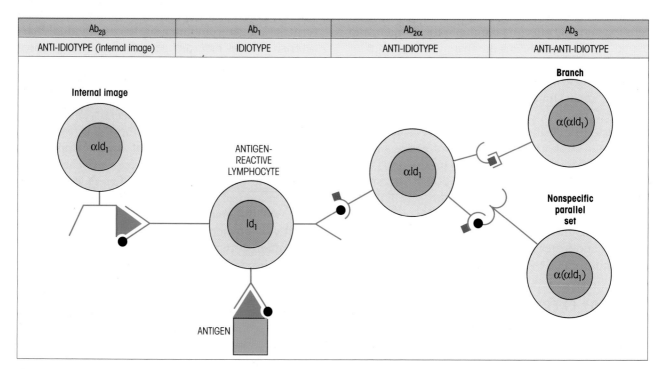

Figure 9.2 Elements in an idiotypic network in which the antigen receptors on one lymphocyte reciprocally recognize an idiotype on the receptors of another. T–T interactions could occur through direct recognition of one T-cell receptor (TCR) by the other, or more usually by recognition of a processed TCR peptide associated with major histocompatibility complex (MHC). One of the anti-idiotype sets, $Ab_2\beta$, may bear an idiotype of similar shape to (i.e. provides an **internal image** of) the antigen.

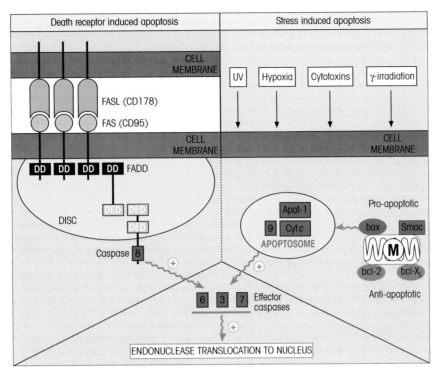

Figure 9.3 Activation-induced cell death. Receptor-based induction of apoptosis involves the trimerization of Fas by FasL (Fas-ligand). This brings together cytoplasmic death domains (DD) which can recruit a number of death effector domain (DED)-containing adapter molecules, such as FADD (Fas-associated protein with death domain) to form the death-inducing signaling complex (DISC). The DISC induces the cleavage of inactive procaspase 8 into active caspase 8, with subsequent activation of downstream effector caspases. A second pathway of apoptosis induction, often triggered by cellular stress, involves a number of mitochondria-associated proteins including cytochrome c, Smac/DIABLO and the bcl-2 family member bax. Caspase 9 activation is the key event in this pathway and requires association of the caspase with a number of other proteins including the cofactor Apaf-1 (apoptosis activating factor-1); the complex formed incorporates cytochrome c and is referred to as the apoptosome. The activated caspase 9 then cleaves procaspase 3. Although the death receptor and mitochondrial pathways are shown as initially separate in the figure, there is some crosstalk between them. Thus, caspase 8 can cleave the bcl-2 family member bid (not shown), a process which promotes cytochrome c release from mitochondria. Other members of the bcl-2 family, such as bcl-2 itself and bcl-X_L, inhibit apoptosis, perhaps by preventing the release of pro-apoptotic molecules from the mitochondria. M, mitochondrion; UV, ultraviolet.

In the CD95 system, Fas (CD95) expressed on the surface of all lymphoid cells interacts with its ligand, which is expressed on T-cells after they are activated. The FasL (Fas ligand) may combine with numerous Fas molecules on the same or on neighboring cells and even on B-cells resulting in their death. FasL binds an intracellular protein called FADD (Fas-associated death domain) which recruits the inactive form of caspase 8 and cleaves this into an active form. The activated caspase 8 now cleaves downstream caspases ultimately leading to endonuclease digestion of DNA, resulting in nuclear fragmentation and cell death. Details are shown in figure 9.3.

In the mitochondrial pathway, cytochrome c is released from the mitochondria into the cytoplasm where, together with a protein called Apaf-1 (apoptosis activating factor-1), it activates caspase 9 resulting in apoptosis. Like many other biologic systems, apop-

tosis needs to be regulated. Several gene products inhibit apoptosis and these belong mainly to the bcl-2 family. Those bcl-2 family members with anti-apoptotic activity probably do so by controlling the release of cytochrome c.

The cytokine interleukin-2 (IL-2) plays an important role in activation-induced cell death. Early in the immune response IL-2 acts as an important T-cell growth promoter. However, as the response develops and levels of this cytokine increase, it develops growth inhibitory effects by rendering T-cells more sensitive to the induction of apoptosis.

Activated T-cells exchange CD28 for cytotoxic T-lymphocyte antigen-4 (CTLA-4)

Early in the response, B7 molecules bind to CD28, which is important for T-cell activation. After activation, however, CTLA-4 is induced on T-cells and this competes with CD28 for B7 on the antigen-presenting cell (APC). Cytotoxic T-lymphocyte antigen-4 inhibits the transcription of IL-2 and subsequent T-cell proliferation, which will cause a decline of the immune response.

Regulatory T-cells

For many years immunologists have demonstrated the presence of suppressor or regulatory cells that could modulate a variety of humoral and cellular responses. We now recognize that when T-cells are activated they develop high levels of IL-2 receptor (CD25) on their surface, and that a population of these activated CD4+ CD25+ cells have regulatory activity on T-cell responses. It is thought that regulation is mediated by immunosuppressive cytokines which inhibit proliferation of other T-cells. These cytokines include IL-10 and transforming growth factor-β (TGFβ) which control the expansion of specific T-cells, and, by inhibiting interferon γ (IFNγ) production by the T-cells, will bring activated APCs back to their resting state. Other populations of CD4+CD25+ regulatory T-cells appear to act via a poorly defined cytokine-independent, but cell contact-dependent, mechanism.

THE INFLUENCE OF GENETIC AND OTHER FACTORS

Some genes affect general responsiveness

Mice can be selectively bred for high or low antibody responses through several generations to yield two lines, one of which consistently produces high-titer antibodies to a variety of antigens (high responders), and the other antibodies of relatively low titer (low responders). Out of the several different genetic loci involved, some give rise to a higher rate of B-cell proliferation and differentiation, whilst others affect macrophage behavior.

There was much excitement when it was first discovered that the antibody responses to a number of thymus-dependent antigenically simple substances are determined by genes mapping to the major histocompatibility complex (MHC) and three mechanisms have been proposed to account for MHC-linked high and low responsiveness.

1 *Defective processing and presentation.* In a high responder, processing of antigen and its recognition by a corresponding T-cell lead to lymphocyte triggering and clonal expansion (figure 9.4a). Sometimes, the

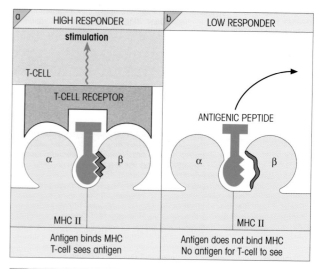

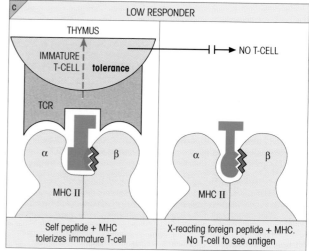

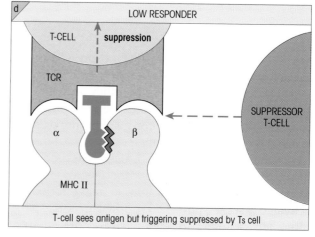

Figure 9.4 Different mechanisms can account for low T-cell response to antigen in association with major histocompatibility complex (MHC) class II. TCR, T-cell receptor; Ts, T-suppressor.

natural processing of an antigen in a given individual does not produce a peptide that fits well into their MHC molecules. Furthermore, it is known that variation in certain key residues of the MHC influence the binding to individual peptides. If a given MHC is unable to bind the peptide then obviously it cannot present antigen to the reactive T-cell (figure 9.4b).

2 *Defective T-cell repertoire.* T-cells with moderate to high affinity for self MHC molecules and their complexes with processed self antigens will be rendered unresponsive (cf. tolerance induction), so creating a "hole" in the T-cell repertoire. If there is a cross-reaction, i.e. similarity in shape at the T-cell recognition level between a foreign antigen and a self molecule which has already induced unresponsiveness, the host will lack T-cells specific for the foreign antigen and therefore be a low responder (figure 9.4c).

3 *T-suppression.* Major histocompatibility complex-restricted low responsiveness has been observed to relatively complex antigens containing several different epitopes. Such observations support the notion that low responder status can arise as an expression of regulatory cell activity (figure 9.4d).

Psychoimmunology

Attention has been drawn increasingly to interactions between immunologic and neuroendocrine systems generating the subject of "psychoimmunology." There is now extensive evidence that psychosocial stress can result in immune modulation resulting in detrimental changes in health. Many of the studies have examined immune function in individuals facing psychosocial stress such as students taking examinations, people providing long-term care to a spouse with Alzheimer's disease, or recently bereaved individuals. In all these groups depressed immune function was documented. Depressive symptoms in human immunodeficiency virus (HIV) infected men have been associated with decreased CD4$^+$ counts and a more rapid immune decline. Individuals with generalized anxiety disorders showed reduced natural killer (NK) cell activity and decreased IL-2 receptor expression on activated T-cells, but an increase in production of proinflammatory cytokines such as IL-6 and tumor necrosis factor-α (TNFα). Stress influenced the response of medical students to hepatitis B vaccinations in that those students who were less stressed mounted an antibody response earlier than those who were more anxious. It is likely therefore that the immune response to infectious agents will be reduced in this latter group. There are also studies documenting that wound heal-

ing is impeded by stress and this will enhance the risk for wound infection after surgery or trauma.

It is likely that many of the immunologic effects of stress are mediated via the endocrine system. Social stress has been shown to elevate hormones such as catecholamines and cortisol which have multiple immunomodulatory effects.

The secretion of glucocorticoids is a major response to stress induced by a wide range of stimuli such as extreme changes of temperature, fear, hunger and physical injury. Steroids are also released as a consequence of immune responses and limit those responses in a neuroendocrine feedback loop. Thus, IL-1, IL-6 and TNFα are capable of stimulating glucocorticoid synthesis and do so through the hypothalamic–pituitary–adrenal axis. This in turn leads to downregulation of Th1 and macrophage activity, so completing the negative feedback circuit (figure 9.5).

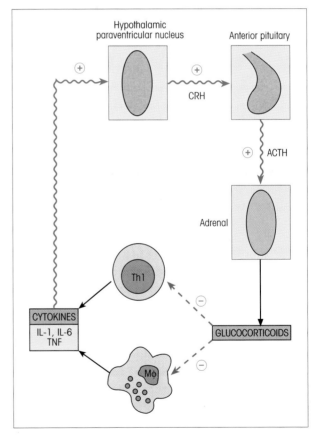

Figure 9.5 Glucocorticoid negative feedback on cytokine production. Cells of the immune system in both primary and secondary lymphoid organs can produce hormones and neuropeptides, while classical endocrine glands as well as neurones and glial cells can synthesize cytokines and appropriate receptors. ACTH, adrenocorticotropic hormone; CRH, corticotropin-releasing hormone; IL, interleukin; Mϕ, macrophage; TNF, tumor necrosis factor.

Sex hormones come into the picture

Estrogen is said to be the major factor influencing the more active immune responses in females relative to males. Women have higher serum Igs and secretory IgA levels, a higher antibody response to T-independent antigens, relative resistance to T-cell tolerance and greater resistance to infections. Females are also far more susceptible to autoimmune disease, an issue that will be discussed in greater depth in Chapter 17, but here let us note that oral contraceptives can induce flares of the autoimmune disorder systemic lupus erythematosus (SLE).

Decreased immune response in the elderly (immunosenescence)

Aging is associated with complex changes in many parts of the normal immune response (table 9.1), which accounts for the relative susceptibility of the elderly to viral and bacterial infections. Looking at early events in the response, the phagocytic and microbicidal activity of neutrophils is significantly diminished in later life. The reduced ability to phagocytose *Staphylococcus aureus* is of particular importance because of the increased susceptibility to this pathogen in the elderly. Although NK cell numbers are increased in this population they have decreased cytotoxic activity.

T-cell function and number are significantly altered with increasing age. T-cells, particularly the CD8 component, decrease significantly, probably due to an increase in apoptotic activity. This is associated with impairment of many T-cell functions including expression of CD28, proliferation, cytotoxicity, IL-2 secretion and delayed hypersensitivity reactions. It is primarily the Th1 subset that diminishes in the aged, and there is an increase in cytokine production by the Th2 subset. Therefore, levels of IL-6 are raised in the elderly population whilst IL-2 levels are decreased (figure 9.6).

Humoral immunity is less affected by age, although there is an increase in autoantibody levels. Circulating IgG and IgA levels are generally increased. However, the primary antibody response is diminished in the elderly, resulting in lower antibody levels that decrease far sooner after reaching their peak than in younger people.

Healthy elderly individuals show evidence of low-grade inflammatory activity in their blood with high circulating levels of TNFα, IL-6 and the IL-1 receptor antagonist (IL-1Ra). Although the cause of this is unclear, these proinflammatory cytokines may play a role in the pathogenesis of age-related diseases such as

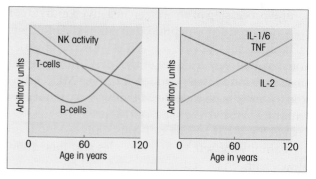

Figure 9.6 Age trends in some immunological parameters. IL, interleukin; NK, natural killer; TNF, tumor necrosis factor. (Based on C., Franceschi, D., Monti, P., Sansoni & A., Cossarizza. (1995) *Immunology Today* **16**, 12.)

Alzheimer's disease, Parkinson's disease and certainly atherosclerosis. The high levels of cytokines also contribute to muscle breakdown, which is found in the elderly, and increased osteoclastic activity resulting in osteoporosis. The low-grade inflammation may also play a role in the depressed cell-mediated immune responses by inhibiting T-cell activity through long-term activation. Aging therefore is associated with impaired cellular immunity combined with low-grade chronic inflammation.

Table 9.1 Immune deficiencies observed in normal elderly individuals.

NEUTROPHILS
Decreased phagocytic activity
Decreased microbicidal activity
CELL-MEDIATED IMMUNITY
Decreased CD3+ cells
Increased Th2 subset and decreased Th1 subset
Decreased lymphocyte proliferation
Decreased CD28 expression
Decreased delayed type hypersensitivity
Increased production of pro-inflammatory cytokines
HUMORAL IMMUNITY
Increased autoantibodies
Decreased ability to generate primary immune responses
NATURAL KILLER CELLS
Increased percentage
Decreased cytotoxic activity

Malnutrition diminishes the effectiveness of the immune response

The greatly increased susceptibility of undernourished individuals to infection can be attributed to many factors including a stressful lifestyle, poor sanitation and personal hygiene, overcrowding and inadequate health education. But, in addition, there are gross effects of protein calorie malnutrition on immunocompetence. The widespread atrophy of lymphoid tissues and the 50% reduction in circulating CD4 T-cells underlies serious impairment of cell-mediated immunity. Antibody responses may be intact but they are of lower affinity; phagocytosis of bacteria is relatively normal but the subsequent intracellular destruction is defective.

It should be remembered that undernutrition is very common amongst the elderly and further depresses cell-mediated immunity including lymphocyte proliferation, cytokine synthesis and decreased antibody responses to vaccine. The immunosuppression of the elderly is further enhanced by zinc deficiency, which is extremely frequent in aged individuals.

REVISION

Control by antigen

• Immune responses are largely antigen driven and as the level of exogenous antigen falls, so does the intensity of the response.

Feedback control by antibody

• Immunoglobulin G (IgG) antibodies inhibit responses via the Fcγ receptor on B-cells.

T-cell regulation

• Activated T-cells express Fas and FasL (Fas ligand) which can restrain unlimited clonal expansion.
• The costimulatory molecule CD28 is replaced by the inhibitory molecule CTLA-4 (cytotoxic T-lymphocyte antigen-4) following T-cell activation.
• During the immune response regulatory T-cells emerge which suppress T-helpers, presumably as feedback control of excessive T-helper cell (Th) expansion.

Idiotype networks

• Antigen-specific receptors on lymphocytes can interact with the idiotypes on the receptors of other lymphocytes to form a network (Jerne).

Genetic factors influence the immune response

• A number of genes control the overall antibody response to complex antigens: some affect macrophage antigen processing and microbicidal activity and some the rate of proliferation of differentiating B-cells.

Immunoneuroendocrine networks

• Immunologic, neurologic and endocrinologic systems can all interact.
• The field of psychoimmunology examines the state of the immune system in individuals living through acute or chronic stressful episodes.
• Stress may result in diminished natural killer (NK) cell activity, antibody production and cellular immunity, resulting in increased susceptibility to infection and depressed would healing.
• Estrogens may be largely responsible for the more active immune responses in females relative to males.

Effects of aging and diet on immunity

• Protein–calorie malnutrition grossly impairs cell-mediated immunity and phagocyte microbicidal potency.
• The elderly exhibit impaired immune responses to infectious agents.
• The pattern of cytokines produced by peripheral blood cells changes with age, interleukin-2 (IL-2) decreasing and tumor necrosis factor-α (TNFα), IL-1 and IL-6 increasing.

See the accompanying website (**www.roitt.com**) for multiple choice questions

FURTHER READING

Bruunsgaard, H., Pederson, M. & Pederson, B.K. (2001) Aging and proinflammatory cytokines. *Current Opinion in Hematology*, **8**, 131–6.

Chandra, R.K. (1998) Nutrition and the immune system. In: *Encyclopedia of Immunology* (eds P.J. Delves & I.M. Roitt), 2nd edn, pp. 1869–71. Academic Press, London. [See also other relevant articles in the *Encyclopedia*: "Cinader, B. Aging and the immune system," pp. 4559–61; "Cohen, N., Moynihan, J.A., Ader, R. Behavioural regulation of immunity," pp. 336–40; "Yamamoto, N. Vitamin D and the immune response," pp. 2494–9.]

Lesourd, B.M., Mazari, L. & Ferry, M. (1998) The role of nutrition in immunity in the aged. *Nutrition Reviews*, **56**, S113–25.

Padgett, D.A. & Glaser, R. (2003) How stress influences the immune response. *Trends in Immunology*, **24**, 444–8.

Selin, L.K. (ed.) (2004) Section on lymphocyte effector function. *Current Opinion in Immunology*, **16**, 257–83.

Swain, S.L. & Cambier, J.C. (eds) (1996) Lymphocyte activation and effector functions. *Current Opinion in Immunology*, **8**, 309–418.

Ontogeny

THE MULTIPOTENTIAL HEMATOPOIETIC STEM CELL GIVES RISE TO THE FORMED ELEMENTS OF THE BLOOD

Hematopoiesis originates in the early yolk sac and, as embryogenesis proceeds, this function is taken over by the fetal liver and finally by the bone marrow where it continues throughout life. The hematopoietic stem cell which gives rise to the formed elements of the blood (figure 10.1) can be shown to be multipotent, to seed other organs and to have a relatively unlimited capacity to renew itself through the creation of further stem cells. Thus, an animal can be completely protected against the lethal effects of high doses of radiation by injection of stem cells which will repopulate its lymphoid and myeloid systems. This forms the basis of human bone marrow transplantation.

We have come a long way towards the goal of isolating highly purified populations of hematopoietic stem cells, although not all agree that we have yet achieved it. CD34 is a marker of an extremely early cell but there is some debate as to whether this identifies the holy pluripotent stem cell itself. The stem cells differentiate within the microenvironment of stromal cells which produce various growth factors such as interleukin-3 (IL-3), IL-4, IL-6, IL-7, granulocyte-macrophage colony-stimulating factor (GM-CSF) and others (figure 10.1).

THE THYMUS PROVIDES THE ENVIRONMENT FOR T-CELL DIFFERENTIATION

The thymus is organized into a series of lobules based upon meshworks of epithelial cells which form well-defined cortical and medullary zones (figure 10.2). This framework of epithelial cells provides the microenvironment for T-cell differentiation. There are subtle interactions between the extracellular matrix proteins and a variety of integrins on different lymphocyte subpopulations which, together with chemokines and chemokine receptor expression, play a role in the homing of progenitors to the thymus and their subsequent migration within the gland. In addition, the epithelial cells produce a series of peptide hormones including thymulin, thymosin α_1, thymic humoral factor (THF) and thymopoietin, which are capable of promoting the appearance of T-cell differentiation markers.

The specialized large epithelial cells in the outer cortex are known as "nurse" cells because they can each be associated with large numbers of lymphocytes which appear to be lying within their cytoplasm. The epithelial cells of the deep cortex have branched dendritic processes rich in class II major histocompatibility complex (MHC). They connect through desmosomes to form a network through which cortical lymphocytes must pass on their way to the medulla (figure 10.2). The cortical lymphocytes are densely packed compared

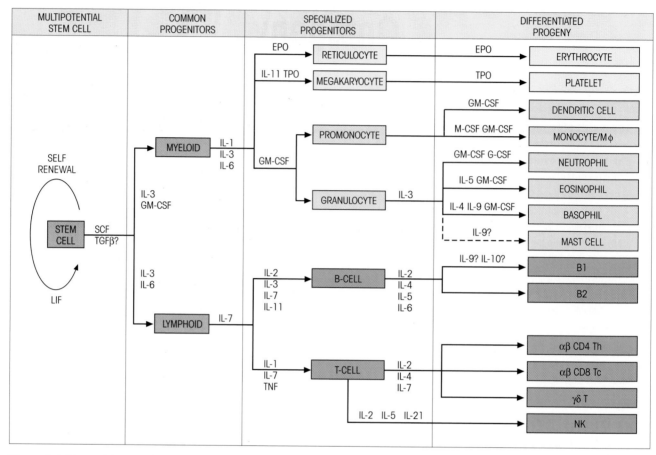

Figure 10.1 The multipotential hematopoietic stem cell and its progeny which differentiate under the influence of a series of growth factors within the microenvironment of the bone marrow. EPO, erythropoietin; G-CSF, granulocyte colony-stimulating factor; GM-CSF, granulocyte-macrophage colony-stimulating factor, so called because it promotes the formation of mixed colonies of these two cell types from bone marrow progenitors either in tissue culture or on transfer to an irradiated recipient where they appear in the spleen; IL-3, interleukin-3, often termed the multi-CSF because it stimulates progenitors of platelets, mast cells and all the other types of myeloid and erythroid cells; LIF, leukemia inhibitory factor; Mφ, macrophage; M-CSF, macrophage colony-stimulating factor; NK, natural killer; SCF, stem cell factor; TGFβ, transforming growth factor-β; TNF, tumor necrosis factor; TPO, thrombopoietin.

with those in the medulla, many are in division and large numbers are undergoing apoptosis as a result of positive and negative selection (see later). A number of bone marrow-derived interdigitating dendritic cells (DCs) are present in the medulla and the epithelial cells have broader processes than their cortical counterparts and express high levels of both class I and class II MHC.

In the human, thymic involution commences within the first 12 months of life, reducing by around 3% a year to middle age and by 1% thereafter. The size of the organ gives no clue to these changes because there is replacement by adipose tissue. In a sense, the thymus is progressively disposable because, as we shall see, it establishes a long-lasting peripheral T-cell pool which enables the host to withstand loss of the gland without catastrophic failure of immunologic function, witness the minimal effects of thymectomy in the adult compared with the **dramatic influence in the neonate**.

T-CELL ONTOGENY

Differentiation is accompanied by changes in surface markers

T-lymphocytes originate from hematopoietic stem cells which express a number of chemokine receptors and are attracted to the thymus by chemokines secreted by the thymic stromal cells. The T-cell precursors stain positively for CD34 and for the enzyme terminal deoxynucleotidyl transferase (TdT) (figure 10.3), which inserts nontemplated ("N-region") nucleotides

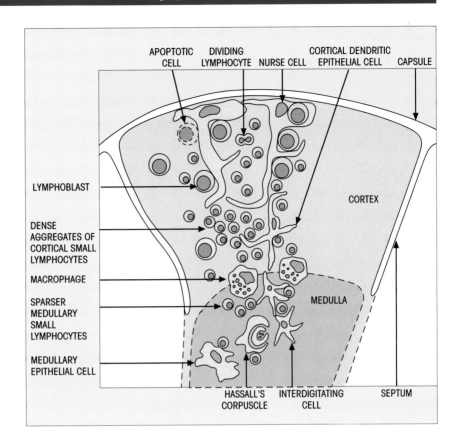

Figure 10.2 Cellular features of a thymus lobule. See text for description. (Adapted from L.E. Hood, I.L. Weissman, W.B. Wood & J.H. Wilson (1984) *Immunology*, 2nd edn, p. 261. Benjamin Cummings, California.)

at the junctions between the V, D and J variable region segments to increase diversity of the T-cell receptors (TCRs). Under the influence of IL-1 and tumor necrosis factor (TNF) the T-cell precursors differentiate into prothymocytes, committed to the T-lineage. At this stage the cells begin to express various TCR chains and are then expanded, ultimately synthesizing CD3, the invariant signal-transducing complex of the TCR, and becoming **double-positive** for CD4$^+$ and CD8$^+$. Finally, under the guiding hand of chemokines, the cells traverse the cortico-medullary junction to the medulla, where they appear as separate immunocompetent populations of **single-positive CD4$^+$ T-helpers** and **CD8$^+$ cytotoxic T-cell precursors**. The γδ cells remain double-negative, i.e. CD4$^-$8$^-$, except for a small subset which express CD8.

Receptor rearrangement

The development of TCRs

The earliest T-cell precursors have TCR genes in the germ-line configuration, and the first rearrangements to occur involve the γ and δ loci. The αβ receptors are only detected a few days later. The $V\beta$ is first rearranged in the double-negative CD4$^-$8$^-$ cells and associates with an invariant pre-α-chain and the CD3 molecules to form a single "pre-TCR." Expression of this complex leads the pre-T-cells to proliferate and become **double-positive** CD4$^+$8$^+$ cells. Further development now requires rearrangement of the $V\alpha$ gene segments so allowing formation of the mature αβ TCR, and the cells are now ready for subsequent bouts of positive and negative receptor editing, as will be discussed shortly. Rearrangement of the $V\beta$ genes on the sister chromatid is suppressed by a process called **allelic exclusion** so that each cell only expresses a single TCR β chain.

Cells are positively selected for self MHC restriction in the thymus

The ability of T-cells to recognize antigenic peptides in association with self MHC is developed in the thymus gland. A small proportion of the double-positive (CD4$^+$8$^+$) T-cells bearing their TCR will bind with low avidity to MHC molecules expressed on thymic cortical epithelial cells and will be **positively selected** to complete their progress to mature T-cells. The rest of the cells that do not recognize their own MHC are

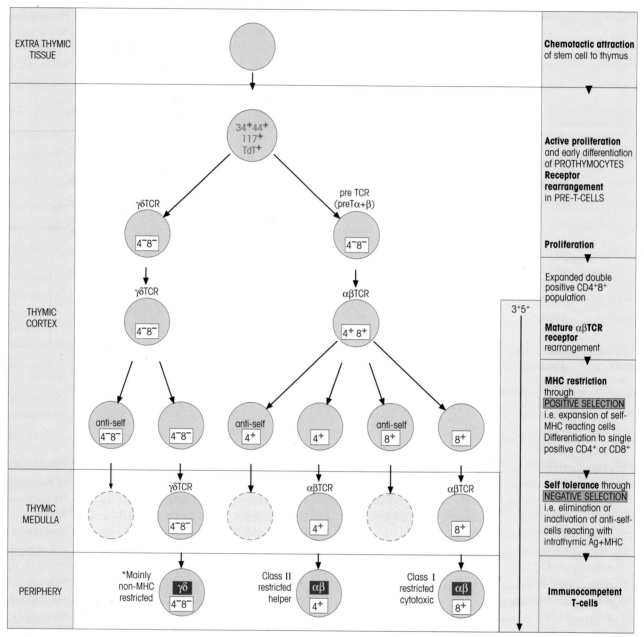

Figure 10.3 Differentiation of T-cells within the thymus. Numbers refer to CD designation. TdT, terminal deoxynucleotidyl transferase. Negatively selected cells in gray. The diagram is partly simplified for the sake of clarity. *γδ cells mainly appear to recognize antigen directly, in a manner analogous to the antibody molecule on B-cells, although some may be restricted by major histocompatibility complex (MHC) class I or II.

eliminated and will die in 3 or 4 days. Another feature of this selection phase of T-cell development is that CD4+8+ cells bearing TCR which recognize self MHC on the epithelial cells are positively selected for differentiation to CD4+8− or CD4−8+ single-positive cells. A cell coming into contact with self MHC class I molecules will mature as a CD8+ cell, whereas if contact is made with MHC class II molecules the cells will develop as CD4+ T-cells. In the rare immunodeficiency disorder called the **bare lymphocyte syndrome**, MHC molecules do not appear on the surface of cells. As a result CD8+ cells will not develop in those cases which lack class I MHC, while CD4+ cells fail to appear in those cases without class II MHC molecules.

Self-reactive cells are removed in the thymus by negative selection

Many of the cells that survive positive selection have receptors for self antigen and if allowed to mature would produce immune responses to autoantigens. These thymocytes therefore undergo **negative selection**, which is crucial for maintaining tolerance to self antigens. In this process self antigens are presented to the maturing thymocytes by DCs or macrophages, and any cell responding with high avidity is eliminated by the induction of apoptosis. The result of positive and negative selection is that all mature T-cells in the thymic medulla will recognize foreign peptide only in the context of self MHC, and will not have the potential to mount immune responses against self antigens and in the case of αβ TCR cells, will either be CD4 or CD8 positive.

T-CELL TOLERANCE

The induction of immunologic tolerance is necessary to avoid self-reactivity

In essence, lymphocytes recognize foreign antigens through complementarity of shape mediated by the intermolecular forces we have described previously. To a large extent the building blocks used to form microbial and host molecules are the same, so it is the assembled shapes of *self* and *nonself* molecules which must be discriminated by the immune system if potentially disastrous autoreactivity is to be avoided. Many self-reacting T-cells are eliminated by apoptosis during negative selection in the thymus and others are tolerized in the periphery; for example, by being made anergic (functionally inactivated) following contact with self antigens in a "nonstimulatory" context. The restriction of each lymphocyte to a single specificity makes the job of establishing self-tolerance that much easier, simply because it just requires a mechanism which functionally deletes self-reacting cells and leaves the remainder of the repertoire unscathed. The most radical difference between self and nonself molecules lies in the fact that, in early life, the developing lymphocytes are surrounded by self and normally only meet nonself antigens at a later stage and then within the context of the adjuventicity and cytokine release characteristic of infection. With its customary efficiency, the blind force of evolution has exploited these differences to establish the mechanisms of **immunologic tolerance to host constituents**.

Dendritic cells are important in the induction of T-cell tolerance

We have previously described how DCs, when encountering foreign antigens or cytokines from an inflamed site, become activated and develop costim-

ulatory molecules important in the activation of T-cells. In the absence of microorganisms or inflammation, DCs will capture the remains of cells that die physiologically and present these to autoreactive T-cells. However, because they are not activated they will present tissue antigens without costimulatory molecules resulting in **T-cell anergy** rather than T-cell activation.

DEVELOPMENT OF B-CELL SPECIFICITY

The B-lymphocyte precursors, pro-B-cells, are present in the fetal liver by 8–9 weeks gestation. Production of B-cells by liver gradually wanes and is mostly taken over by bone marrow for the remainder of life.

The sequence of immunoglobulin gene rearrangements

Stage 1 Initially, the *D–J* segments on both heavy chain coding regions (one from each parent) rearrange (figure 10.4).

Stage 2 A *V–DJ* recombinational event now occurs on one heavy chain. If this proves to be a *nonproductive* rearrangement (i.e. adjacent segments are joined in an incorrect reading frame or in such a way as to generate a termination codon downstream from the splice point), then a second *V–DJ* rearrangement will occur on the sister heavy chain region. If a productive rearrangement is not achieved, we can wave the pre-B-cell a fond farewell.

Stage 3 Assuming that a productive rearrangement is made, the pre-B-cell can now synthesize μ heavy chains. At around the same time, two genes, V_{preB} and λ_5, with homology for the V_L and C_L segments of λ-light chains respectively, are temporarily transcribed to form a "pseudo light chain," which associates with the μ chains to generate a surface surrogate "immunoglobulin M (IgM)" receptor together with the Ig-α and Ig-β chains conventionally required to form a functional B-cell receptor. This surrogate receptor closely parallels the pre-Tα/β receptor on pre-T-cell precursors of αβ TCR-bearing cells.

Stage 4 The surface receptor is signaled, perhaps by a stromal cell, to suppress any further rearrangement of heavy chain genes on a sister chromatid. This is termed **allelic exclusion**.

Stage 5 It is presumed that the surface receptor now initiates the next set of gene rearrangements which

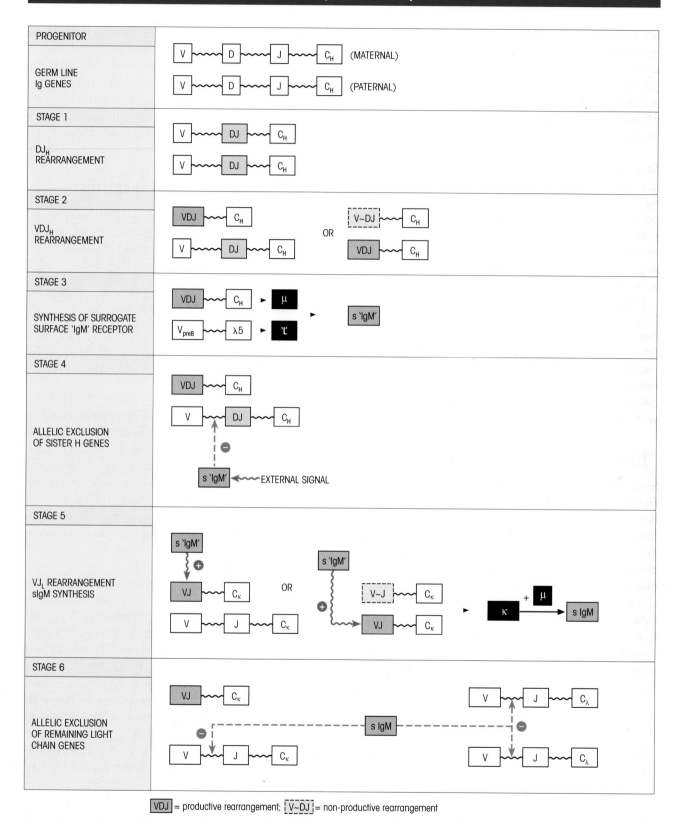

VDJ = productive rearrangement; V~DJ = non-productive rearrangement

Figure 10.4 Postulated sequence of B-cell gene rearrangements and mechanism of allelic exclusion (see text).

occur on the κ light chain gene loci. These involve *V–J* recombinations on first one and then the other κ allele until a productive V_κ–*J* rearrangement is accomplished. Were that to fail, an attempt would be made to achieve productive rearrangement of the λ alleles. Synthesis of conventional surface IgM (sIgM) now proceeds.

Stage 6 The sIgM molecule now prohibits any further gene shuffling by allelic exclusion of any unrearranged light chain genes. The further addition of surface IgD now marks the readiness of the virgin (naive) B-cell for priming by antigen. B-cells bearing self-reactive receptors of moderately high affinity are eliminated by a negative selection process akin to that operating on autoreactive T-cells in the thymus.

Following encounter with specific antigen, the naive B-cell can develop into an IgM-secreting plasma cell, or can undergo class switching in which case the surface IgM and IgD will be replaced with, usually, a single class of immunoglobulin (IgG, IgA or IgE). At the terminal stages in the life of a fully mature plasma cell only the secreted version of the Ig molecule is made with virtually no sIg present.

The importance of allelic exclusion

Since each cell has chromosome complements derived from each parent, the differentiating B-cell has four light- and two heavy-chain gene clusters to choose from. We have described how once a productive *VDJ* DNA rearrangement has occurred within one heavy-chain cluster, and a productive *VJ* rearrangement in one light-chain cluster, the *V* genes on the other four chromosomes are held in the germ line configuration by an allelic exclusion mechanism. Thus, the cell is able to express only one light and one heavy chain. This is essential for clonal selection to work since the cell is then programmed only to make the one antibody it uses as a cell surface receptor to recognize antigen.

NATURAL KILLER (NK) CELL ONTOGENY

The precise lineage of NK cells is still to be established. They share a common early progenitor with T-cells and express the CD2 molecule which is also present on T-cells. Furthermore, they have IL-2 receptors, are driven to proliferate by IL-2 and produce interferon γ. However, they do not develop in the thymus and their TCR *V* genes are not rearranged. The current view is therefore that they separate from the T-cell lineage very early on in their differentiation.

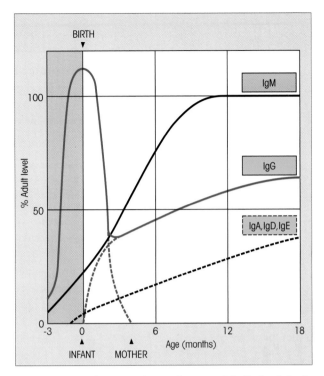

Figure 10.5 Development of serum immunoglobulin levels in the human. (After J.R. Hobbs (1969) In: *Immunology and Development* (ed. M. Adinolfi), p. 118. Heinemann, London.)

THE OVERALL RESPONSE IN THE NEONATE

Lymph node and spleen remain relatively underdeveloped in the fetus except where there has been intrauterine exposure to antigens, as in congenital infections with rubella or other organisms. The ability to reject grafts and to mount an antibody response is reasonably well developed by birth, but the immunoglobulin levels, with one exception, are low, particularly in the absence of intrauterine infection. The exception is IgG, which is acquired by placental transfer from the mother, a process dependent upon Fc structures specific to this Ig class. Maternal IgG is catabolized with a half-life of approximately 30 days so that serum levels fall over the first 3 months, accentuated by the increase in blood volume of the growing infant. Thereafter the rate of synthesis overtakes the rate of breakdown of maternal IgG and the overall concentration increases steadily. The other immunoglobulins do not cross the placenta and the low but significant levels of IgM in cord blood are synthesized by the baby (figure 10.5). Immunoglobulin M reaches adult levels by 9 months of age. Only trace levels of IgA, IgD and IgE are present in the circulation of the newborn.

REVISION

Multipotential stem cells from the bone marrow give rise to all the formed elements of the blood
- Expansion and differentiation are driven by soluble growth (colony-stimulating) factors and contact with reticular stromal cells.

The differentiation of T-cells occurs within the microenvironment of the thymus
- Precursor T-cells arising from stem cells in the marrow need to travel to the thymus under the influence of chemokines. There they become immunocompetent T-cells.
- Numerous lymphocytes undergo apoptosis either due to not being positively selected or due to negative selection.
- Thymic involution commences within the first 12 months of life.

T-cell ontogeny
- Differentiation to immunocompetent T-cell subsets is accompanied by changes in the surface phenotype which can be recognized with monoclonal antibodies.
- CD34 positive stem cells differentiate into prothymocytes and begin expressing various T-cell receptor (TCR) chains and CD3.
- Double-negative CD4$^-$8$^-$ pre-T-cells are expanded to become double-positive CD4$^+$8$^+$.
- As the cells traverse the cortico-medullary junction under the influence of chemokines, they become either CD4$^+$ or CD8$^+$.

Receptor rearrangement
- The first TCR rearrangement involves the γ and δ loci.
- Rearrangements of first the $V\beta$ locus and later the $V\alpha$ locus form the mature $\alpha\beta$ TCR.

T-cells are positively and negatively selected in the thymus
- The thymus epithelial cells positively select CD4$^+$8$^+$ T-cells with avidity for their major histocompatibility complex (MHC) haplotype so that single-positive CD4$^+$ or CD8$^+$ T-cells develop that are restricted to the recognition of antigen in the context of the epithelial cell haplotype.

- The rest of the cells that do not recognize their own MHC are eliminated.
- Cells that have receptors for self antigen undergo negative selection and are also eliminated.

T-cell tolerance
- The induction of immunological tolerance is necessary to avoid self-reactivity.
- Many T-cells reacting with self antigens are eliminated by negative selection in the thymus. Others are tolerized in the periphery when they come into contact with self antigens in the absence of costimulatory molecules, as when they are presented by non-activated dendritic cells (DCs).

Development of B-cell specificity
- The sequence of immunoglobulin (Ig) heavy chain variable gene rearrangements is D to J and then V to DJ.
- VDJ transcription produces μ chains which associate with V_{preB}. λ_5 chains to form a surrogate surface IgM-like receptor.
- This receptor signals allelic exclusion of unrearranged heavy chains.
- If the rearrangement at any stage is unproductive, i.e. does not lead to an acceptable gene reading frame, the allele on the sister chromosome is rearranged.
- The next set of gene rearrangements is V to J on the κ light gene, or, if this fails, on the λ light chain gene.
- The cell now develops a commitment to producing a particular class of antibody.
- The mechanisms of allelic exclusion ensure that each lymphocyte is programmed for only one antibody (figure 10.4).

The overall response in the neonate
- Maternal IgG crosses the placenta and provides a high level of passive immunity at birth.

See the accompanying website (**www.roitt.com**) for multiple choice questions

FURTHER READING

Banchereau, J., Paezesny, S., Blanco, P. *et al.* (2003) Dendritic cells: Controllers of the immune system and a new promise for immunotherapy. *Annals of the New York Academy of Sciences*, **987**, 180–7.

von Boehmer, H. (2000) T-cell lineage fate: Instructed by receptor signals? *Current Biology*, **10**, R642–5.

Hardy, R.R. & Hayakawa, K. (2001) B cell development pathways. *Annual Review of Immunology*, **19**, 595–621.

Herzenberg, L.A. (2000) B-1 cells, the lineage question revisited. *Immunological Reviews*, **175**, 9–22.

Kamradt, T. & Mitchison, N.A. (2001) Tolerance and autoimmunity. *New England Journal of Medicine*, **344**, 655–64.

Phillips, R.L., Ernst, R.E., Brunk, B. *et al.* (2000) The genetic program of hematopoietic stem cells. *Science*, **288**, 1635–40.

Adversarial strategies during infection

We are engaged in constant warfare with the microbes that surround us, and the processes of mutation and evolution have tried to select microorganisms with the means of evading our defense mechanisms. In this chapter, we look at the varied, often ingenious, adversarial strategies which our enemies and we have developed over very long periods of time.

INFLAMMATION REVISITED

The acute inflammatory process involves a protective influx of white cells, complement, antibody and other plasma proteins into a site of infection or injury and was discussed in broad outline in the introductory chapters.

Mediators of inflammation

A complex variety of mediators are involved in acute inflammatory responses. Some act directly on the smooth muscle wall surrounding the arterioles to alter blood flow. Others act on the venules to cause contraction of the endothelial cells with transient opening of the inter-endothelial junctions and consequent transudation of plasma. The migration of leukocytes from the bloodstream is facilitated by cytokines, such as interleukin-1 (IL-1) and tumor necrosis factor (TNF), which upregulate the expression of adherence molecules on both endothelial and white cells, and chemokines, which lead the leukocytes to the inflamed site.

Initiation of the acute inflammatory response

A very early event in inflammation is the upregulation of the adhesion molecules E-selectin on endothelium and L-selectin on leukocytes. Engagement of P-selectin with ligands on polymorphonuclear neutrophils (PMNs) causes a leukocyte adhesion cascade. The cells are tethered to the endothelium and then roll along it, followed by firm adhesion and migration through the endothelium. Inflammatory mediators also increase surface expression of the integrins LFA-1 (named lymphocyte function-associated antigen-1, but in fact found on all leukocytes) and Mac-1. Under the influence of cytokines, ICAM-1 (intercellular adhesion molecule-1) is induced on endothelial cells and binds the various integrins on the PMN surface causing PMN arrest (figure 11.1). Exposure of the PMN to IL-8 from endothelial cells and to various cytokines produced at the site of infection will also cause activation of the PMN. This makes them more responsive to chemotactic agents, and they will exit from the circulation under the influence of C5a, leukotriene-B4 and chemokines (*chemo*tactic cyto*kines*; table 11.1). They move purposefully through the gap between endothelial cells, across the basement membrane (**diapedesis**)

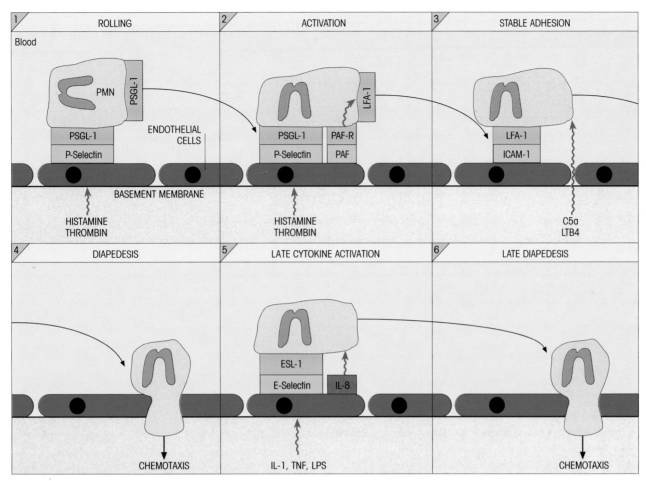

Figure 11.1 Early events in inflammation affecting neutrophil margination and diapedesis. Induced upregulation of P-selectin on the vessel walls plays the major role in the initial leukocyte–endothelial interaction (rolling) by interaction with ligands on the neutrophil such as the mucin-like P-selectin glycoprotein ligand-1 (PSGL-1, CD162). Recognition of extracellular gradients of the chemotactic mediators by receptors on the polymorphonuclear neutrophil (PMN) surface triggers intracellular signals which generate motion. The cytokine-induced expression of E-selectin, which is recognized by the glycoprotein E-selectin ligand-1 (ESL-1) on the neutrophil, occurs as a later event. Chemotactic factors such as interleukin-8 (IL-8), which is secreted by a number of cell types including the endothelium itself, are important mediators of the inflammatory process. ICAM-1, intercellular adhesion molecule-1; LFA-1, lymphocyte function-associated antigen-1; LPS, lipopolysaccharide; PAF, platelet activating factor; TNF, tumor necrosis factor.

and up the chemotactic gradient to the inflammation site.

The ongoing inflammatory process

During the inflammatory process, not only are leukocytes recruited from the blood but also cells such as macrophages and mast cells, which are pre-stationed in the tissue, will become activated. Mast cells respond early to anaphylatoxins (C3a and C5a) produced by the complement cascade and to bacteria and their products. They will release histamine, platelet activating factor (PAF), TNF, newly synthesized cytokines and various **chemokines**. Tissue macrophages under the stimulus of local infection or injury secrete an imposing array of mediators. These include the cytokines IL-1 and TNFα that stimulate the endothelial cells to upregulate the adhesion molecule E-selectin, and a group of chemokines such as IL-8, which are highly effective PMN chemotaxins. In general, chemokines of the C-X-C subfamily (defined in table 11.1) such as IL-8 are specific for neutrophils and, to varying extents, lymphocytes, whereas chemokines with the C-C motif are chemotactic for monocytes and natural killer (NK) cells, basophils and eosinophils. Eotaxin (CCL11) is highly specific for eosinophils and the presence of significant concentrations of this mediator together with RANTES (*r*egulated *u*pon *a*ctivation, *n*ormal *T*-cell

Table 11.1 Chemokines: leukocyte chemo-attractant specificities.

Chemokine	Chemoattractant specificity					
	Neutrophils	Basophils	Eosinophils	NK cells	Monocytes	Lymphocytes
ENA-78 (CXCL5)	+					
IL-8 (CXCL8)	+	+				+
IP-10 (CXCL10)				+		+
NAP-2 (CXCL7)	+					
Eotaxin-1 (CCL11)		+	+			+
MCP-1 (CCL2)		+		+	+	+
MCP-2 (CCL8)		+		+	+	+
MCP-3 (CCL7)		+	+	+	+	+
MIP-1α (CCL3)			+	+	+	+
MIP-1β (CCL4)				+	+	+
RANTES (CCL5)		+	+	+	+	+
Lymphotactin (XCL1)						+
Fractalkine (CX3CL1)				+	+	+

C, lacks first and third cysteines of the motif; except for IP-10, the CXC motif is preceded by the amino acids E-L-R; CC, no intervening residue; CXC, chemokine with any amino acid X intervening between the first and second conserved cysteines of the four which characterize the chemokine structural motif; ENA-78, epithelial derived neutrophil attractant-78; IP-10, interferon-inducible protein-10; MCP, monocyte chemotactic proteins; MIP, macrophage inflammatory protein; NAP-2, neutrophil activating protein-2; RANTES, regulated upon activation normal T-cell expressed and secreted.

(Data summarized from Schall T.J. & Bacon K.B. (1994) *Current Opinion in Immunology* **6**, 865.)

expressed and secreted) in mucosal surfaces, could account for the enhanced population of eosinophils in those tissues.

Clearly this whole operation serves to focus the immune defenses around the invading microorganisms. These become coated with antibody, C3b and certain acute phase proteins and are ripe for phagocytosis by the activated PMN and macrophages.

Of course it is beneficial to recruit lymphocytes to sites of infection and we should remember that endothelial cells in these areas express VCAM-1 (vascular cell adhesion molecule-1), which acts as a homing receptor for VLA-4 (very late antigen-4) -positive activated memory T-cells. In addition, the endothelial cells themselves, when activated, release the chemokines IL-8 and lymphotactin, which will attract lymphocytes to the site of the inflammatory response.

Regulation and resolution of inflammation

With its customary prudence, evolution has established regulatory mechanisms to prevent inflammation from getting out of hand. The complement system is controlled by a series of complement regulatory proteins such as C1 inhibitor, the C3 control proteins factors H and I, complement receptor CR1, and decay accelerating factor (DAF). Regulation of inflammatory cells is mediated by prostaglandin E_2 (PGE$_2$), transforming growth factor-β (TGFβ), IL-10 and other cytokines, which were discussed more fully in Chapter 8. Prostaglandin E_2 is a potent inhibitor of lymphocyte proliferation and cytokine production by T-cells and macrophages. Transforming growth factor-β and IL-10 deactivate macrophages by inhibiting the production of reactive oxygen intermediates and downregulating major histocompatibility complex (MHC) class II expression. Most importantly these cytokines inhibit the release of TNF and other proinflammatory cytokines.

Endogenous glucocorticoids produced via the hypothalamic–pituitary–adrenal axis exert their anti-inflammatory effects both through the repression of a number of genes, including those for proinflammatory cytokines and adhesion molecules, and the induction of inhibitors of inflammation such as lipocortin-1, secretory leukocyte proteinase inhibitor and IL-1 receptor antagonist (IL-1Ra). Once the inflammatory agent has been cleared, these regulatory processes will normalize the site. When the inflammation traumatizes tissues through its intensity and extent, TGFβ plays a major role in the subsequent wound healing by stimulating fibroblast division and the laying down of new extracellular matrix elements forming scar tissue.

Chronic inflammation

If an inflammatory agent persists, either because of its resistance to metabolic breakdown or through the inability of a deficient immune system to clear an infectious microbe, the character of the cellular response changes. The site becomes dominated by macrophages with varying morphology: many have an activated appearance, some form arrays of what are termed "epithelioid" cells and others fuse to form giant cells. Collectively these macrophages produce the characteristic **granuloma** which walls off the persisting agent from the remainder of the body (see section on type IV hypersensitivity in Chapter 14, and figure 14.13). If an adaptive immune response is involved, lymphocytes in various guises will also be present.

EXTRACELLULAR BACTERIA SUSCEPTIBLE TO KILLING BY PHAGOCYTOSIS AND COMPLEMENT

Bacterial survival strategies

The variety and ingenuity of escape mechanisms demonstrated by bacteria are most intriguing and, as with virtually all infectious agents, if you can think of a possible avoidance strategy, some microbe will already have used it.

A common mechanism by which virulent forms escape phagocytosis is by synthesis of an outer **capsule**. This does not adhere readily to phagocytic cells and covers carbohydrate molecules on the bacterial surface that could otherwise be recognized by phagocyte receptors. Other organisms have actively **antiphagocytic** cell surface molecules, and some go as far as to secrete **exotoxins**, which actually poison the leukocytes. Many organisms have developed mechanisms to resist complement activation and lysis. For example, Gram-positive organisms have evolved thick peptidoglycan layers which prevent the insertion of the lytic C5b–9 membrane attack complex into the bacterial cell membrane, and certain strains of group B streptococci actually produce a C5a-ase which cleaves and inactivates C5a.

The host counterattack

The defense mechanisms exploit the specificity and variability of the antibody molecule. Antibodies can defeat these devious attempts to avoid engulfment by neutralizing the antiphagocytic molecules and by binding to the surface of the organisms to focus the site for fixation of complement, so "opsonizing" the organisms for ingestion by polymorphs and macrophages or preparing them for the terminal membrane attack complex.

Most antigen-presenting cells (APCs) have receptors on their surface, which detect bacterial components such as lipopolysaccharide. These receptors include CD14 and Toll-like receptor 4 (TLR4) which when activated lead to the expression of a broad range of proinflammatory genes. These include IL-1, IL-6, IL-12 and TNF and the B7.1 (CD80) and B7.2 (CD86) costimulatory molecules. A related receptor TLR2 recognizes Gram-positive bacterial cell wall components.

Toxin neutralization

Circulating antibodies neutralize the soluble antiphagocytic molecules and other exotoxins released by bacteria. These antibodies, which in this context are also called **antitoxins**, inhibit the binding of the toxin to specific receptors on target cells and thereby prevent the toxin from damaging tissue.

Opsonization of bacteria

Mannose-binding lectin (MBL) is a molecule with a similar ultrastructure to C1q which can bind to terminal mannose on the bacterial surface and can lead to complement activation. Mannose-binding lectin does this by interacting with two MBL-associated serine proteases called MASP-1 and MASP-2 which are homologous in structure to C1r and C1s. This leads to antibody-independent activation of the classical pathway. Encapsulated bacteria which resist phagocytosis become extremely attractive to polymorphs and macrophages when coated with antibody and C3b, and their rate of clearance from the bloodstream is strikingly enhanced (figures 11.2 & 11.3). Furthermore, complexes containing C3b may show immune adherence to the CR1 complement receptors on red cells to provide aggregates which are transported to the liver for phagocytosis.

Some elaboration on **complement receptors** may be pertinent at this stage. The CR1 receptors for C3b are also present on neutrophils, macrophages, B-cells and

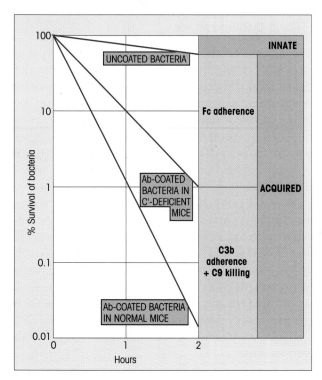

Figure 11.2 Effect of opsonizing antibody and complement on rate of clearance of virulent bacteria from the blood. The uncoated bacteria are phagocytosed rather slowly (innate immunity) but, on coating with antibody, adherence to phagocytes is increased many-fold (acquired immunity). The adherence is less effective in animals temporarily depleted of complement. This is a hypothetical but realistic situation; the natural proliferation of the bacteria has been ignored. Ab, antibody.

follicular dendritic cells in lymph nodes. Together with the CR3 receptor, they have the main responsibility for clearance of complexes containing C3.

CR2 receptors, which bind to various breakdown products of C3 such as C3dg and iC3b, are present on B-cells and follicular dendritic cells and transduce accessory signals for B-cell activation, especially in the germinal centers. Their affinity for the Epstein–Barr virus (EBV) provides the means for entry of the virus into the B-cell.

CR3 receptors on polymorphs, macrophages and NK cells all bind the inactivated form of C3b called C3bi.

The secretory immune system protects the external mucosal surfaces

We have earlier emphasized the critical nature of the mucosal barriers, particularly in the gut where there is a potentially hostile interface with the gut flora. With a huge surface area of around $400 \, m^2$, the epithelium of the adult mucosae represents the most frequent portal of entry for common infectious agents, allergens and carcinogens. The need for well-marshalled, highly effective mucosal immunity is glaringly obvious.

The mucosal surfaces are defended by both antigen-specific and nonantigen-specific mechanisms. The latter include a group of antibacterial peptides called **defensins** which are produced by neutrophils,

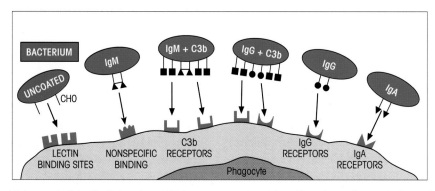

Figure 11.3 Coating with immunoglobulin (Ig) and complement greatly increase the adherence of bacteria (and other antigens) to macrophages and polymorphs. Uncoated bacteria adhere to lectin-like sites, including the mannose receptor. There are no specific binding sites for IgM (▲▲) but there are high-affinity receptors for IgG (Fc) (●) and iC3b (■: CR1 and CR3 types) on the macrophage surface which considerably enhance the strength of binding. The augmenting effect of complement is due to the fact that two adjacent IgG molecules can fix many C3b molecules, thereby increasing the number of links to the macrophage. Although IgM does not bind specifically to the macrophage, it promotes adherence through complement fixation. Specific receptors for the Fcα domains of IgA have also been defined.

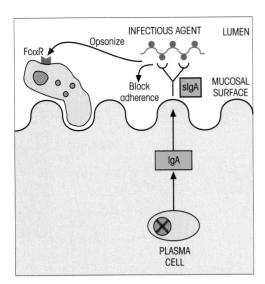

Figure 11.4 Defense of the mucosal surfaces. Immunoglobulin A (IgA) opsonizes organisms and prevents adherence to the mucosa. sIgA, secretory IgA.

macrophages and mucosal epithelium. The production of these antibacterial substances is upregulated by cytokines such as IL-1 and TNF. Specific immunity is provided by secretory immunoglobulin A (IgA) and IgM. The size of the task is highlighted by the fact that 80% of the Ig-producing B-cells in the body are present in the secretory mucosae and exocrine glands. Immunoglobulin A antibodies afford protection in the external body fluids, tears, saliva, nasal secretions and those bathing the surfaces of the intestine and lung, by coating bacteria and viruses and preventing their adherence to the epithelial cells of the mucous membranes. In addition high-affinity Fc receptors for this Ig class have been identified on macrophages and polymorphs and can mediate phagocytosis (figure 11.4).

If an infectious agent succeeds in penetrating the IgA barrier, it comes up against the next line of defense of the secretory system which is manned by IgE antibodies. It is worth noting that most serum IgE arises from plasma cells in mucosal tissues and in the lymph nodes that drain them. Although present in low concentration, IgE is bound very firmly to the Fc receptors of the mast cell. Contact with antigen leads to the release of mediators which effectively generate a local acute inflammatory reaction. Thus, histamine, by increasing vascular permeability, causes the transudation of IgG and complement into the area, while chemotactic factors for neutrophils and eosinophils attract the effector cells needed to dispose of the infectious organism coated with specific IgG and with C3b. Engagement of the Fcγ and C3b receptors on local macrophages by such complexes will lead to secretion of cytokines and chemokines which further reinforce these vascular permeability and chemotactic events.

Where the opsonized organism is too large for phagocytosis, it can be killed by antibody-dependent cellular cytotoxicity (ADCC), discussed earlier (p. 23). This is particularly important in controlling parasitic infections.

BACTERIA THAT GROW IN AN INTRACELLULAR HABITAT

Cell-mediated immunity is crucial for the control of intracellular organisms

Some strains of bacteria, such as the tubercle and leprosy bacilli and *Listeria* and *Brucella* organisms, escape the immune system by taking up residence inside macrophages (figure 11.5). Entry of opsonized bacteria is facilitated by phagocytic uptake after attachment to

Figure 11.5 Evasion of phagocytic death by intracellular bacteria. Mφ, macrophage.

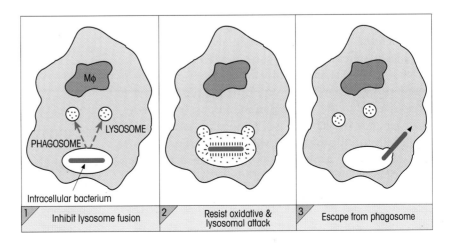

Fcγ and C3b receptors but, once inside, many of them defy the mighty macrophage by subverting the innate killing mechanisms.

In an elegant series of experiments, Mackaness demonstrated the importance of cell-mediated immunity (CMI) reactions for the killing of these intracellular parasites and the establishment of an immune state. Animals infected with moderate doses of *Mycobacterium tuberculosis* overcome the infection and are immune to subsequent challenge with the bacillus. The immunity can be transferred to a normal recipient by means of T-lymphocytes but not macrophages or serum from an immune animal. Supporting this view, that specific immunity is mediated by T-cells, is the greater susceptibility of patients with T-cell defects such as human immunodeficiency virus (HIV) infection to infection with mycobacteria or other intracellular organisms.

Activated macrophages kill intracellular parasites

Resting macrophages can be activated in several stages, but the ability to kill obligate intracellular microbes only comes after stimulation by macrophage activating factor(s) such as interferon γ (IFNγ) released from stimulated cytokine-producing T-cells or NK cells. Primed T-cells react with processed antigen derived from the intracellular bacteria present on the surface of the infected macrophage in association with MHC class II. The activated T-cells express CD40L (CD40 ligand) which reacts with CD40 on the macrophage, and, in the presence of IFNγ, the macrophage is activated and endowed with the ability to kill the organisms it has phagocytosed (figure 11.6). Foremost amongst the killing mechanisms which are upregulated, are those mediated by reactive oxygen intermediates and nitric oxide (NO). The **activated macrophage** is undeniably a remarkable and formidable cell, capable of secreting a vast array of cytokines and microbicidal substances which are concerned in chronic inflammatory reactions (figure 11.7).

Where the host has difficulty in effectively eliminating these organisms, the chronic CMI response to local antigen leads to the accumulation of densely packed macrophages, which release angiogenic and fibrogenic factors and stimulate the formation of granulation tissue and ultimately fibrosis. The activated macrophages, perhaps under the stimulus of IL-4, transform to epithelioid cells and fuse to become giant cells. As suggested earlier, the resulting granuloma represents an attempt by the body to isolate a site of persistent infection.

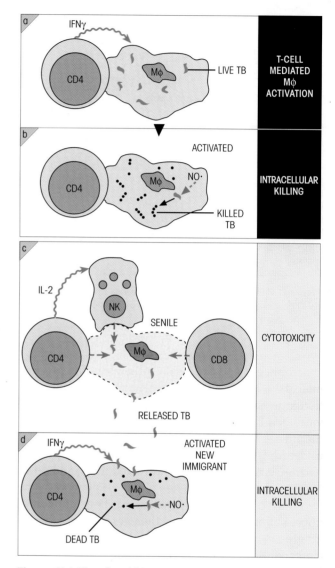

Figure 11.6 The "cytokine connection": nonspecific murine macrophage killing of intracellular bacteria triggered by a specific T-cell-mediated immune reaction. (a) Specific CD4 Th1 cell recognizes mycobacterial peptide associated with major histocompatibility complex (MHC) class II and releases macrophage (Mφ)-activating interferon γ (IFNγ). (b) The activated Mφ kills the intracellular tubercle bacilli (TB), mainly through generation of toxic nitric oxide (NO). (c) A "senile" Mφ, unable to destroy the intracellular bacteria, is killed by CD8 and CD4 cytotoxic cells and possibly by interleukin-2 (IL-2) -activated natural killer (NK) cells. The Mφ then releases live TB, which are taken up and killed by newly recruited Mφ susceptible to IFNγ activation.

IMMUNITY TO VIRAL INFECTION

Innate immune mechanisms

Early in the infection, before the primary antibody response has developed, the rapid production of type 1 interferons (IFNα and IFNβ) by infected cells is the most significant mechanism used to counter the viral

Figure 11.7 The role of the activated macrophage in the initiation and mediation of chronic inflammation with concomitant tissue repair, and in the killing of microbes and tumor cells. It is possible that macrophages differentiate along distinct pathways to subserve these different functions. The electron micrograph shows a highly activated macrophage with many lysosomal structures, which have been highlighted by the uptake of thorotrast; one (arrowed) is seen fusing with a phagosome containing the protozoan *Toxoplasma gondii*. (Photograph kindly supplied by Professor C. Jones.) IFNγ, interferon γ; IL-1, interleukin-1; NO, nitric oxide; TNF, tumor necrosis factor.

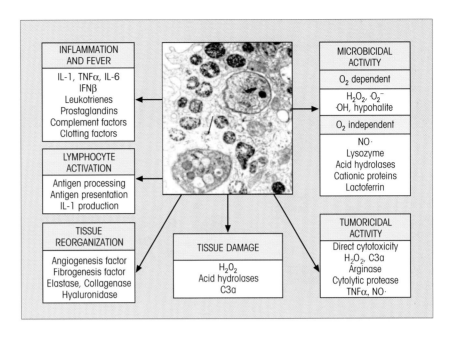

infection. The production of IFNα during viral infection not only protects surrounding cells but also activates NK cells and upregulates MHC expression on the adjacent cells. The surface of a virally infected cell undergoes modification, probably in its surface carbohydrate structures, making it an attractive target for NK cells. As described previously, NK cells possess two families of surface receptors. One binds to the novel structures expressed by infected cells and the other recognizes specificities common to several MHC class I alleles. The first activates killing but the recognition of class I delivers an inhibitory signal to the NK cell and protects normal cells from NK attack. Thus, the sensitivity of the target cell is closely related to self MHC class I expression. Virally infected cells, by inhibiting protein synthesis, may block production of class 1 MHC molecules, thereby turning off the inhibitory signal and allowing NK cells to attack. Therefore, whereas T-cells search for the presence of foreign shapes, NK cells survey tissues for the absence of self as indicated by aberrant or absent expression of MHC class I, which might occur in tumorigenesis or viral infections.

Protection by serum antibody

The antibody molecule can neutralize viruses by a variety of means. It may stereochemically inhibit combination with the receptor site on cells, thereby preventing penetration and subsequent intracellular multiplication . The protective effect of antibodies to influenza virus is an example of this. Antibody may destroy a free virus particle directly through activation of the classical complement pathway or it may produce aggregation, enhanced phagocytosis and intracellular death by mechanisms already discussed. With some viral diseases, such as influenza and the common cold, there is a short incubation time as the final target organ for the virus is the same as the portal of entry. Antibody, as assessed by the serum titer, seems to arrive on the scene much too late to be of value in aiding recovery. However, antibody levels may be elevated in the local fluids bathing the infected surfaces, for example nasal mucosa and lung, despite low serum titers, and it is the production of antiviral antibody (most prominently IgA) by locally deployed immunologically primed cells which is of major importance for the prevention of subsequent infection. Unfortunately, in so far as the common cold is concerned, a subsequent infection is likely to involve an antigenically unrelated virus so that general immunity to colds is difficult to achieve.

Cell-mediated immunity gets to the intracellular virus

In Chapter 2 we emphasized the general point that antibody dealt with extracellular infective agents and CMI with intracellular ones. The same holds true for viruses which have established themselves in an intracellular habitat. Local or systemic antibodies can block the spread of cytolytic viruses released from the host cell that they have just killed. Antibodies alone, how-

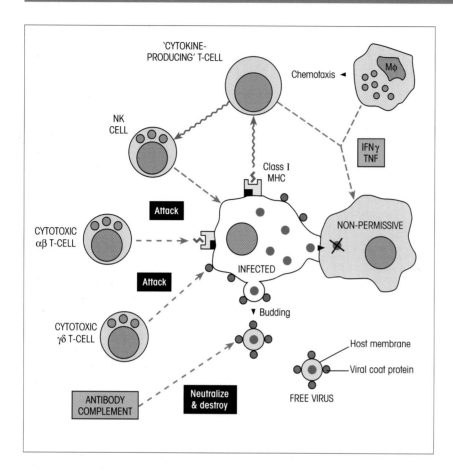

Figure 11.8 Control of infection by "budding" viruses. Free virus released by budding from the cell surface is neutralized by antibody. Specific cytotoxic T-cells kill virally infected targets directly. Interaction with a (separate?) subpopulation of T-cells releases cytokines, which attract macrophages, prime contiguous cells with interferon γ (IFNγ) and tumor necrosis factor (TNF) to make them resistant to viral infection, and activate cytotoxic natural killer (NK) cells. Natural killer cells are powerful producers of IFNγ. They recognize a lack of major histocompatibility complex (MHC) class 1 on the infected cell membrane. They can also lyse cells by antibody-dependent cellular cytotoxicity (ADCC) if antibody to viral coat protein is bound to the infected cell. Mφ, macrophage; TCR, T-cell receptor.

ever, are usually inadequate in controlling those viruses which bud off from the surface as infectious particles because they may spread to adjacent cells without becoming exposed to antibody (figure 11.8). The importance of CMI for recovery from infection with these agents is underlined by the inability of children with primary T-cell immunodeficiency to cope with such viruses, whereas patients with Ig deficiency but intact CMI are not troubled in this way.

Cytotoxic T-cells (Tc) are crucial elements in immunity to infection by budding viruses

T-lymphocytes from a sensitized host are directly cytotoxic to cells infected with viruses, the new MHC-associated peptide antigens on the target cell surface being recognized by specific αβ receptors on the aggressor CD8⁺ cytotoxic T-cells. Although γδ T-cells, which recognize native viral coat protein (e.g. herpes simplex virus glycoprotein) on the cell surface may play a role in controlling viral infection, most cytotoxic T-cells are CD8⁺ αβ T-cells (figure 11.8). Specific Tc cells

undergo significant proliferation during a viral infection. They can usually be detected in the peripheral blood in 3–4 days and then decline as the infection is controlled. Studies on volunteers, showing that high levels of cytotoxic activity before challenge with live influenza correlated with low or absent shedding of virus, speak in favor of the importance of Tc in human viral infection.

Cytokines recruit effectors and provide a "cordon sanitaire"

CD4⁺ T-cells also play an important role in antiviral defence by producing cytokines such as IFNγ that has antiviral activity, and IL-2 which recruits and activates CD8⁺ cells. Cytokines can also be produced by CD8 cells themselves, an activity that may well be crucial when viruses escape the cytotoxic mechanism and manage to sidle laterally into an adjacent cell. T-cells stimulated by viral antigen release cytokines such as IFNγ and macrophage or monocyte chemokines. The mononuclear phagocytes attracted to the site will be activated to secrete TNF, which will synergize with the IFNγ to render the contiguous cells nonpermissive for the replication of any virus acquired by intercellular transfer (figure 11.8). In this way, a cordon of resistant cells can surround the site of infection. Like IFNα, IFNγ may also increase the nonspecific cytotoxicity of NK cells for infected cells. This generation of "immune interferon" (IFNγ) and TNF in response to nonnucleic acid viral components provides a valuable back-up mechanism when dealing with viruses which are intrinsically poor stimulators of interferon synthesis.

After a natural infection, both antibody and Tc cells are generated; subsequent protection is long lived without reinfection. By contrast, injection of killed influenza produces antibodies but no Tc and protection is only short term.

IMMUNITY TO FUNGI

Many fungal infections become established in immunocompromised hosts or when the normal commensal flora is upset by prolonged administration of broad-spectrum antibiotics. Patients with neutrophil deficiency or neutrophil dysfunction such as in chronic granulomatous disease are particularly susceptible to *Candida albicans* and other fungi. Cell-mediated immunity is crucial in the defence against fungi as evidenced by the high opportunistic fungal infection rate in patients with HIV infection. T-cells function primarily by activating macrophages containing ingested organisms, but some T-cells and NK cells can exert a direct cytotoxic effect on a number of organisms such as *Cryptococcus neoformans* and *Candida albicans*.

IMMUNITY TO PARASITIC INFECTIONS

The consequences of infection with the major parasitic organisms could be at one extreme a lack of immune response leading to overwhelming superinfection, and at the other an exaggerated life-threatening immunopathologic response. Such a response may occur when parasites persist chronically in the face of an immune reaction which frequently produces tissue-damaging reactions. One example is the immune complex-induced nephrotic syndrome of Nigerian children associated with quartan malaria. Another example is the liver damage resulting from IL-4-mediated granuloma formation around schistosome eggs. Cross-reaction between parasite and self may give rise to autoimmunity, and this has been proposed as the basis for the cardiomyopathy in Chagas' disease. It is also pertinent that the nonspecific immunosuppression that is so widespread in parasitic diseases tends to increase susceptibility to superimposed bacterial and viral infections.

The host responses

A wide variety of defensive mechanisms are deployed by the host but the rough generalization may be made that a humoral response develops when the organisms invade the bloodstream (e.g. malaria, trypanosomiasis), whereas parasites which grow within the tissues (e.g. cutaneous leishmaniasis) usually elicit CMI.

Humoral immunity

Antibodies of the right specificity present in adequate concentrations and affinity are reasonably effective in providing protection against blood-borne parasites such as *Trypanosoma brucei* and the sporozoite and merozoite stages of malaria. Thus, individuals receiving IgG from solidly immune adults in malaria endemic areas are themselves temporarily protected against infection, the effector mechanisms being phagocytosis of opsonized organisms, and complement-dependent lysis.

A marked feature of the immune reaction to helminthic infections such as *Trichinella spiralis* is the eosinophilia and the high level of IgE antibody produced. Serum levels of IgE can rise from normal values of around 100 ng/ml to as high as 10 000 ng/ml. These changes have all the hallmarks of a response to Th2-type cytokines, and it is notable that in animals infected with helminths, injection of anti-IL-4 greatly reduces IgE production and anti-IL-5 suppresses the eosinophilia. It is relevant to note that schistosomules, the early immature form of the schistosome, can be killed in cultures containing both specific IgG and eosinophils by the ADCC mechanism.

Cell-mediated immunity

Just like mycobacteria, many parasites have adapted to life within the macrophage despite the possession by that cell of potent microbicidal mechanisms including NO·. Intracellular organisms such as *Toxoplasma gondii*, *Trypanosoma cruzi* and *Leishmania* spp. use a variety of ploys to subvert the macrophage killing systems but again, as with mycobacterial infections, cytokine-producing T-cells are crucially important for the stimulation of macrophages to release their killing power and dispose of the unwanted intruders.

In vivo, the balance of cytokines produced may be of

the utmost importance. Infection of mice with *Leishmania major* is instructive in this respect: the organism produces fatal disease in susceptible mice but other strains are resistant. In susceptible mice there is excessive stimulation of Th2 cells producing IL-4, whereas resistant strains are characterized by the expansion of Th1 cells which secrete IFNγ in response to antigen presented by macrophages harboring *living* protozoa.

Organisms such as malarial plasmodia, rickettsiae and chlamydiae that live in cells, which are not professional phagocytes, may be eliminated through activation of intracellular defense mechanisms by IFNγ released from CD8+ T-cells or even by direct cytotoxicity.

When it comes to worm infection, a vigorous response by Th2 cells will release a variety of cytokines which are responsible for the high IgE levels and the eosinophilia observed in these patients. This Th2 response is necessary for protection against these worms and to suppress Th1 cytokine induced immunopathology. In numerous mouse experiments it has been shown that IL-4 and IL-13 are crucial for expulsion of gastrointestinal worms, and that IL-5 and the eosinophils that it promotes are important in destroying larval forms of some worms as they migrate through the body. Human worm infections are also associated with Th2 cytokine responses including eosinophilia, mastocytosis and high levels of serum IgE (figure 11.9). Th2 cytokines also appear to protect against ectoparasites such as ticks, probably by degranulation of mast cells, thereby initiating inflammation and skin edema which prevent the tick from locating a host blood vessel.

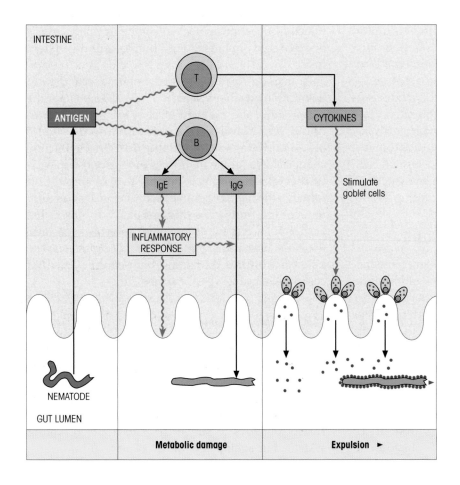

Figure 11.9 The expulsion of nematode worms from the gut. The parasite is first damaged by immunoglobulin G (IgG) antibody passing into the gut lumen, perhaps as a consequence of IgE-mediated inflammation and possibly aided by accessory antibody-dependent cellular cytotoxicity (ADCC) cells. Cytokines released by antigen-specific triggering of T-cells stimulate proliferation of goblet cells and secretion of mucous materials, which coat the damaged worm and facilitate its expulsion from the body by increased gut motility induced by mast cell mediators, such as leukotriene-D4, and diarrhea resulting from inhibition of glucose-dependent sodium absorption by mast cell-derived histamine and prostaglandin E_2 (PGE_2). B, B-cell; T, T-cell.

REVISION

Immunity to infection involves a constant battle between the host defenses and the mutant microbes trying to evolve evasive strategies. Specific acquired responses amplify and enhance innate immune mechanisms.

Inflammation revisited

• Inflammation is a major defensive reaction initiated by infection or tissue injury.

The acute inflammatory response

• The mediators released upregulate adhesion molecules such as P-selectin on endothelial cells. These pair with ligands on leukocytes, initially causing rolling of leukocytes along the vessel wall and then passage across the blood vessel up the chemotactic gradient to the site of inflammation.

• Under the influence of interleukin-1 (IL-1) and tumor necrosis factor (TNF), ICAM-1 (intercellular adhesion molecule-1) is induced on endothelial cells and binds to integrins on polymorphonuclear neutrophil (PMN) surfaces causing their arrest.

• Macrophages and mast cells present in the inflamed tissue are activated and release a variety of mediators, cytokines and chemokines. Endothelial cells themselves may release cytokines and chemokines.

• Activated granulocytes and macrophages easily phagocytose organisms coated with antibody and complement proteins.

• Cytokines such as transforming growth factor-β (TGFβ) and IL-10 are powerful regulators of inflammation and endogenous glucocorticoids.

• When tissue is severely traumatized, TGFβ may stimulate fibroblasts to lay down collagen forming scar tissue, which is the end result of many inflammatory events.

• Inability to eliminate the initiating agent leads to a chronic inflammatory response dominated by macrophages and often forming granulomas.

Extracellular bacteria susceptible to killing by phagocytosis and complement

• Bacteria try to evade the immune response by surrounding themselves with capsules to avoid phagocytosis, secreting exotoxins which kill phagocytes or impede inflammatory reactions, resisting insertion of the complement membrane attack complex, or by secreting enzymes which destroy C5.

• Antibody combats these tricks by neutralizing the toxins, and by overcoming the antiphagocytic nature of the capsules by opsonizing them with immunoglobulin G (IgG) and C3b.

• Antigen-presenting cells (APCs) have receptors for microorganisms, such as the Toll-like receptors (TLRs), which when activated lead to the production of proinflammatory cytokines.

• Mannose binding lectin (MBL) binds to mannose on bacterial surfaces. In association with MASP-1 and MASP-2 it leads to a further pathway of complement activation.

• Complement activation is controlled by a number of inhibitory proteins and by various complement receptors.

Protection of mucosal surfaces

• Defensins are antimicrobial proteins produced by macrophages and mucosal cells. Their production is upregulated by proinflammatory cytokines.

• The secretory immune system protects the external mucosal surfaces. Immunoglobulin A inhibits adherence of bacteria and can opsonize them.

• Immunoglobulin E bound to mast cells can be found in mucosal tissue. In contact with antigen it will cause degranulation of the mast cells. This initiates release of mediators which generate a local inflammatory reaction.

Bacteria which grow in an intracellular habitat

• Intracellular bacteria such as tubercle and leprosy bacilli grow within macrophages.

• They are killed by cell-mediated immunity (CMI): specifically sensitized T-cells become activated and release interferon γ (IFNγ) which activates the macrophage to kill the organisms.

• When intracellular organisms are not destroyed, a chronic inflammatory reaction will lead to the formation of a macrophage rich granuloma.

Immunity to viral infection

• Infected cells release type 1 interferons which have antiviral activity.

• Natural killer (NK) cells are activated by IFNγ and IL-2. They can now attack virally infected cells which have

(continued)

downregulated major histocompatibility complex (MHC) class 1 expression.

- Antibody neutralizes free virus and is particularly effective when the virus has to travel through the bloodstream before reaching its final target.
- Antibody is important in preventing reinfection.
- "Budding" viruses that can invade lateral cells without becoming exposed to antibody are combated by CMI. Infected cells express a processed viral antigen peptide on their surface in association with MHC class I.
- Rapid killing of the cell by cytotoxic $\alpha\beta$ T-cells prevents viral multiplication.
- Cytokines produced by CD4$^+$ and CD8$^+$ cells activate APCs and control the replication of virus particles.
- Natural infection generates specific antibody and T-cytotoxic (Tc) cells with subsequent long-term protection against reinfection.

Immunity to fungi

- Fungal infections are common in individuals with neutrophil dysfunction and in patients with defective CMI.

Immunity to parasitic infections

- Chronic parasitic infection can cause exaggerated immune responses leading to severe tissue injury.

- Antibodies are usually effective against the blood-borne parasitic diseases.
- Most parasitic infections stimulate a Th2 response, with IgE production and eosinophilia. These are important in destruction of parasites such as schistosomes, which when coated with IgG or IgE are killed by adherent eosinophils through the mechanism of antibody-dependent cellular cytotoxicity (ADCC).
- Organisms such as *Leishmania* spp., *Trypanosoma cruzi* and *Toxoplasma gondii* hide from antibodies inside macrophages and use the same strategies as intracellular parasitic bacteria to survive. Like them, they are killed when the macrophages are activated by cytokines produced during CMI responses.
- Cytokines produced by Th2 cells are important in the expulsion of gastrointestinal worms and in destroying larval forms. They may also protect against ectoparasites such as ticks by degranulating mast cells.

See the accompanying website (**www.roitt.com**) for multiple choice questions

FURTHER READING

Bloom, B. & Zinkernagel, R. (1996) Immunity to infection. *Current Opinion in Immunology*, **8**, 465–6.

Brandtzaeg, P. (1995) Basic mechanisms of mucosal immunity: A major adaptive defense system. *The Immunologist*, **3**, 89–96.

Finkelman, F.D. & Urban, J.F. (2001) The other side of the coin: The protective role of the Th2 cytokines. *Journal of Allergy and Clinical Immunology*, **107**, 772–80.

Ley, K. (2002) Integration of inflammatory signals by rolling neutrophils. *Immunological Reviews*, **186**, 8–18.

Nathan, C. (2002) Points of control in inflammation. *Nature*, **420**, 846–52.

Price, D.A., Klenerman, P., Booth, B.L., Phillips, R.E. & Sewell, A.K. (1999) Cytotoxic T lymphocytes, chemokines and antiviral immunity. *Immunology Today*, **20**, 212–16.

Rappuoli, R., Pizza, M., Douce, G. & Dougan, G. (1999) Structure and mucosal adjuvanticity of cholera and *Escherichia coli* heat-labile enterotoxins. *Immunology Today*, **20**, 493–500.

Prophylaxis

Immunization against infectious disease represents one of science's greatest triumphs. Many of the epidemic diseases of the past are now controlled and all but eliminated in developed countries, and new vaccines promise protection against a variety of more recently recognized infectious diseases including the various forms of hepatitis, Lyme disease and hopefully human immunodeficiency virus (HIV) infection. Modern vaccine biology is now targeting not only infectious diseases but also autoimmune and malignant disease. This chapter will review various procedures for stimulating antibody production or activating T-cell responses against defined prophylactically administered antigens.

PASSIVELY ACQUIRED IMMUNITY

Temporary protection against infection can be established by giving preformed antibody from another individual of the same or a different species (table 12.1). The advantage of this form of therapy is that humoral immunity is acquired immediately. The disadvantage is that the administered antibodies are rapidly utilized by combination with antigen or catabolized in the normal way. Therefore protection is quite quickly lost and memory is not conferred. An additional problem with passive immunotherapy is the potential transmission of infectious agents present in donor serum.

In the past, horse globulins containing antitetanus and antidiphtheria toxins were extensively employed prophylactically, but with the advent of antibiotics the requirement for such antisera has diminished. One complication of this form of therapy was **serum sickness** developing in response to the foreign protein. Although horse serum is now seldom used in modern medical practice, monoclonal antibodies produced in mice and humanized monoclonal antibodies are being increasingly utilized.

Maternally acquired antibody

In the first few months of life, protection is afforded by maternally derived antibodies acquired by placental transfer and by intestinal absorption of colostral immunoglobulins (Igs). The major Ig in both colostrum and milk is secretory IgA (sIgA), which is not absorbed by the baby but remains in the intestine to protect the mucosal surfaces. The surface IgA antibodies are directed against bacterial and viral antigens often present in the intestine, and it is presumed that in the mother, IgA-producing cells, responding to gut antigens, migrate and colonize breast tissue where the antibodies they produce appear in the milk.

Pooled human gammaglobulin

Regular injection of pooled human adult gammaglobulin collected from the plasma of normal donors is an essential treatment for patients with long-standing humoral immunodeficiency. Preparations containing

Table 12.1 Passive immunotherapy with antibody.

INFECTION	SOURCE OF ANTIBODY		USE
	HORSE	HUMAN	
Tetanus Diphtheria	√	√	Prophylaxis Treatment
Botulism Gas gangrene Snake or scorpion bite	√	–	Treatment
Varicella zoster	–	√	Treatment immunodeficiency
Rabies	–	√	Post-exposure to vaccine
Hepatitis B	–	√	Treatment
Hepatitis A	–	√	Prophylaxis (Travel)
Measles	–	√	Treatment
Cytomegalovirus	–	√	Prophylaxis in patients receiving immunosuppression
RSV*		√	Treatment

*A humanized monoclonal antibody is also available.
RSV, respiratory syncytial virus.

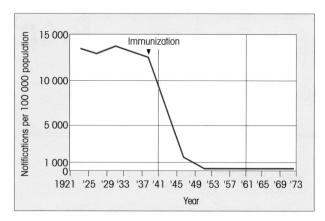

Figure 12.1 Notification of diphtheria in England and Wales per 100 000 population showing a dramatic fall after immunization. (Reproduced from G. Dick (1980) *Immunisation.* Leiden University Press, Leiden, The Netherlands, with kind permission of the author and publishers.)

high titers of antibodies to specific antigens may be used to modify the effects of respiratory syncytial virus (RSV) infection, chickenpox or measles especially in patients with defective immune responses due to prematurity, protein malnutrition, steroid treatment or leukemia. Contacts of infectious hepatitis patients may also be afforded protection by gammaglobulin, especially when the material is derived from the serum of individuals vaccinated some weeks previously. Cytomegalovirus (CMV) human immune globulin is now administered to recipients of organ transplants taken from CMV-positive donors, and rabies immune globulin may be given together with active immunization to patients bitten by a potentially rabid animal. It is of interest that pooled gammaglobulin is being increasingly used as immune-modulating therapy in the treatment of autoimmune diseases such as idiopathic thrombocytopenic purpura although the mechanism behind the beneficial effect is currently unclear. The bioengineering of custom-designed antibodies is of increasing importance (see Chapter 3).

VACCINATION

Herd immunity

In the case of tetanus, active immunization is of benefit to the individual but not to the community since it will not eliminate the organism, which persists in the soil as highly resistant spores. Where a disease depends on

human transmission, immunity in just a proportion of the population can help the whole community if it leads to a fall in the reproduction rate (i.e. the number of further cases produced by each infected individual) to less than one. Under these circumstances the disease will die out. An example of this is the disappearance of diphtheria from communities in which around 75% of the children have been immunized (figure 12.1) In contrast, focal outbreaks of poliomyelitis have occurred in communities that object to immunization on religious grounds, raising an important point for parents in general.

Strategic considerations

The objective of vaccination is to provide effective immunity by establishing adequate levels of appropriate immune effector mechanisms, together with a primed population of memory cells which can rapidly expand on renewed contact with antigen and so provide protection against infection. Sometimes, as with polio infection, a high blood titer of antibody is required; in mycobacterial diseases such as tuberculosis (TB), a macrophage-activating cell-mediated immunity (CMI) is most effective, whereas with influenza virus infection, antibodies and cytotoxic T-cells (Tc) play a significant role. The site of the immune response evoked by vaccination may also be most important. For example in cholera, antibodies need to be in the gut lumen to inhibit adherence to and colonization of the intestinal wall.

In addition to an ability to engender effective immunity, a number of mundane but nonetheless crucial

Table 12.2 Factors required for a successful vaccine.

FACTOR	REQUIREMENTS
Effectiveness	Must evoke protective levels of immunity: at the appropriate site of relevant nature (Ab, Tc, Th1, Th2) of adequate duration
Availability	Readily cultured in bulk or accessible source of subunit
Stability	Stable under extreme climatic conditions, preferably not requiring refrigeration
Cheapness	What is cheap in the West may be expensive in developing countries but WHO tries to help
Safety	Eliminate any pathogenicity

Ab, antibody; WHO, World Health Organization.

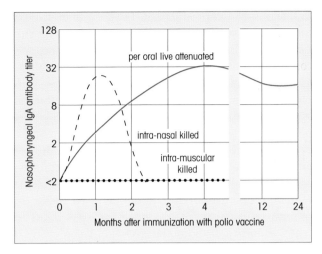

Figure 12.2 Local immunoglobulin A (IgA) response to polio vaccine. Local secretory antibody synthesis is confined to the specific anatomical sites, which have been directly stimulated by contact with antigen. (Data from P.L. Ogra *et al.* (1975) In: *Viral Immunology and Immunopathology* (ed. A.L. Notkins), p. 67. Academic Press, New York.)

conditions must be satisfied for a vaccine to be considered successful (table 12.2). The antigens must be readily available, the preparation should be stable on storage, and it should be cheap, easy to administer and, certainly, safe.

KILLED ORGANISMS AS VACCINES

The simplest way to destroy the ability of microbes to cause disease yet maintain their antigenicity is to prevent their replication by killing in an appropriate manner, such as with formaldehyde treatment. Parasitic worms and, to a lesser extent, protozoa are extremely difficult to grow up in bulk to manufacture killed vaccines. This problem does not arise for many bacteria and viruses and, in these cases, the inactivated microorganisms have generally provided safe antigens for immunization. Examples are typhoid, cholera and killed poliomyelitis (Salk) vaccines. Care has to be taken to ensure that important protective antigens are not destroyed in the inactivation process.

LIVE ATTENUATED ORGANISMS HAVE MANY ADVANTAGES AS VACCINES

The objective of attenuation is to produce a modified organism that mimics the natural behavior of the original microbe without causing significant disease. In many instances the immunity conferred by killed vaccines, even when given with adjuvant (see below), is often inferior to that resulting from infection with live organisms. This must be partly because the replication of the living microbes confronts the host with a **larger and more sustained dose of antigen** and that, with budding viruses, infected cells are required for

the establishment of good **Tc memory**. Another significant advantage of using live organisms is that the **immune response takes place largely at the site of the natural infection**. This is well illustrated by the nasopharyngeal IgA response to immunization with polio vaccine. In contrast with the ineffectiveness of parenteral injection of killed vaccine, intra-nasal administration evoked a good local antibody response that declined over a period of 2 months. Oral immunization with *live attenuated* virus produced an even better response with a persistently high IgA antibody level (figure 12.2).

Classical methods of attenuation

The objective of attenuation, that of producing an organism that causes only a very mild form of the natural disease, can be equally well attained by employing heterologous strains which are virulent for another species, but avirulent in humans. The best example of this was Jenner's seminal demonstration that cowpox infection would protect against smallpox. Since then, a truly remarkable global effort by the World Health Organization, combining extensive vaccination and selective epidemiological control methods, **has completely eradicated the human disease**—a wonderful achievement.

Attenuation itself can be achieved by modifying the conditions under which an organism grows. Pasteur first achieved the production of live but nonvirulent forms of chicken cholera bacillus and anthrax by culturing at higher temperatures and under anaerobic conditions. A virulent strain of *Mycobacterium tuberculosis* became attenuated by chance in 1908 when Calmette and Guérin at the Institut Pasteur, Lille, added bile to the culture medium in an attempt to achieve dispersed growth. After 13 years of culture in bile-containing medium, the strain remained attenuated and was used successfully to vaccinate children against tuberculosis. The same organism, BCG (bacille bilié de Calmette–Guérin), is widely used today for immunization of tuberculin-negative individuals in many countries. It should be stressed that an individual receiving BCG immunization will convert from being tuberculin skin test-negative to the positive state. Although the immunization often confers protection, the feeling in the USA is that a negative skin test is important in excluding a diagnosis of TB, and BCG negates the use of the skin test. For this reason, therefore, BCG is not employed in the USA.

Attenuation of viruses usually requires cultivation in nonhuman cells where after many rounds of culture the viruses develop multiple random genetic mutations, some of which lead to a loss of ability to infect human cells. Unfortunately on very rare occasions pathogenicity may return by further mutations of the organism, as was seen with the polio virus vaccine where reversions to the wild type resulted in clinical cases of the disease occurring in vaccinated children. Another problem with live attenuated vaccines is the risk to immunocompromised patients in whom they may behave as opportunistic pathogens.

Attenuation by recombinant DNA technology

Instead of the random mutations achieved by classic attenuation procedures, genetic modification techniques are now being used to develop various attenuated strains of viruses.

Microbial vectors for other genes

An ingenious trick is to use a virus as a "piggyback" for genes from another virus, particularly one that cannot be grown successfully, or which is inherently dangerous. Large DNA viruses, such as vaccinia, can act as carriers for one or many foreign genes while retaining infectivity for animals and cultured cells. The proteins encoded by these genes are appropriately expressed *in vivo*, and are processed for major histocompatibility complex (MHC) presentation by the infected cells,

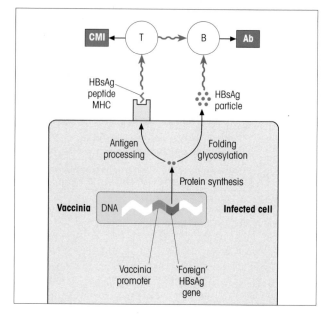

Figure 12.3 Hepatitis B surface antigen (HBsAg) vaccine using an attenuated vaccinia virus carrier. The HBsAg protein is synthesized by the machinery of the host cell: some is secreted to form the HBsAg 22 nm particle which stimulates antibody (Ab) production, and some follows the antigen processing pathway to stimulate cell-mediated immunity (CMI) and T-helper activity. B, B-cell; T, T-cell.

thus effectively endowing the host with both humoral and CMI.

A wide variety of genes have been expressed by vaccinia virus vectors including hepatitis B surface antigen (HBsAg), which has protected chimpanzees against the clinical effects of hepatitis B virus (figure 12.3). Spectacular neutralizing antibody titers were produced by a construct with the gene encoding rabies virus glycoprotein, which protected animals against intra-cerebral challenge. Since approximately 10% of the poxvirus genome can be replaced by foreign DNA, the potential exists for producing multivalent vaccines in these vectors.

Another approach is to employ attenuated bacteria such as BCG or *Salmonella* as vehicles for antigens required to evoke CD4-mediated T-cell immunity. BCG is avirulent, has a low frequency of serious complications, can be administered any time after birth, has strong adjuvant properties, gives long-lasting CMI after a single injection and is inexpensive. The use of *Salmonella* is particularly interesting because these bacteria elicit **mucosal responses by oral immunization**. It is possible therefore that the oral route of immunization may be applicable to develop gut mucosal immunity and perhaps systemic protection.

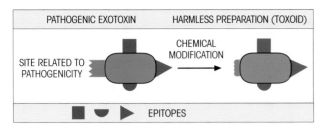

PATHOGENIC EXOTOXIN   HARMLESS PREPARATION (TOXOID)

CHEMICAL MODIFICATION

SITE RELATED TO PATHOGENICITY

EPITOPES

Figure 12.4 Modification of toxin to harmless toxoid without losing many of the antigenic determinants. Thus, antibodies to the toxoid will react well with the original toxin.

SUBUNIT VACCINES CONTAINING INDIVIDUAL PROTECTIVE ANTIGENS

A whole parasite or bacterium usually contains many antigens that are not concerned in the protective response of the host but may provoke hypersensitivity. Vaccination with the isolated protective antigens may avoid these complications, and identification of these antigens then opens up the possibility of producing them synthetically.

Bacterial exotoxins such as those produced by diphtheria and tetanus bacilli have long been used as immunogens. First, they must of course be detoxified and this is achieved by formaldehyde treatment, which fortunately does not destroy the major immunogenic determinants (figure 12.4). Immunization with the resulting **toxoid** will therefore provoke the formation of protective antibodies, which neutralize the toxin by stereochemically blocking the active site. The toxoid is generally given after adsorption to aluminum hydroxide, which acts as an adjuvant and produces higher antibody titers.

Other isolated protective antigens include purified extracts of some component of the organism such as the subunit acellular pertussis vaccine or the subunit influenza vaccine. Soluble capsular material, such as is found in the pneumococcal or hemophilus influenza vaccines, stimulate significant protection but are suboptimal in young children and therefore are conjugated to carrier proteins such as tetanus or diphtheria toxoids.

Use of transgenic plants

Viral and bacterial antigens such as HBsAg, rabies glycoprotein and *Escherichia coli* enterotoxin may be produced in transgenic plants. The advantage of such an approach is the low cost and the possibility that the person may only have to eat the transgenic plant to be immunized. In addition to antigens, specific antibodies called plantibodies are being produced in plants. Studies with antibodies produced in this way against *Streptococcus mutans* (the cause of dental caries) show promising results, and numerous other plantibodies are now available.

Antigens can be synthesized through gene cloning

The emphasis now is to move towards gene cloning of individual proteins once they have been identified immunologically and biochemically. Recombinant DNA technology enables us to make genes encoding part or the whole of a protein peptide chain almost at will, and to express them in an appropriate vector. This approach has been used to produce a commercial hepatitis vaccine employing the product secreted by yeast cells expressing the *HBsAg* gene. A similar approach has been used to produce a vaccine against *Borrelia burgdorferi,* the cause of Lyme disease. The potential of gene cloning is clearly vast and, in principle, economical, but there are sometimes difficulties in identifying a good expression vector and in obtaining correct folding of the peptide chain to produce an active protein.

One restriction to gene cloning has been that carbohydrate antigens cannot be synthesized directly by recombinant DNA technology. However, the glycosylation pathway in the yeast *Pichia pastoris* has recently been humanized by replacing the endogenous yeast glycosylation pathways with their eukaryotic equivalents, thereby permitting the synthesis of complex carbohydrates.

The naked gene itself acts as a vaccine

It has recently been appreciated that injected DNA functions as a source of immunogen and can induce strong immune responses, both humoral and cell-mediated. The gene is stitched in place in a DNA plasmid with appropriate promoters and enhancers and injected into muscle where it can give prolonged expression of protein. The plasmids may even be introduced into the body using a biolistics gun which delivers gold microspheres coated with plasmids of the gene encoding the vaccine antigen. As mentioned above, DNA has also been placed into microorganisms such as vaccinia, adenovirus or *Salmonella* spp. Broad immune responses are observed including induction of Tc cells, presumably reflecting the cytosolic expression of the protein and its processing with MHC class I.

DNA for this procedure can be obtained directly from current clinical material without having to select specific mutant strains. Altogether, the speed and simplicity mean that the 2 years previously needed to make a recombinant vaccine can be reduced to months. DNA vaccines do not need the cumbersome and costly protein synthesis and purification procedures that subunit formulations require; they can be prepared in a highly stable powder and, above all, they are incredibly cheap. Before there is widespread use in humans, however, a number of safety considerations, such as the possibility of permanent incorporation of a plasmid into the host genome, need to be addressed.

ADJUVANTS

For practical and economic reasons, prophylactic immunization should involve the minimum number of injections and the least amount of antigen. We have referred to the undoubted advantages of replicating attenuated organisms in this respect, but nonliving organisms, and especially purified products, frequently require an adjuvant. This is a substance that by definition is incorporated into or injected simultaneously with antigen and potentiates the immune response (Latin *adjuvare*, to help). The mode of action of adjuvants involves a number of mechanisms, one of which is to counteract the dispersion of free antigen and localize it, either at an extracellular location or within macrophages. The most common adjuvants of the type used in humans are **aluminum compounds** (phosphate and hydroxide). Virtually all adjuvants stimulate antigen-presenting cells (APCs) and improve their immunogenicity by the provision of accessory costimulatory signals to direct lymphocytes towards an immune response rather than tolerance, and by the secretion of soluble stimulatory factors (e.g. interleukin-1 (IL-1)), which influence the proliferation of lymphocytes.

CURRENT VACCINES

The established vaccines in current use and the schedules for their administration are set out in table 12.3.

Because of the pyrogenic reactions and worries about possible hypersensitivity responses to the whole-cell component of the conventional pertussis vaccine, a new generation of vaccines containing one or more purified components of *Bordetella pertussis*, and therefore termed "acellular" vaccines, has been licensed in the USA. The combination of diphtheria and tetanus toxoids with acellular pertussis (DTP) is recommended for the later fourth and fifth "shots" and for children at increased risk for seizures. Children under 2 years of age make inadequate responses to the T-independent *Haemophilus influenzae* capsular poly-

Table 12.3 Current vaccination practice.

VACCINE		ADMINISTRATION		
		UK	USA	OTHER COUNTRIES
CHILDREN				
Triple (DTP) vaccine: diphtheria, tetanus, pertussis	Primary	2–6 mo (3x/4 weekly)		Japan: 2 yr
	Boost DT	3–5yr	15 mo/4 yr DT every 10 yr	
Polio: live	Primary	Concomitant with DTP		
	Boost	4/6 yr	15 mo, 4 yr high-risk adult	
killed		Immunocompromised		
MMR vaccine: measles, mumps rubella	Primary	12–15 mo		Africa: 6 mo
	Boost	4–5 yr 10–14 yr seronegative girls selectively with rubella		
BCG (TB, leprosy)		10–14 yr	high risk only	Tropics: at birth
Haemophilus		Concomitant with DTP		
Varicella		Neonates at risk, immunocompromised		
ELDERLY				
Pneumococcal polysaccharide serotypes		Aged & high risk		
Influenza		Aged & high risk		
SPECIAL GROUPS				
Hepatitis B		Travelers, high risk groups		
Hepatitis A Meningitis (A+C)		Travelers to endemic areas		
Yellow fever Typhoid		Travelers to endemic areas		Tropics: infants Yellow fever: boost residents and frequent visitors every 10 yr
Rabies		Prophylactically in high risk groups Post-exposure to contacts in endemic areas		

saccharide, so they are now routinely immunized with the antigen conjugated with tetanus or diphtheria toxoids.

A resurgence of measles outbreaks in recent years has prompted recommendations for the reimmunization of children, at the age of school entry or at the change to middle (secondary) school, with measles vaccine. The considerable morbidity and mortality associated with hepatitis B infection, its complex epidemiology and the difficulty in identifying high-risk individuals have led to recommendations for vaccination in the 6–18-month age group.

Relevant information about protocols for immunization and immunization-related problems are available at the web site of the Centers for Disease Control and Prevention (http://www.cdc.gov/nip)

and the UK Health Protection Agency (http://www.hpa.org.uk).

Immunization in transplant patients

Many common infections produce a more severe clinical picture in immunosuppressed patients than in normal individuals. It is important therefore to immunize these patients wherever possible. However, the immunosuppression associated with transplantation presents a number of special immunization problems for patients, especially children. Immunization with live viral vaccines may lead to vaccine-associated disease, and are not usually administered after transplantation. Children, therefore, who have not been immunized, should receive immunizations before the transplant takes place. Inactivated vaccines do not replicate and therefore do not cause vaccine-associated disease. However, due to the immunosuppression, immune responses are suboptimal and multiple booster immunizations are required.

Immunization in adults

Many childhood immunizations do not last a lifetime and adults need to be reimmunized against tetanus, diptheria and other illnesses. Adults need to be protected against chickenpox if they have not had the disease or the vaccine, and a measles, mumps and rubella (MMR) vaccine may be indicated if they have an unreliable history of being previously immunized. Adults over the age of 50 years should be immunized annually against current influenza strains, and individuals aged 65 years and older should receive the pneumococcal vaccine.

REVISION

Passively acquired immunity
• Horse antisera have been extensively used in the past but their use is now more restricted because of the danger of serum sickness.
• Passive immunity can be acquired by maternal antibodies or from homologous pooled gammaglobulin.
• Sera containing high-titer antibodies against a specific pathogen are useful in treating or preventing various viral diseases such as severe chickenpox, cytomegalovirus (CMV) infection or rabies.

Vaccination
• Active immunization provides a protective state through contact with a harmless form of the organism.
• A good vaccine should be based on antigens that are easily available, cheap, stable under extreme climatic conditions and nonpathogenic.

Killed organisms as vaccines
• Killed bacteria and viruses have been widely used.

Live attenuated organisms
• The advantages are that replication of organisms produces a bigger dose, and the immune response is produced at the site of the natural infection.
• Attenuated vaccines are produced by altering the conditions under which organisms are cultivated.
• Recombinant DNA technology is now used to manufacture attenuated strains.
• Attenuated vaccinia can provide a "piggyback" carrier for genes from other organisms that are difficult to attenuate.
• BCG is a good vehicle for antigens requiring CD4 T-cell immunity, and Salmonella constructs may give oral and systemic immunity. Intra-nasal immunization is fast gaining popularity.
• Risks are reversion to the virulent form and danger to immunocompromised individuals.

Subunit vaccines
• Whole organisms have a multiplicity of antigens, some of which are not protective, may induce hypersensitivity or might even be frankly immunosuppressive.
• It makes sense in these cases to use purified components.
• Toxoids are exotoxins treated with formaldehyde that destroys the pathogenicity of the organism but leaves antigenicity intact.
• There is greatly increased use of recombinant DNA technology to produce these antigens.
• Microbial antigens can be produced in transgenic plants and plantibodies are specific antibodies also produced in plants.
• Naked DNA encoding the vaccine subunit can be inject-

(continued)

ed directly into muscle, where it expresses the protein and produces immune responses. The advantages are stability, ease of production and cheapness.

Adjuvants

• Adjuvants work by producing depots of antigen, and by activating antigen-presenting cells (APCs); they sometimes have direct effects on lymphocytes.

Current vaccines

• Children in the USA and UK are routinely immunized with diphtheria and tetanus toxoids and pertussis (DTP triple vaccine) and attenuated strains of measles, mumps and rubella (MMR) and polio. BCG is given at 10–14 years in the UK.

• Subunit forms of pertussis lacking side effects are being introduced.

• The capsular polysaccharide of *Haemophilus influenzae* has to be linked to a carrier.

• Vaccines for hepatitis A and B, meningitis, yellow fever, typhoid, cholera and rabies are available for travelers and high-risk groups.

Immunization in transplant patients

• Transplant patients are highly susceptible to common infections and should be protected wherever possible.

• Live attenuated vaccines are generally not administered to these patients because of the concern of vaccine-associated disease.

• Killed vaccines are safe in transplanted individuals but multiple booster immunizations may be required

Immunization in adults and the elderly

• Childhood vaccine effects do not last a lifetime and adults should receive booster vaccines at regular intervals.

• Influenza vaccine for people over the age of 50 years and pneumococcal vaccine for those over 65 years is recommended.

See the accompanying website (**www.roitt.com**) for multiple choice questions

FURTHER READING

Ada, G. (2001) Advances in immunology: Vaccines and vaccination. *New England Journal of Medicine*, **345**, 1042–53.

Dietrich, G., Gentschev, I., Hess, J. *et al*. (1999) Delivery of DNA vaccines by attenuated intracellular bacteria. *Immunology Today*, **20**, 251–3.

Faix, R. (2002) Immunization during pregnancy. *Clinical Obstetrics and Gynecology*, **45**, 42–58.

Kumar, V. & Sercarz, E. (1996) Genetic vaccination: The advantages of going naked. *Nature Medicine*, **2**, 857–9.

Moylett, E.H. & Hanson, I.C. (2003) Immunization. *Journal of Allergy and Clinical Immunology*, **111**, S754–65.

Sherwood, J.K., Zeitlin, L., Whaley, K.J. *et al*. (1996) Controlled release of antibodies for long-term topical passive immunoprotection of female mice against genital herpes. *Nature Biotechnology*, **14**, 468–71.

Immunodeficiency

PRIMARY IMMUNODEFICIENCY STATES IN THE HUMAN

A multiplicity of immunodeficiency states in humans that are **not secondary** to environmental factors have been recognized. We have earlier stressed the manner in which the interplay of complement, antibody and phagocytic cells constitutes the basis of a tripartite defense mechanism against pyogenic (pus-forming) infections. Hence it is not surprising that deficiency in any one of these factors may predispose the individual to repeated infections of this type. Patients with T-cell deficiency of course present a markedly different pattern of infection, being susceptible to those viruses, intracellular bacteria, fungi and parasites that are normally eradicated by cell-mediated immunity (CMI).

The following sections examine various forms of these primary immunodeficiencies.

DEFICIENCIES OF INNATE IMMUNE MECHANISMS

Phagocytic cell defects

Primary defects in neutrophil number are rare as most cases of neutropenia are due to treatment with cytotoxic drugs usually associated with malignant disease. As would be expected, neutropenic patients are generally prone to pyogenic bacterial infections but not to parasitic or viral infections. A number of primary immunodeficiency disorders involve qualitative defects of phagocytic cells:

Chronic granulomatous disease (CGD) is a rare disease in which the monocytes and neutrophils fail to produce reactive oxygen intermediates (figure 13.1) required for the intracellular killing of phagocytosed organisms. This results in severe recurrent bacterial and fungal infections, which when unresolved may lead to granulomas that can obstruct the gastrointestinal and urogenital systems. Curiously, the range of infectious pathogens that trouble these patients is relatively restricted. The most common pathogen is *Staphylococcus aureus* but certain Gram-negative bacilli and fungi such as *Aspergillus fumigatus* and *Candida albicans* are frequently involved.

The disease is a heterogeneous disorder due to defects in any one of four subunits of NADPH (nicotinamide adenine dinucleotide phosphate) oxidase which is crucial for the formation of hydrogen peroxide.

Prophylactic daily treatment with antibiotics considerably reduces the frequency of infections. Interferon γ (IFNγ) has been shown to stimulate the production of superoxide by CGD neutrophils resulting in considerably fewer infectious episodes. Because CGD results from a single gene defect in phagocytic cells, the ideal treatment of the disease would be the transfer of the correct gene into the bone marrow stem cells. Initial work in this area is encouraging. Some patients have

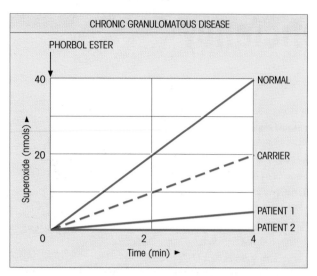

Figure 13.1 Defective respiratory burst in neutrophils of patients with chronic granulomatous disease (CGD). The activation of the NADP (nicotinamide adenine dinucleotide phosphate)/cytochrome oxidase is measured by superoxide anion ($\cdot O_2^-$; cf. figure 1.6) production following stimulation with phorbol myristate acetate. Patient 2 has a $p92^{phox}$ mutation which prevents expression of the protein, whilst patient 1 has the variant $p92^{phox}$ mutation producing very low but measurable levels. Many carriers of the X-linked disease express intermediate levels, as in the individual shown who is the mother of patient 2. (Data from R.M. Smith & J.T. Curnutte (1991) *Blood*, **77**, 673–86.)

been effectively treated by bone marrow transplantation from a normal major histocompatibility complex (MHC) -matched sibling, but the significant mortality of this procedure needs to be weighed against the much-improved quality of life that patients can now expect from conservative treatments with antibiotics and IFNγ.

Chediak–Higashi disease is a rare autosomal recessive disease due to various mutations in a gene called the *CHS* gene. In this condition, neutrophils, monocytes and lymphocytes contain giant lysosomal granules which result from increased granule fusion. This gives rise to phagocytic cells which are defective in chemotaxis, phagocytosis and microbicidal activity, and to natural killer (NK) cells which lack cytotoxic activity. In addition to increasing susceptibility to pyogenic infections, these lysosomal defects affect melanocytes causing albinism and platelets giving rise to bleeding disorders.

Leukocyte adhesion deficiency results from lack of the CD18 β-subunit of the β_2-integrins, which include LFA-1 (lymphocyte function-associated antigen-1). Children with this defect suffer from repeated pyogenic infections because phagocytic cells do not bind

to intercellular molecules on endothelial cells and therefore cannot emigrate through the vessel walls to the infected tissue. Patients also have problems with wound healing, and delayed separation of the umbilical cord is often the earliest manifestation of this defect. Fortunately, bone marrow transplantation has resulted in restoration of neutrophil function and is now the treatment of choice.

Defects in the IFNγ–interleukin-12 (IL-12) axis. Normally initiators of the Th1 cytokine pathway, mycobacteria induce macrophages and dendritic cells (DCs) to secrete IL-12, which then activates both NK cells and Th1-cells; these then produce IFNγ, which switch on macrophage killing mechanisms providing protection against pathogenic mycobacteria.

An interesting group of patients who are selectively susceptible to poorly pathogenic mycobacterial species and other intracellular bacteria have defects in this Th1 cytokine pathway. These patients have mutations in the IFNγ receptor, the IL-12 receptor or IL-12 itself, resulting in defective activation of macrophages and inability to control intracellular infections.

Complement system deficiencies

As we have seen previously, activation of the complement system plays an important role in host defense against bacterial infections and is also crucial for the clearance of immune complexes from the circulation. Genetic deficiencies in almost all the complement proteins have now been described and, as would be expected, these result in either recurrent infections or failure to clear immune complexes.

Deficiency in the mannose-binding lectin (MBL) pathway results in recurrent infection

The MBL pathway is an important system for activating complement and for depositing complement fragments on microorganisms where they facilitate phagocytosis and initiate inflammatory reactions. It is therefore not surprising that a deficiency of MBL is associated with susceptibility to infections and with the development of immunological diseases particularly in children. This suggests that it is important for opsonin production during the interval between the loss of passively acquired maternal immunity and the time of development for a mature immune system. Recently a patient with MBL-associated serine protease-2 (MASP-2) deficiency has been described who also shows significant recurrent bacterial infections.

Deficiency of early classical pathway proteins results in increased susceptibility to immune-complex disease

This has been observed in patients with deficiency of the C1 proteins, C2 or C4 who have some increase in susceptibility to infection but also have an unusually high incidence of a systemic lupus erythematosus (SLE) -like disease. Although the reason for this is unclear, it could be due to a decreased ability to mount an adequate host response to infection with a putative etiologic agent or, more probably, to eliminate antigen–antibody complexes effectively.

Deficiency of C3 or the control proteins factor H or factor I, results in severe recurrent infections

Although deficiency of C3 is rare, the clinical picture seen in these patients is instructive in emphasizing the crucial role of C3 in both the classical and alternative pathways. Complete absence of this component causes a block in both pathways resulting in defective opsonizing and chemotactic activities. Factor H or factor I deficiency produce a similar clinical picture, because there is inability to control C3b. This results in continuous activation of the alternative pathway through the feedback loop, leading to consumption of C3, the levels of which may fall to zero.

Permanent deficiencies in C5, C6, C7 and C8 result in susceptibility to Neisseria infection

Many of the individuals with these rare disorders are quite healthy and not particularly prone to infection apart from an increased susceptibility to disseminated *Neisseria gonorrhoeae* and *N. meningitidis* infection. Presumably the host requires a complete and intact complement pathway with its resulting cytolytic activity to destroy these particular organisms.

Deficiency of the C1 inhibitor causes hereditary angioedema

C1INH acts on the classical complement system by inhibiting the binding of C1r and C1s to C1q, and it also inhibits factor XII of the clotting system (figure 13.2). Absence of C1INH leads to recurring episodes of acute circumscribed noninflammatory edema mediated by the unrestricted production of the vasoactive C2 fragment. Lack of C1INH also leads to an increase in generation of bradykinin, which adds to the increased

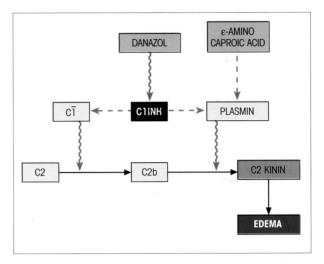

Figure 13.2 C1 inhibitor deficiency and angioedema. C1 inhibitor stoichiometrically inhibits C1, plasmin, kallikrein and activated Hageman factor and deficiency leads to formation of the vasoactive C2 kinin by the mechanism shown. The synthesis of C1 inhibitor can be boosted by methyltestosterone or preferably the less masculinizing synthetic steroid, danazol; alternatively, attacks can be controlled by giving ε-aminocaproic acid to inhibit the plasmin.

permeability of small vessels causing the edema associated with this disease. These patients therefore present with recurrent episodes of swelling of the skin, acute abdominal pain due to swellings of the intestine, and obstruction of the larynx which may rapidly cause complete laryngeal obstruction. The majority of cases (type 1) are due to a mutant gene leading to markedly suppressed amounts of C1INH whereas a less common form of the disease (type 2) is due to a dysfunctional C1INH protein.

Attacks are precipitated by trauma or excessive exercise and can be controlled by anabolic steroids such as danazol, which for unknown reasons suppress the symptoms of hereditary angioedema.

GPI (glycosylphosphatidylinositol) -anchor protein deficiencies

A mutation in the *PIG-A* glycosyltransferase gene leads to an inability to synthesize the GPI-anchors for the complement regulatory proteins decay accelerating factor (DAF, CD55), homologous restriction factor (HRF, CD59), and membrane cofactor protein (MCP, CD46). The absence of these proteins from the erythrocyte surface results in a condition known as paroxysmal nocturnal hemoglobinuria due to the inability to inactivate bound C3b generated from spontaneous hydrolysis of fluid phase C3.

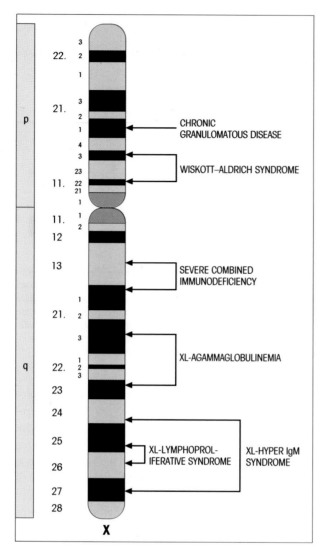

Figure 13.3 Loci of the X-linked (XL) immunodeficiency syndromes.

IMMUNOGLOBULIN DEFICIENCIES

X-linked agammaglobulinemia (XLA) is one of several immunodeficiency syndromes that have been mapped to the X-chromosome (figure 13.3). The defect is due to mutations in the **Bruton's tyrosine kinase (Btk) gene**, which is expressed early in B-cell development and which is crucial for maturation of the B-cell series from pre-B cells. Over 100 different Btk mutations are now recorded in the XLA mutation registry. Early B-cells are generated in the bone marrow but fail to mature, and the production of immunoglobulin in affected males is grossly depressed. B-cells are reduced or absent in the peripheral blood and there are few lymphoid follicles or plasma cells in the lymph nodes.

Affected boys are usually well for the first few months of life as they are protected by transplacentally acquired maternal antibody. They are then subject to repeated infection by pyogenic bacteria—*Staphylococcus aureus, Streptococcus pyogenes* and *pneumoniae, Neisseria meningitidis, Haemophilus influenzae*—and by *Giardia lamblia* which chronically infects the gastrointestinal tract. Resistance to viruses and fungi, which depends on T-lymphocytes, is normal, with the exception of hepatitis and enteroviruses. Therapy involves the repeated administration of human gammaglobulin to maintain adequate concentrations of circulating immunoglobulin.

Immunoglobulin A (IgA) deficiency due to a failure of IgA-bearing lymphocytes to differentiate into plasma cells is encountered with relative frequency. Many of these individuals are clinically asymptomatic but those with symptoms have sinopulmonary and gastrointestinal infections. An increased frequency of autoimmune and allergic disorders is noted in these patients who are at risk for developing anti-IgA antibodies on receipt of blood products.

Common variable immunodeficiency (CVID) is the most common form of primary immunodeficiency but the least well characterized. It is a heterogeneous disease usually appearing in adult life and is associated with a high incidence of autoimmune disorders and malignant disease, particularly of the lymphoid system. It probably results from inadequate T-cell signal transduction, which causes imperfect interactions between T- and B-cells. In the absence of suitable T-cell interactions, there is defective terminal differentiation of B-lymphocytes into plasma cells in some cases or defective ability to secrete antibody in others. Although some patients with CVID have a homozygous partial deletion of the *ICOS* gene (the "inducible costimulator" on activated T cells), the genetic basis of this disease in most patients is still unknown.

X-linked hyper-IgM syndrome is a rare disorder characterized by recurrent bacterial infections, very low levels or absence of IgG, IgA and IgE, and normal to raised concentrations of serum IgM and IgD. The disease is due to point mutations, usually single amino acid substitutions in the CD40L (CD40 ligand) expressed by CD4+ T-cells. Such defects will interfere with the normal interaction between CD40L and its counter-receptor CD40 on B-cells, a reaction which is crucial for the generation of memory B-cells and for Ig class-switching. Furthermore, it has been shown that interaction between CD40L on activated T-cells and CD40 on macrophages will stimulate IL-12 secretion, which is important in eliciting an adequate immune response against intracellular pathogens. This may ex-

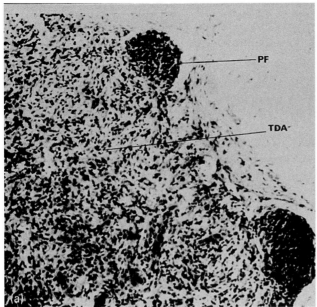

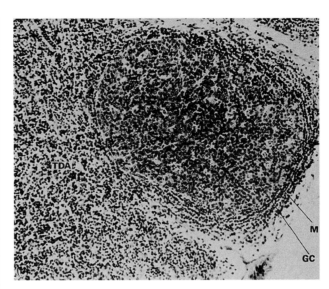

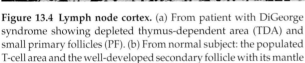

Figure 13.4 Lymph node cortex. (a) From patient with DiGeorge syndrome showing depleted thymus-dependent area (TDA) and small primary follicles (PF). (b) From normal subject: the populated T-cell area and the well-developed secondary follicle with its mantle of small lymphocytes (M) and pale-staining germinal center (GC) provide a marked contrast. (DiGeorge material kindly supplied by Dr D. Webster; photograph by Mr C.J. Sym.)

plain why these patients are also unduly susceptible to the intracellular organism *Pneumocystis carinii*.

Transient hypogammaglobulinemia of infancy is associated with an abnormal delay in the onset of Ig synthesis, which can extend into the second or third year of life. It is characterized by recurrent respiratory infections, and low IgG levels which return to normal by 4 years of age.

PRIMARY T-CELL DEFICIENCY

DiGeorge syndrome is characterized by a failure of the thymus to develop normally from the third and fourth pharyngeal pouches during embryogenesis. These children also lack parathyroids and have severe cardiovascular abnormalities, and most show microdeletion of specific DNA sequences from chromosome 22q11.2. Consequently, stem cells cannot differentiate to become T-lymphocytes and the "thymus-dependent" areas in lymphoid tissue are sparsely populated; in contrast lymphoid follicles are seen but even these are poorly developed (figure 13.4). Cell-mediated immune responses are undetectable, and, although the infants can deal with common bacterial infections, they may be overwhelmed by vaccinia (figure 13.5) or measles, or by BCG (bacille bilié de Calmette–Guérin)

if given by mistake. Humoral antibodies can be elicited but the response is subnormal, presumably reflecting the need for the cooperative involvement of T-cells. Transplantation of cultured, mature thymic epithelial cells has successfully reconstituted immune function in these patients and is considered as the treatment of choice. Partial hypoplasia of the thymus is more frequent than total aplasia, and immunologic treatment is usually not indicated.

PRIMARY T-CELL DYSFUNCTION

A number of syndromes due to abnormal T-cell function have been described. These differ from severe combined immunodeficiency (SCID; see below) by having T-cells in the peripheral blood. They include patients with mutations in the genes encoding the γ or ε chain of the CD3 molecule resulting in T-cells with defective function. Another group have a defective form of ZAP-70, a tyrosine kinase crucial for T-cell signal transduction, and a further subset of patients have abnormal IL-2 production resulting from an IL-2 gene transcription failure. The clinical picture produced by these defects is similar to that seen in patients with SCID, and bone marrow transplantation offers the only hope of long-term cure.

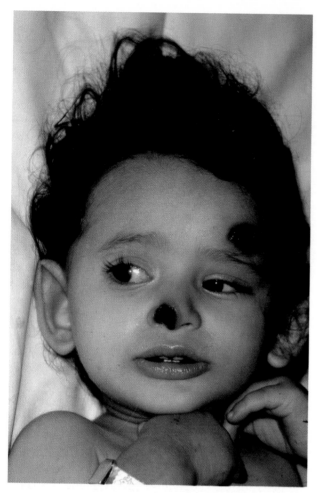

Figure 13.5 A child with severe combined immunodeficiency (SCID) showing skin lesions due to infection with vaccinia gangrenosum resulting from smallpox immunization. Lesions were widespread over the whole body. (Reproduced by kind permission of Professor R.J. Levinsky and the Medical Illustration Department of the Hospital for Sick Children, Great Ormond Street, London.)

SEVERE COMBINED IMMUNODEFICIENCY (SCID)

Severe combined immunodeficiency is a heterogeneous group of diseases involving T-cell immunodeficiency with or without B-cell or NK-cell immunodeficiency, resulting from any one of several genetic defects. The cases are characterized by severe lymphopenia with deficient cellular and humoral immunity. These children suffer recurrent infections early in life. Prolonged diarrhea resulting from gastrointestinal infections and pneumonia due to *Pneumocystis carinii* are common; *Candida albicans* grows vigorously in the mouth or on the skin. If vaccinated with attenuated organisms (figure 13.5) these children usually die of progressive infection, and most will not

survive the first year of life unless their immune systems are reconstituted by hematopoietic stem cell transplantation.

Mutation in the common cytokine receptor γ_c chain is the commonest cause of SCID

Severe combined immunodeficiency occurs in both an X-linked recessive and an autosomal form, but 50–60% of the cases are X-linked (X-SCID) and derive from **mutations in the common γ chain** of the IL-2, IL-4, IL-7, IL-9, IL-15 and IL-21 receptors. A number of mutations of this gene have been described and each results in a complex association of defects in the six affected cytokine/cytokine receptor systems.

Severe combined immunodeficiency can be due to mutations in purine salvage pathway enzymes

Many SCID patients with the autosomal recessive form of the disease have a genetic deficiency of the purine degradation enzymes, especially **adenosine deaminase** (ADA) and less commonly **purine nucleoside phosphorylase** (PNP). This results in the accumulation of metabolites that are toxic to lymphoid stem cells. Enzyme replacement therapy with injections of polyethylene glycol-modified adenosine deaminase results in clinical and immunologic improvement, and gene therapy using transfer of the *ADA* gene into either peripheral blood lymphocytes or hematopoietic stem cells has also met with some success. Bone marrow transplantation remains the treatment of choice.

Other SCID variants

A variety of other rare defects have been identified in individual SCID patients. These include mutations in the *RAG* genes, which initiate *VDJ* recombination events, and in another gene called the *Artemis* gene, which is crucial for repairing DNA after double-stranded cuts have been made by the *RAG* genes. Severe combined immunodeficiency will also result from mutations of the gene encoding JAK3 kinase, which is crucial for transducing the signal when IL-2 and other cytokines bind their receptors. Other patients with SCID have mutations of the CD45 common leukocyte antigen surface protein, which is normally required to regulate the Src kinase required for T- and B-cell antigen receptor signal transduction. There are also patients with a defect in the *CD3δ* gene who show a complete block in the development of T-cells. In the **bare lymphocyte syndrome** there is an MHC class II deficiency; few CD4$^+$ cells developing in the thymus, and those that do are inadequately stimulated by antigen-presenting cells lacking class II molecules. Because MHC class I molecules are normal, CD8$^+$ cells are present. The condition is due to mutations in one of a number of genes that regulate class II MHC expression rather than in the class II MHC genes themselves. Rare patients with mutations in TAP1 or TAP2 have MHC class I deficiency and are also prone to recurrent infections. Interaction between MHC class I molecules on thymic cells is essential for CD8$^+$ cell maturation, and therefore these patients have very low or absent CD8$^+$ cells but normal numbers of functioning CD4$^+$ cells.

OTHER COMBINED IMMUNODEFICIENCY DISORDERS

Wiskott–Aldrich syndrome (WAS) is an X-linked disease characterized by thrombocytopenia, type I hypersensitivity and immunodeficiency. This results in bleeding, eczema and recurrent infections. The condition is due to mutations of the gene encoding the so-called Wiskott–Aldrich syndrome protein (WASP) that is important in the organization of the cytoskeleton of both lymphocytes and platelets. This accounts for the disorganization of the cytoskeleton and loss of microvilli seen in T-cells from these patients, a feature that can be used to diagnose these cases prenatally. In numerous patients the platelet and immunologic abnormalities have been corrected by allogeneic stem cell transplantation. Gene therapy is likely to be the treatment of the future, and in *in vitro* studies retroviral infection of WASP-negative cells with WASP can restore normal function.

Ataxia telangiectasia is an autosomal recessive disorder of childhood characterized by progressive cerebellar ataxia due to degeneration of Purkinje cells, associated with vascular malformations (telangiectasia), increased incidence of malignancy and defects of both T- and B-cells. These patients also display a hypersensitivity to X-rays, which, together with the unduly high incidence of cancer, has been laid at the door of a defect in DNA repair mechanisms.

X-linked lymphoproliferative disease, also called Duncan's syndrome, is an immunodeficiency syndrome associated with infection by the Epstein–Barr virus (EBV). The condition is due to a mutation of the gene encoding SAP (SLAM-associated protein), which regulates signal transduction from the "signaling lymphocyte activation molecule" (SLAM) present on the surfaces of T and B-cells. Since activation of SLAM enhances IFNγ production by T-cells and proliferation of B-cells, significant immune deficiency results from this mutation.

A summary of the various primary immunodeficiency states is shown in Table 13.1.

RECOGNITION OF IMMUNODEFICIENCIES

Defects in humoral immunity can be assessed by quantitative Ig estimations and by measuring the antibody responses that follow active immunization with diphtheria, tetanus, pertussis and killed poliomyelitis. B-cells can be enumerated by flow cytometry using antibodies against CD19, CD20 and CD22.

Enumeration of T-cells is most readily achieved by flow cytometry using CD3 monoclonal antibody or other antibodies directed against T-cells such as CD2, CD5, CD7 or CD4 and CD8. Patients with T-cell deficiency will be hyporeactive or unreactive in skin tests to such antigens as tuberculin, *Candida*, tricophytin, streptokinase/streptodornase and mumps, and their lymphocytes demonstrate reduced cytokine production when stimulated by phytohemagglutinin (PHA) or other nonspecific mitogens.

In vitro tests for complement and for the bactericidal and other functions of polymorphs are available, while the reduction of nitroblue tetrazolium (NBT) or the stimulation of superoxide production provides a measure of the oxidative enzymes associated with active phagocytosis and bactericidal activity.

SECONDARY IMMUNODEFICIENCY

Immune responsiveness can be depressed nonspecifically by many factors. Cell-mediated immunity in particular may be impaired in states of malnutrition, even of the degree which may be encountered in urban areas of the more affluent regions of the world.

Viral infections are not infrequently immunosuppressive, and the depressed CMI, which accompanies measles infection, has been attributed to suppression of IL-12 production by the virus. The most notorious immunosuppressive virus, human immunodeficiency virus (HIV), is elaborated upon below.

Many therapeutic agents such as X-rays, cytotoxic drugs and corticosteroids may have dire effects on the immune system. **B-lymphoproliferative disorders** like chronic lymphocytic leukemia, myeloma and Waldenström's macroglobulinemia are associated with varying degrees of hypogammaglobulinemia and impaired antibody responses. These patients are susceptible to infections with common pyogenic bacteria, in contrast to the situation in Hodgkin's disease where the patients display all the hallmarks of

Table 13.1 Summary of primary immunodeficiency states.

DEFECTIVE GENE PRODUCT(S)	DISORDER
COMPLEMENT DEFICIENCES	
MBL, MASP-2	Recurrent bacterial infections
C1, C2, C4	Immune complex disease (SLE)
C1 inhibitor	Angioedema
PIG-A glycosyltransferase	Paroxysmal nocturnal hemoglobinuria
C3, Factor H, Factor I	Recurrent pyogenic infections
C5, C6, C7, C8	Recurrent *Neisseria* infections
PHAGOCYTIC DEFECTS	
NADPH oxidase	Chronic granulomatous disease
CD18 (β_2-integrin β chain)	Leukocyte adhesion deficiency
CHS	Chediak–Higashi disease
IFNγR1/2, IL-12p40, IL-12Rβ1	Mendelian susceptibility to mycobacterial infection
PRIMARY B-CELL DEFICIENCY	
Bruton's tyrosine kinase	X-linked agammaglobulinemia
?	IgA deficiency
ICOS	Common variable immunodeficiency
?	Transient infant hypogammaglobulinemia
PRIMARY T-CELL DEFICIENCY	
?	DiGeorge and Nezelof syndromes; failure of thymic development
RAG-1/2	Omenn's syndrome; partial *VDJ* recombination
MHC class II promoters	Bare lymphocyte syndrome
Atm	Ataxia telangiectasia; defective DNA repair
CD154 (CD40L)	Hyper-IgM syndrome
CD3 ϵ and γ chains, ZAP-70	Severe T-cell deficiency
COMBINED IMMUNODEFICIENCY	
?	Reticular dysgenesis; defective production of myeloid and lymphoid precursors
IL-7Rα	SCID due to defective IL-7 signaling
γ_c, JAK3	SCID due to defective cytokine signaling
RAG-1/2	Complete failure of *VDJ* recombination
ADA	Adenosine deaminase deficiency; toxic to early lymphoid stem cells
PNP	Purine nucleoside phosphorylase deficiency toxic to T-cells
SAP	X-linked lymphoproliferative disease; defective cell signaling
WASP	Wiskott–Aldrich syndrome; defective cytoskeletal regulation

Ig, immunoglobulin; IL-7, interleukin-7; SCID, severe combined immunodeficiency; SLE, systemic lupus erythematosus.

defective CMI—susceptibility to tubercle bacillus, *Brucella*, *Cryptococcus* and herpes zoster virus.

ACQUIRED IMMUNODEFICIENCY SYNDROME (AIDS)

Acquired immunodeficiency syndrome is due to the human immunodeficiency virus (HIV) of which there are two main variants called HIV-1 and HIV-2. The virus is transmitted inside infected CD4 T cells and macrophages, and the disease is therefore spread sexually or through blood or blood products such as encountered by intravenous drug users. The virus may also be transmitted from an infected mother to her infant, in which case babies born with a high viral load progress more rapidly than those with lower viral

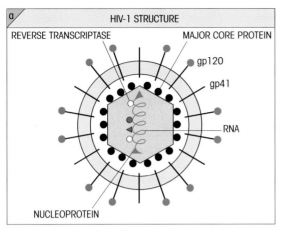

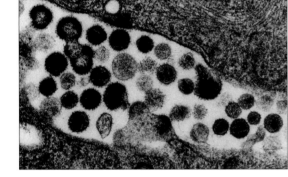

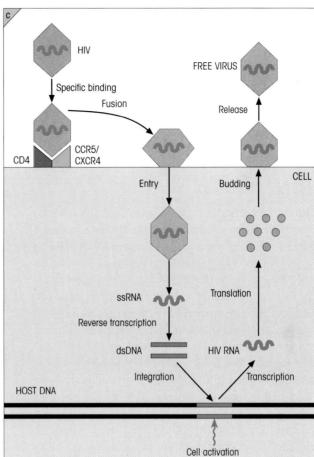

Figure 13.6 Characteristics of the HIV-1 acquired immunodeficiency syndrome (AIDS) virus. (a) HIV-1 structure. (b) Electron micrograph of mature and budding HIV-1 particles at the surface of human phytohemagglutinin (PHA) blasts. (c) Intracellular life cycle of human immunodeficiency virus (HIV). (Photograph kindly supplied by Dr C. Upton and Professor S. Martin.)

loads. The disease causes widespread immune dysfunction, with a protracted latent period but progressive decrease in CD4 cells leading eventually to severely depressed CMI. Once the absolute CD4 count falls below 200 cells/cu mm an individual becomes susceptible to opportunistic infections. These involve most commonly, *Pneumocystis carinii*, cytomegalovirus, EBV, herpes simplex virus, fungi such as *Candida*, *Aspergillus* and *Cryptococcus*, and the protozoan *Toxoplasma*; additionally, there is exceptional susceptibility for Kaposi's sarcoma induced by human herpesvirus 8 (HHV-8).

Characteristics of HIV

Transmission of the disease is usually through infection with blood or semen containing the HIV-1 virus or the related HIV-2. Sexual transmission occurs via mucosal surfaces followed by spread throughout the lymphatic system. HIV-1/2 are members of the lentivirus group, which are budding viruses (figure 13.6b) whose genome is relatively complex and tightly compressed. The many virion proteins (figure 13.6a) are generated by RNA splicing and cleavage by the viral protease.

The infection of cells by HIV

Infection takes place when envelope glycoprotein gp120 of HIV **binds avidly to cell-surface CD4** molecules on helper T-cells, macrophages, DCs and microglia. Dendritic cells populate the human mucosa and project their dendrites through the epithelial cells so that they are directly exposed on the mucosal surface. The binding to the CD4 molecule initiates the fusion of gp41 on the viral membrane to various chemokine co-receptors on the host cell (figure 13.6c). (It is worth noting that a new very successful anti-HIV drug (Enfuvirtide) acts by specifically inhibiting this fusion.) Early in infection the viruses utilize the CCR5 co-receptor present on memory T-cells, macrophages and DCs, and later infect resting T-cells using the CXCR4 co-receptor. It is interesting that mutations or complete absence of the CCR5 receptor have been described in 1% of Caucasians, and are associated with increased resistance to infection. Such mutations have not been described in people of African or Japanese descent.

Human immunodeficiency virus is an RNA retrovirus, which utilizes a **reverse transcriptase** to convert its genetic RNA into the corresponding DNA. This is integrated into the host genome where it can remain latent for long periods (figure 13.6c). Stimulation of latently infected T-cells or macrophages activates HIV replication through an increase in the intracellular concentration of NFκB (nuclear factor-kappa B) dimers, which bind to consensus sequences in the HIV enhancer region. This initiation of HIV gene transcription occurs when the host cells are activated by cytokines or by specific antigen. It is significant that tumor necrosis factor-α (TNFα), which upregulates HIV replication through this NFκB pathway, is present in elevated concentrations in the plasma of HIV-infected individuals, particularly in the advanced stage when they are infected with multiple organisms. Perhaps also, the more rapid progression of HIV infection in Africa may be linked to activation of the immune system through continual microbial insult.

The AIDS infection depletes helper T-cells

Natural history of the disease

The sequence of events following HIV-1 infection is charted in figure 13.7. The virus normally enters the body by infecting Langerhans' cells in the rectal or vaginal mucosa and then moves to local lymph nodes where it replicates. The virus is then disseminated by a viremia, which is associated with an acute early syndrome of fever, myalgia and arthralgia. A dominant nucleocapsid viral antigen, p24, can be detected in the blood during this phase. This phase is eventually controlled by activation of CD8 T-cells and by circulating antibodies to p24 and the envelope proteins gp120 and gp41. The efficacy of cytotoxic T-cells in controlling the virus is seen by a decline in level of virus, associated with a rebound of CD4$^+$ cells. This immune response leads to **sequestration of HIV in lymphoid tissue**, which becomes the major reservoir of HIV during the next stage of the disease, which is regarded as the clinically latent phase. Within the lymphoid follicles infectious virus becomes concentrated in the form of immune complexes held by follicular dendritic cells (FDCs). Although only low levels of virus are produced during the latent phase, destruction of CD4$^+$ cells continues within the lymphoid tissue. Eventually **circulating CD4 T-cell numbers fall progressively**, but it may take many years before CD4 cell loss leads to the chronic progressive phase of the disease. The patient is now wide open to life-threatening infections with normally nonpathogenic (opportunistic) agents.

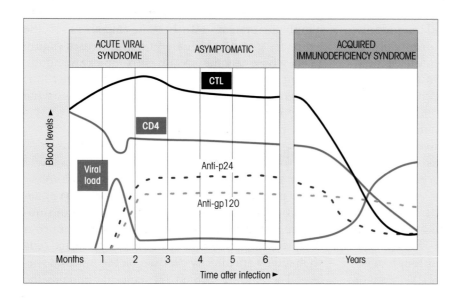

Figure 13.7 The natural history of HIV-1 infection. The changes in p24 antigen and antibody shown late in the disease are seen in some but not all patients. CTL, cytotoxic T-lymphocyte.

Mechanisms of CD4 cell depletion

The major immunologic feature of AIDS is the destruction of CD4 cells, a phenomenon that cannot be solely explained by the direct cytopathic effect of HIV. There is certainly no shortage of hypotheses to account for CD4 depletion with the corresponding change in the CD4 : CD8 ratio. These include:

1 A direct cytopathic effect by the virus either on single cells or through the formation of multinucleate syncytia between infected and noninfected CD4 cells.

2 Human immunodeficiency virus sensitizes CD4$^+$ T cells for activation-induced apoptosis. Stimulation of CD4 T-cells in HIV-infected individuals leads to apoptosis. This may explain the deterioration that follows other infections and the subsequent cytokine production that is so common in these patients. There is some evidence that HIV-infected cells are particularly sensitive to Fas-induced apoptosis, and this may relate to the expression of Fas on infected or uninfected T-cells induced by gp120 and tat proteins produced by HIV.

3 Cytotoxic CD8 cells are crucial in reducing viral load early in the HIV infection. They expand rapidly in infected patients and may play an important role in lysing infected CD4-positive cells.

4 Antibodies against HIV proteins may bind to infected cells which may then be destroyed by antibody-dependent cellular cytotoxicity (ADCC).

5 Human immunodeficiency virus infection is often associated with defective production or maturation of new T-cells from the thymus or bone marrow.

It is likely that a combination of several of these mechanisms ultimately act to tip the balance in favor of the virus.

Human immunodeficiency virus has strategies that allow it to evade the immune response

Human immunodeficiency virus employs a number of strategies to evade immune attack but most important is the high mutation rate of the virus that allows it to evade specific antibodies and cytotoxic T-cells. In fact immune responses against the virus may cause selection pressure that favors survival of the most genetically variable virus strains. Also, by depleting CD4 cells, especially HIV specific T-cells, HIV infection results in a severely compromised immune system. In addition, an HIV protein called Nef has the ability to downregulate the expression of MHC class 1 molecules, a process that could impair cytotoxic activity by CD8 cells.

Laboratory diagnosis of AIDS

Patients with HIV infection will demonstrate the presence of viral antibodies within a few weeks of infection. CD4 levels decrease rapidly after infection as is shown by a reversal of the normal CD4 : CD8 ratio. **Quantitative HIV-RNA plasma viral load** measurement is now routinely employed to evaluate and monitor patients with HIV infection. It includes measuring the baseline of viral load prior to initiation of antiretroviral therapy and assessing the efficacy of antiviral drug treatment. Quantitative HIV-RNA measurements are also the best indicator of the development of AIDS-defining opportunistic infections and subsequent progression of the disease. Associated with the decline in CD4 cells many tests of CMI will show defects, including the delayed hypersensitivity skin response to recall antigens.

Treatment of HIV disease

Therapeutic options for treating HIV are expanding with the development of numerous new drugs. The management of patients, however, has become highly complex due to the emergence of drug resistance and recognition of long-term toxicity of antiretroviral agents. Prolonged survival depends on the use of antiretroviral agents, immunization and chemoprophylaxis, and aggressive treatment of infectious and malignant complications when they occur. An increasing number of antiretroviral agents have been developed and these include both nonnucleoside and nucleoside reverse transcriptase inhibitors and protease inhibitors. Usually these are given as triple-drug therapy (HAART or highly active antiretroviral drug therapy) to reduce the development of mutated forms of the virus. Although the optimal time to initiate these therapies is controversial, they should always be used in symptomatic patients and in any infected person with a CD4 count below 500 mm^{-3} or with a viral load >50 000 copies/ml. The major drawback of these drugs is their enormous expense, which limits their use in those communities of the world where they are most needed. The ideal solution is to produce both prophylactic and therapeutic vaccines against HIV, but despite a huge effort an effective vaccine remains elusive.

REVISION

Primary immunodeficiency states

- These occur in the human, albeit somewhat rarely, as a result of a defect in almost any stage of differentiation in the whole immune system.
- Rare X-linked mutations produce disease in males.
- Defects in phagocytic cells, the complement pathways or the B-cell system lead in particular to infection with bacteria, which are disposed of by opsonization and phagocytosis.
- Patients with T-cell deficiencies are susceptible to viruses and fungi, which are normally eradicated by cell-mediated immunity (CMI).

Deficiencies of innate immune mechanisms

- Chronic granulomatous disease results from mutations in the NADPH (nicotinamide adenine dinucleotide phosphate) oxidase of phagocytic cells.
- Chediak–Higashi leukocytes contain giant lysosomal granules which interfere with their function.
- Leukocyte adhesion deficiency involves mutations in the CD18 subunit of β_2-integrins.
- Deficiency of one of the early components of the classical complement pathway may result in immune complex disease.
- Deficiency of C3 results in severe recurrent pyogenic infections.
- Deficiency of the late complement components results in increased susceptibility to recurrent *Neisseria* infections.
- Lack of C1 inhibitor leads to hereditary angioedema.
- Deficiencies in C1, C4 or C2 are associated with systemic lupus erythematosus (SLE) -like syndromes.

Primary B-cell deficiency

- Congenital X-linked agammaglobulinemia (XLA) (Bruton), involving differentiation arrest at the pre-B stage, is caused by mutations in the Bruton's tyrosine kinase (*Btk*) gene.
- Patients with immunoglobulin A (IgA) deficiency are susceptible to infections of the respiratory and gastrointestinal tract.
- In common variable immunodeficiency the B-cells fail to secrete antibody, probably due to abnormal interactions with T-cells.
- Mutations in the T-cell CD40L (CD40 ligand) gene provide the basis for hyper-IgM syndrome.

Primary T-cell deficiency

- DiGeorge syndrome results from failure of thymic development.

Primary T-cell dysfunction

- This group of patients have circulating T-cells, but their function is abnormal due a variety of genetic defects.

Severe combined immunodeficiency (SCID)

- Fifty to sixty percent of the patients with SCID have mutations in the gene for the γ chain common to receptors for IL-2, IL-4, IL-7, IL-9, IL-15 and IL-21.
- Many SCID patients have a genetic deficiency of the purine degradation enzymes adenosine deaminase (ADA) and purine nucleoside phosphorylase (PNP), which leads to accumulation of toxic products. Patients with ADA deficiency are being corrected by gene therapy.
- The bare lymphocyte syndrome is due to defective expression of major histocompatibility complex (MHC) class II molecules.

Other combined immunodeficiency disorders

- Wiskott–Aldrich males have a syndrome characterized by thrombocytopenia, eczema and immunodeficiency.
- Defective DNA repair mechanisms are found in patients with ataxia telangiectasia.

Recognition of immunodeficiencies

- Humoral immunodeficiency can be assessed initially by quantitation of immunoglobulins in the blood.
- B- and T-cell numbers can be enumerated by flow cytometric analysis.

Secondary immunodeficiency

- Immunodeficiency may arise as a secondary consequence of malnutrition, lymphoproliferative disorders, agents such as X-rays and cytotoxic drugs, and viral infections.

Acquired immunodeficiency syndrome (AIDS)

- AIDS results from infection by the RNA retroviruses HIV-1 and HIV-2.
- Human immunodeficiency virus (HIV) infects T-helper cells through binding of its envelope gp120 to CD4 with the help of a cofactor molecule, CXCR4 and other similar cytokine receptors. It also infects macrophages, microglia, T-cell-stimulating dendritic cells (DCs) and follicular dendritic cells (FDCs), the latter through a CD4-independent pathway.
- Within the cell, the RNA is converted by the reverse transcriptase to DNA, which can be incorporated into the host's genome where it lies dormant until the cell is activated by stimulators such as tumor necrosis factor-α

(TNFα) which increase NFκB (nuclear factor-kappa B) levels.

- There is usually a long asymptomatic phase after the early acute viral infection has been curtailed by an immune response, and the virus is sequestered to the FDC in the lymphoid follicles where it progressively destroys the DC meshwork.

- A disastrous fall in CD4 cells destroys cell-mediated defenses and leaves the patient open to life-threatening infections through opportunist organisms such as *Pneumocystis carinii* and cytomegalovirus.

- There is a tremendous battle between the immune system and the virus, with extremely high rates of viral destruction and CD4 T-cell replacement.

- CD4 T-cell depletion may eventually occur as a result of direct pathogenicity, apoptosis, antibody-dependent cellular cytotoxicity (ADCC), direct cytotoxicity by CD8 cells or disruption of normal T-cell production.

- AIDS is diagnosed in an individual with opportunistic infections, by low CD4 but normal CD8 T-cells in blood, poor delayed-type skin tests, positive tests for viral antibodies and p24 antigen, lymph node biopsy and isolation of live virus or demonstration of HIV genome by polymerase chain reaction (PCR).

See the accompanying website (**www.roitt.com**) for multiple choice questions

FURTHER READING

Ballow, M. (2002) Primary immunodeficiency disorders: Antibody deficiency. *Journal of Allergy and Clinical Immunology*, **109**, 581–91.

Buckley, R.H. (2002) Primary cellular immunodeficiencies. *Journal of Allergy and Clinical Immunology*, **109**, 74–57.

Buckley, R.H. (2000) Primary immunodeficiency diseases due to defects in lymphocytes. *New England Journal of Medicine*, **343**, 1313–24.

Cohen, O.J. (1997) Host factors in the pathogenesis of HIV disease. *Immunological Reviews*, **159**, 31–48.

Conley, M.E. (ed.) (2003) Section on immunodeficiency. *Current Opinion in Immunology*, **15**, 567–98.

Gandhi, R.T. & Walker, B.D. (2002) Immunologic control of HIV-1. *Annual Review of Medicine*, **53**, 149–72.

Lekstrom-Himes, J.A. & Gallin, J.I. (2000) Immunodeficiency diseases caused by defects in phagocytes. *New England Journal of Medicine*, **343**, 1703–14.

Ochs, H.D., Smith, C.I.E. & Puck, J.M. (eds) (2000) *Primary Immunodeficiency Diseases—A Molecular and Genetic Approach*. Oxford University Press, New York & Oxford.

Stebbing, J., Gazzard, B. & Douek, D.C. (2004) Where does HIV live? *New England Journal of Medicine*, **350**, 1872–80.

Hypersensitivity

INAPPROPRIATE IMMUNE RESPONSES CAN LEAD TO TISSUE DAMAGE

When an individual has been immunologically primed, further contact with antigen leads to secondary boosting of the immune response. However, the reaction may be excessive and lead to tissue damage (hypersensitivity). It should be emphasized that the mechanisms underlying these inappropriate reactions are those normally employed by the body in combating infection, as discussed in Chapter 11. Coombs and Gell defined four types of **hypersensitivity**. Types I, II and III depend on the interaction of antigen with humoral antibody, whereas type IV involves T-cell recognition. Because of the longer time course this has in the past been referred to as "delayed-type hypersensitivity."

TYPE I: ANAPHYLACTIC HYPERSENSITIVITY

Type 1 allergic disease, often referred to as atopic disease, is a group of conditions occurring in people with a hereditary predisposition to produce immunoglobulin E (IgE) antibodies against common environmental antigens (allergens). These conditions include some of the commonest causes of ill health including allergic rhinitis, asthma and atopic eczema.

Type I allergic reactions are due to activation of Th2 cells and the overproduction of IgE antibodies

The reason for this overproduction of IgE antibodies in certain individuals is unclear. There is increasing evidence that lack of exposure to bacteria which stimulate Th1 responses in early life favors the Th2 phenotype with subsequent development of atopy. This "hygiene hypothesis" could explain the lower incidence of allergic disease in individuals who farm or live in rural communities where they are presumably exposed to organisms from livestock. Allergic reactions are initiated by a limited number of allergens which are deposited in low doses on mucosal epithelium or skin. This is a particularly efficient way of activating Th2 cells and inducing IgE responses. Allergic individuals not only have larger numbers of allergen-specific Th2 cells in their blood, but these cells produce greater amounts of interleukin-4 (IL-4) per cell than Th2 cells from normal people. As with other antigens, allergens are processed by Langerhans' or other antigen-presenting cells and are proteolytically cleaved into small peptides and presented to uncommitted Th0 cells. In the case of an allergic response, these cells now differentiate into Th2 lymphocytes, which release various cytokines that inhibit Th1 cell activation and upregulate IgE production. These cytokines, particularly IL-4 and IL-13 together with signals delivered

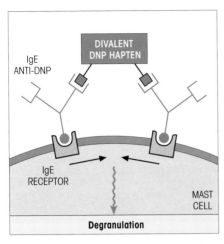

Figure 14.1 Clustering of immunoglobulin E (IgE) receptors by divalent hapten (used as a model for multivalent antigen).

by the B-cell surface molecule CD40, induce isotype switching in newly generated IgM-bearing B-cells from μ to ε resulting in subsequent production of IgE.

There is a strong genetic component to allergic diseases

Genetic susceptibility to allergic reactions has not been clearly defined but high levels of IgE are noted in certain allergic (atopic) families. Human leukocyte antigen (HLA) linkage is associated with allergic responses to a number of allergens including ragweed and house dust mite. A further major genetic locus, which regulates serum IgE levels, has been identified on chromosome 5q in the region containing the genes for IL-4, IL-5 and IL-9, cytokines that are important in regulating IgE synthesis. Polymorphism of the *IL-9* gene is associated with asthma, as is a locus on chromosome 11q13 where the gene encodes the β chain of the IgE receptor.

Clustering of IgE receptors on mast cells through cross-linking triggers anaphylaxis

Mast cells display a high-affinity receptor (FcεRI) for the Cε2:Cε3 junction region of IgE Fc, a property shared with their circulating counterpart, the basophil.

Cross-linking of receptor-bound IgE antibodies by a multivalent antigen will trigger release of the inflammatory mediators responsible for the acute allergic reaction through aggregation of these receptors (figure 14.1). Activation is rapidly followed by the breakdown of phosphatidylinositol to inositol triphosphate (IP3),

the generation of diacylglycerol (DAG) and an increase in intracytoplasmic free calcium. This biochemical cascade allows the granules to fuse with the plasma membrane and release their preformed mediators into the surrounding tissue. It also results in synthesis of lipid mediators including a series of arachidonic acid metabolites formed by the cyclooxygenase and lipoxygenase pathways, and production of a variety of cytokines which are responsible for the late phase of the acute allergic reaction.

Mast cell and basophil mediators

Mast cell degranulation is the major initiating event of the acute allergic reaction. The preformed mediators released from the granules include histamine, heparin, tryptase, neutral protease and various eosinophil and neutrophil chemotactic factors. Histamine itself is responsible for many of the immediate symptoms of allergic reactions including bronchoconstriction, vasodilatation, mucus secretion and edema caused by leakage of plasma proteins from small vessels. These effects can all be reproduced and visualized in the immediate skin test where allergen injected into the skin produces a characteristic wheal and flare reaction with redness, edema and pruritus (itchiness) (cf. figure 14.5a). Tryptase released by mast cells activates receptors on endothelial cells that selectively attract eosinophils and basophils.

Activation of the mast cells also results in the liberation of newly formed lipid mediators, which include the leukotrienes LTB_4, LTC_4 and LTD_4, the prostaglandin D_2 (PGD_2) and platelet activating factor (PAF). Prostaglandin D_2, the leukotrienes and PAF are highly potent bronchoconstrictors, which also increase vascular permeability and are chemotactic for inflammatory cells.

The late phase of the allergic reaction is mediated by cytokines

Mast cells and basophils are responsible for significant production of proinflammatory cytokines including tumor necrosis factor (TNF), IL-1, IL-4 and IL-5, and chemokines such as MIP-1α and MIP-1β. Within 12 h of an acute allergic reaction a late-phase reaction occurs, which is characterized by a cellular infiltrate of $CD4^+$ cells, monocytes and eosinophils. These cells will themselves release a variety of Th2-type cytokines, especially IL-4 and IL-5, which are responsible for further inflammation at the site of the allergen. Macrophages in particular can be activated through an FcεRII receptor leading to significant release of TNF and IL-1. This late reaction, therefore, resembles a delayed hypersensitivity reaction because of the infiltration of T-cells and the effects of the cytokines. A differentiating feature, however, is the presence of eosinophils and Th2 cells in the late phase of the allergic response and their absence from delayed hypersensitivity reactions.

The sudden degranulation of mast cells therefore leads to release of a complex cascade of mediators, which generally results in the symptoms of acute allergic reactions. Under normal circumstances, these mediators help to orchestrate the development of a defensive acute inflammatory reaction. When there is a massive release of these mediators under abnormal conditions, as in atopic disease, their bronchoconstrictive and vasodilatory effects predominate and become distinctly threatening.

Eosinophils are prominent in the allergic reaction

The preferential accumulation of eosinophils is a characteristic feature of allergic diseases and is due to the production of eosinophil chemoattractants from mast cells. These include eotaxin and RANTES (regulated upon activation, normal T-cell expressed and secreted). Interleukin-5, which is produced by Th2 cells, is important in eosinophil activation and also inhibits the natural apoptosis of eosinophils which regulates their lifespan. Under the influence of these cytokines, eosinophils adhere to vascular endothelium via β_2-integrins and move through to the site of the allergic reaction. The eosinophil granules release very basic, highly charged polypeptides. These include major basic protein and eosinophil peroxidase, which cause tissue damage including destruction of the respiratory epithelium in asthmatics. Eosinophils are also an important source of leukotrienes, PAF, cytokines including IL-3 and IL-5, and a variety of eosinophil chemoattractants which further amplify the eosinophil response.

Atopic allergy

Examples of clinical responses to inhaled allergens

Allergic rhinitis. Nearly 10% of the population suffer to a greater or lesser degree from allergies involving localized IgE-mediated anaphylactic reactions to extrinsic allergens such as grass pollens, animal danders, the feces from mites in house dust (figure 14.2) and so on. The most common manifestation is **allergic rhinitis**, often known as hay fever. The target organs are the

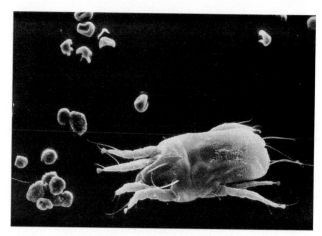

Figure 14.2 House dust mite—a major cause of allergic disease. The electron micrograph shows the rather nasty looking mite, graced by the name *Dermatophagoides pteronyssinus,* and fecal pellets on the bottom left, which are the major source of allergen. The biconcave pollen grains (top left), shown for comparison, indicate the size of particles which can become airborne and reach the lungs. The mite itself is much too large for that. (Reproduced courtesy of Dr E. Tovey.)

mucus membranes of the nose and eyes (figure 14.3) and the allergic inflammation results in congestion, itchiness and sneezing, which is so characteristic of this condition. An increasing number of causative allergens have now been cloned and expressed including **Der p1** and **Der p2** from house dust mites and **Fel d1** from cat dander. Exposure to these and other allergens produces the typical symptoms within minutes.

Asthma. Asthma is a chronic disease characterized by increased responsiveness of the tracheobronchial tree to a variety of stimuli resulting in reversible airflow limitation and inflammation of the airways. It is thought that exposure to indoor allergens early in infancy predisposes to the disease regardless of a family history, but the development of asthma is influenced by multiple genetic and environmental factors. Bronchial biopsy and lavage of asthmatic patients reveals involvement of **mast cells, eosinophils and macrophages** as the major mediator-secreting effector cells, while T-cells provide the microenvironment required to sustain the inflammatory response which is an essential feature of the histopathology (figure 14.4). Cytokines released by all these infiltrating cells give rise to allergic inflammation resulting in edema of the airway wall, mucus hypersecretion, variable airflow obstruction and bronchial hyper-responsiveness. There is also a repair-type response involving the

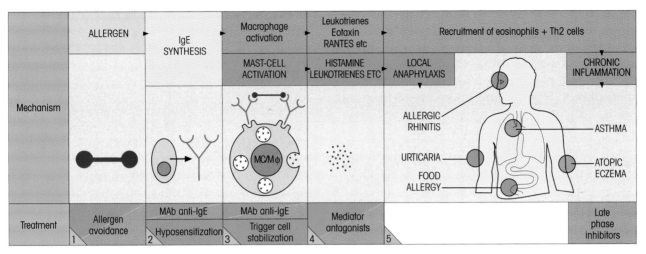

				Leukotrienes Eotaxin RANTES etc	Recruitment of eosinophils + Th2 cells	
	ALLERGEN	IgE SYNTHESIS	Macrophage activation			
Mechanism			MAST-CELL ACTIVATION	HISTAMINE LEUKOTRIENES ETC	LOCAL ANAPHYLAXIS	CHRONIC INFLAMMATION
Treatment	Allergen avoidance	MAb anti-IgE / Hyposensitization	MAb anti-IgE / Trigger cell stabilization	Mediator antagonists		Late phase inhibitors

Figure 14.3 Atopic allergies: sites of local responses and possible therapies. Events and treatments relating to local anaphylaxis in green and to chronic inflammation in red. Mφ, macrophage; MC, mast cell; IgE, immunoglobulin E.

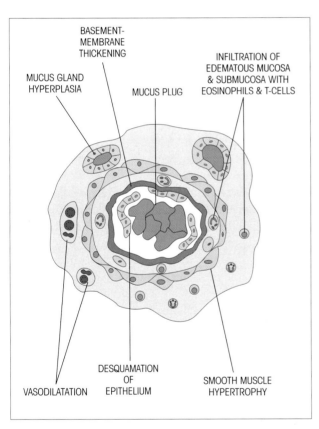

Figure 14.4 Pathologic changes in asthma. Diagram of cross-section of an airway in severe asthma.

production of fibroblast growth factor, transforming growth factor-β (TGFβ) and platelet-derived growth factor (PDGF), which lead to fibrosis and hypertrophy of smooth muscle that further narrows the airways.

Anaphylaxis. The earliest accounts of inappropriate responses to foreign antigens relate to anaphylaxis. The phenomenon can be readily reproduced in guinea pigs which, like humans, are a highly susceptible species. A single injection of 1 mg of an antigen such as egg albumin into a guinea pig has no obvious effect. However, if the injection is repeated 2–3 weeks later, the sensitized animal reacts very dramatically with the symptoms of generalized anaphylaxis; almost immediately the guinea-pig begins to wheeze and within a few minutes dies from asphyxia. Examination shows intense constriction of the bronchioles and bronchi and generally there is contraction of smooth muscle and dilatation of capillaries. Similar anaphylactic reactions can occur in human subjects and comprise laryngeal edema, hypotension and lower-airway obstruction. They may be produced by peanuts, shellfish or other food allergens, or may follow wasp and bee stings or injections of penicillin or other drugs in sensitized individuals. In many instances only a timely injection of epinephrine to counter the hypotension, the smooth muscle contraction and capillary dilatation, can prevent death.

Latex allergy. This is a hypersensitivity reaction to proteins contained in latex, the name given to the sap of the rubber tree. It is often seen in health-care workers and others who have significant exposure to rubber gloves or other rubber-containing materials. The acute allergic reaction may present with skin rashes, itching or redness of the eyes, nasal symptoms or coughing, wheezing and shortness of breath. In severe cases anaphylactic shock may occur. Aerosols of latex may occur when rubber gloves containing powders are removed because the latex can bind to the powder and cause acute respiratory symptoms in allergic individuals. As with other allergies, avoidance of the allergen is crucial. In the case of hospital workers this may entail avoiding all contact with airway masks and straps, anesthesia bags, chest tubes, catheter bags and many other rubber-containing products in the home. There is some evidence that latex-allergic individuals may develop symptoms from various fruits, especially avocado and banana, which contain proteins that cross-react with latex.

Food allergy

Awareness of the importance of IgE sensitization to food allergens in the gut has increased dramatically so that allergy to peanuts or peanut butter is necessitating major changes in school lunch programs. Many foods have been incriminated, especially nuts, shellfish, milk and eggs, and food additives such as sulfiting agents. Sensitization to egg white and cows' milk may even occur in early infancy through breast-feeding, with antigen passing into the mother's milk. Contact of the food with specific IgE on mast cells in the gastrointestinal tract may produce local reactions such as diarrhea and vomiting. It may also allow the allergen to enter the body by changing gut permeability through mediator release resulting in systemic reactions including skin eruptions (urticaria), bronchospasm and anaphylactic shock.

Clinical tests for allergy

Sensitivity is normally assessed by the response to intradermal challenge with antigen. The release of histamine and other mediators rapidly produces a **wheal and flare reaction** at the site (figure 14.5a), maximal within 30 min and then subsiding. This immediate reaction may be followed by the late-phase reaction, which sometimes lasts for 24 h and is characterized by a dense infiltration of eosinophils and T-cells and is more edematous than the early reaction. The similarity to the histopathology of the inflammatory infiltrate in chronic asthma is obvious, and these late-phase reactions can also be seen following challenge of the bronchi and nasal mucosa of allergic subjects.

Allergen-specific serum IgE can also be measured by

an **ELISA type test**, the results of which correlate well with skin test results.

Therapy

If one considers the sequence of reactions from initial exposure to allergen right through to the production of atopic disease, it can be seen that several points in the chain provide legitimate targets for therapy (figure 14.3). Avoidance of contact with environmental allergens is often impractical, but it is possible to avoid contact with incriminating animals, drugs or ingested allergens.

Modulation of the immunologic response. Attempts to desensitize patients immunologically by repeated subcutaneous injections of allergen can lead to worthwhile improvement in certain clinical situations. This is thought to be due to the activation of Th1-type cells rather than Th2, resulting in production of increasing amounts of IgG rather than IgE. The IgG antibody will compete for antigen with IgE and will divert the allergen from contact with tissue-bound IgE. Other strategies attempt to inhibit the binding of IgE to its mast cell receptor using either small blocking peptides or a humanized **monoclonal anti-IgE antibody (Xolair)**. It is noteworthy that this antibody cannot trigger life-threatening anaphylaxis by cross-linking mast cell bound IgE because the epitope is masked through combination with the receptor.

Mast cell stabilization. At the drug level, much relief has been obtained with agents such as inhalant isoprenaline and **sodium cromoglycate**, which render mast cells resistant to triggering. Sodium cromoglycate blocks chloride channel activity and maintains cells in a normal resting physiological state, which probably accounts for its inhibitory effects on a wide range of cellular functions, such as mast cell degranulation, eosinophil and neutrophil chemotaxis and mediator release, and reflex bronchoconstriction. Some or all of these effects are responsible for its anti-asthmatic actions.

Mediator antagonism. Histamine H1-receptor antagonists have for many years proved helpful in the symptomatic treatment of allergic disease. For asthma the long-acting inhaled β_2-**agonists** such as salmeterol and formoterol, which are bronchodilators, protect against bronchoconstriction for over 12 h. Potent **leukotriene antagonists** such as Pranlukast also block constrictor challenges and show striking efficacy in some patients. **Theophylline** has been used in the treatment of asthma for more than 50 years and remains the single most prescribed drug for asthma worldwide. As a **phosphodiesterase (PDE) inhibitor** it increases intra-

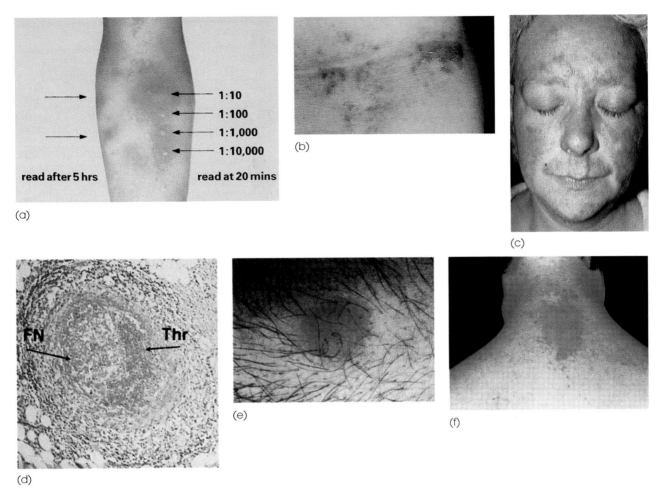

Figure 14.5 Hypersensitivity reactions.

Type I (a) Skin prick tests with grass pollen allergen in a patient with typical summer hay fever. Skin tests were performed 5 h (*left*) and 20 min (*right*) before the photograph was taken. The tests on the right show a typical end-point titration of a type I immediate wheal and flare reaction. The late-phase skin reaction (*left*) can be clearly seen at 5 h, especially where a large immediate response has preceded it. Figures for allergen dilution are given. (b) An atopic eczema reaction on the back of a knee of a child allergic to rice and eggs.

Type III (c) Facial appearance in systemic lupus erythematosus (SLE). Lesions of recent onset are symmetrical, red and edematous. They are often most pronounced on the areas of the face which receive most light exposure, i.e. the upper cheeks and bridge of the nose, and the prominences of the forehead. (d) Histology of acute inflammatory reaction in polyarteritis nodosa associated with immune complex formation with hepatitis B surface (HBs) antigen. A vessel showing thrombus (Thr) formation and fibrinoid necrosis (FN) is surrounded by a mixed inflammatory infiltrate, largely polymorphs.

Type IV (e) Mantoux test showing cell-mediated hypersensitivity reaction to tuberculin, characterized by induration and erythema. (f) Type IV contact hypersensitivity reaction to nickel caused by the clasp of a necklace. ((a), (b) and (e) kindly provided by Professor J. Brostoff; (c) by Dr G. Levene; (d) by Professor N. Woolf; (f) reproduced from British Society for Immunology teaching slides with permission of the Society and Dermatology Department, London Hospital.)

cellular cAMP (cyclic adenosine monophosphate) thereby causing bronchodilatation, inhibition of IL-5-induced prolongation of eosinophil survival and probably suppression of eosinophil migration into the bronchial mucosa. Newer approaches to therapy include the use of leukotriene receptor antagonists, antibodies against IL-4 or the IL-4 receptor, antibodies to endothelial cell adhesion molecules and inhibition of eosinophil activity using antibodies against IL-5.

Attacking chronic inflammation. The triggering of macrophages through allergen interaction with surface-bound IgE is clearly a major initiating factor for late reactions, as discussed above. Resistance to this stimulus can be very effectively achieved with corticosteroids. These drugs play a major role in the treatment of allergic disease by suppressing the transcription of multiple inflammatory genes, especially those encoding cytokine production.

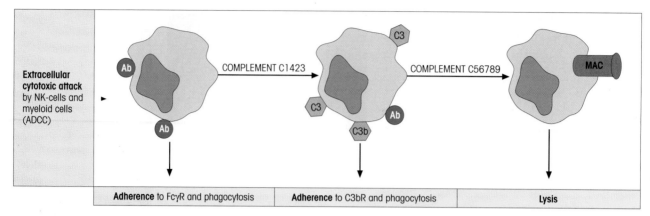

Figure 14.6 Antibody-dependent cytotoxic hypersensitivity (type II). Antibodies directed against cell surface antigens cause cell death not only by C-dependent lysis but also by Fcγ and C3b adherence re-actions leading to phagocytosis, or through nonphagocytic extracellular killing by NK and myeloid cells (antibody-dependent cellular cytotoxicity (ADCC)).

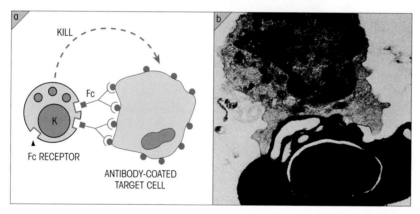

Figure 14.7 Killing of antibody (Ab) -coated target by antibody-dependent cellular cytotoxicity (ADCC). Fcγ receptors bind the effector to the target, which is killed by an extracellular mechanism. Human monocytes and interferon γ (IFNγ) -activated neutrophils kill Ab-coated tumor cells using their FcγRI and FcγRII receptors; natural killer (NK) cells bind to their targets through FcγRIII receptors. (a) Diagram of effector and target cells. (b) Electron micrograph of attack on Ab-coated chick red cell by a mouse NK cell showing close apposition of effector and target and vacuolation in the cytoplasm of the latter. ((b) Courtesy of Dr P. Penfold.)

TYPE II: ANTIBODY-DEPENDENT CYTOTOXIC HYPERSENSITIVITY

This form of hypersensitivity is due to an abnormal antibody directed against a cell or a tissue. Such an antibody attack may activate the **complement** cascade causing target cell destruction by **direct membrane damage** (figure 14.6). Alternatively, antibody may opsonize cells which are then removed by phagocytes. Opsonization may occur directly through the Fc receptor or by **immune adherence** where C3b on the antigen–antibody complex attaches to the CR1 receptor on the phagocytic cell. Target cells coated with low concentrations of IgG antibody can also be killed "nonspecifically" through an extracellular nonphagocytic mechanism involving nonsensitized leukocytes, which bind to the target by their specific receptors for

the Cγ2 and Cγ3 domains of IgG Fc (figure 14.7). This so-called **antibody-dependent cellular cytotoxicity (ADCC)** may be exhibited by both phagocytic cells, such as polymorphs and monocytes, and by nonphagocytic natural killer (NK) cells. Functionally, this extracellular cytotoxic mechanism would be expected to be of significance where the target is too large for ingestion by phagocytosis; for example, large parasites and solid tumors.

Type II reactions between members of the same species (alloimmune)

Transfusion reactions

Of the many different polymorphic constituents of the human red cell membrane, **ABO blood groups** form

Table 14.1 ABO blood groups and serum antibodies.

BLOOD GROUP (PHENOTYPE)	GENOTYPE	ANTIGEN	SERUM ANTIBODY
A	AA, AO	A	ANTI-B
B	BB, BO	B	ANTI-A
AB	AB	A and B	NONE
O	OO	H	ANTI-A ANTI-B

the dominant system. The antigenic groups A and B are derived from H substance by the action of glycosyltransferases encoded by A or B genes respectively. Individuals with both genes (group AB) have the two antigens on their red cells, while those lacking these genes (group O) synthesize H substance only. Antibodies to A or B occur when the antigen is absent from the red cell surface; thus a person of blood group A will possess anti-B and so on. These **isohemagglutinins** are usually IgM and probably belong to the class of "natural antibodies"; they would be boosted through contact with antigens of the gut flora which are structurally similar to the blood group carbohydrates, so that the antibodies formed cross-react with the appropriate red cell type. If an individual is blood group A, they would be tolerant to antigens closely similar to A and would only form cross-reacting antibodies capable of agglutinating B red cells. Similarly an O individual would make anti-A and anti-B (table 14.1). A transfusion of mismatched blood would result in the transfused red cells being coated by the isohemagglutinins and destroyed by complement activation or phagocytic activity giving rise to severe transfusion reactions.

Rhesus (Rh) incompatibility

The **Rh blood groups** form the other major antigenic system, the RhD antigen being of the most consequence for isoimmune reactions. A mother who is RhD-negative (i.e. dd genotype) can readily be sensitized by red cells from a baby carrying RhD antigens (DD or Dd genotype). This sensitization occurs most often at the birth of the first child when a placental bleed can release a large number of the baby's erythrocytes into the mother. The antibodies formed are predominantly of the IgG class and are able to cross the placenta in any subsequent pregnancy. Reaction with the D-antigen on the fetal red cells leads to the latter's destruction through opsonic adherence, giving rise to hemolytic disease of the newborn (figure 14.8). For this reason **RhD-negative mothers are now treated prophylactically** with low doses of avid IgG anti-D at the time of birth of the first child. This coats the baby's red cells in the mother's circulation promoting their phagocytosis and preventing sensitization.

Organ transplant rejection

Hyperacute graft rejection mediated by preformed antibodies in the graft recipient is a classic example of an attack by antibody on target cells. Recipients may develop such antibodies as a result of previous blood transfusions or failed transplants or multiple pregnancies. Following attachment of the blood supply to the new graft these antibodies bind to donor endothelial antigens resulting in thrombosis of vessels in the graft and very rapid hyperacute rejection. Fortunately this complication is not commonly seen, as patients awaiting transplantation are routinely checked for the presence of antibodies.

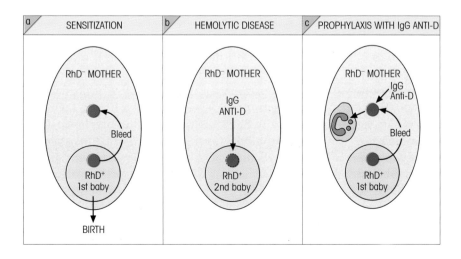

Figure 14.8 Hemolytic disease of the newborn due to rhesus (Rh) incompatibility. (a) RhD-positive red cells from the first baby sensitize the RhD-negative mother. (b) The mother's immunoglobulin G (IgG) anti-D crosses the placenta and coats the erythrocytes of the second RhD-positive baby causing type II hypersensitivity hemolytic disease. (c) Immunoglobulin G anti-D given prophylactically at the first birth removes the baby's red cells through phagocytosis and prevents sensitization of the mother.

Autoimmune type II hypersensitivity reactions

A variety of organ-specific autoimmune diseases result from antibodies directed against various cell or tissue antigens. Autoantibodies to the patient's own red cells are produced in **autoimmune hemolytic anemia**. Red cells coated with these antibodies have a shortened half-life, largely through their adherence to phagocytic cells in the spleen. Antibodies to platelets result in autoimmune thrombocytopenia, and the serum of patients with Hashimoto's thyroiditis contains antibodies which in the presence of complement are directly cytotoxic to thyroid cells. In Goodpasture's syndrome (included here for convenience), antibodies to the basement membranes of kidney glomeruli and lung alveoli are present. Biopsies show these antibodies together with complement components bound to the basement membranes, where the action of the full complement system leads to serious damage (figure 14.9a).

Anti-receptor autoimmune diseases

Autoantibodies directed against cellular receptors may give rise to disease by either blocking or depleting the receptor from the cell surface or by activating the receptor. As will be discussed more fully in Chapter 17, **myasthenia gravis** is a disorder due to an abnormal antibody directed against the acetylcholine receptors resulting in profound muscular weakness. In **Graves' disease (thyrotoxicosis)**, however, the abnormal antibody stimulates the receptor for thyroid-stimulating hormone (TSH) resulting in uncontrolled production of thyroid hormones.

Type II drug reactions

Drugs may become coupled to body components and thereby undergo conversion from a hapten to a full antigen that may sensitize certain individuals. If IgE antibodies are produced, anaphylactic reactions can result. In some circumstances, particularly with topically applied ointments, cell-mediated hypersensitivity may be induced. In other cases where coupling to serum proteins occurs, the possibility of type III immune complex-mediated reactions may arise. In the present context we are concerned with those instances where the drug appears to form an antigenic complex with the surface of a formed element of the blood and evokes the production of antibodies which are cytotoxic for the cell–drug complex. When the drug is withdrawn, the sensitivity is no longer evident.

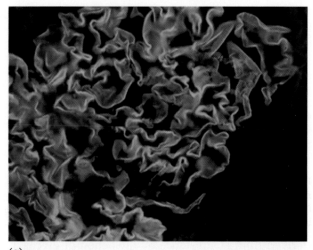

(a)

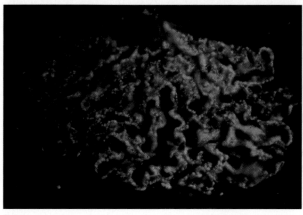

(b)

Figure 14.9 Glomerulonephritis: (a) due to linear deposition of antibody to glomerular basement membrane, here visualized by staining the human kidney biopsy with a fluorescent anti-immunoglobulin G (IgG); and (b) due to deposition of antigen–antibody complexes, which can be seen as discrete masses lining the glomerular basement membrane following immunofluorescent staining with anti-IgG. Similar patterns to these are obtained with a fluorescent anti-C3. (Photographs kindly supplied by Dr S. Thiru.)

Examples of this mechanism have been seen in the **hemolytic anemia** sometimes associated with continued administration of chlorpromazine or phenacetin, in the **agranulocytosis** associated with the taking of aminopyrine or of quinidine, and the now classic situation of **thrombocytopenic purpura** which may be produced by Sedormid, a sedative of yesteryear. In the latter case, freshly drawn serum from the patient will lyse platelets in the presence, but not in the absence, of Sedormid; inactivation of complement by preheating the serum at 56°C for 30 min abrogates this effect.

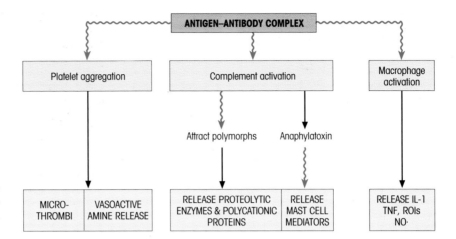

Figure 14.10 Type III immune complex-mediated hypersensitivity. IL, interleukin; NO, nitric oxide; ROIs, reactive oxygen intermediates; TNF, tumor necrosis factor.

TYPE III: IMMUNE COMPLEX-MEDIATED HYPERSENSITIVITY

Under a number of circumstances the body may be exposed to an excess of antigen over a protracted period. The union of such antigens with the subsequently formed antibodies forms insoluble complexes at fixed sites within the body where they may well give rise to acute inflammatory reactions (figure 14.10). When complement is fixed, the anaphylatoxins C3a and C5a will cause release of mast cell mediators resulting in increased vascular permeability. These same chemotactic factors and those released by mast cells will lead to an influx of polymorphonuclear leukocytes, which attempt to phagocytose the immune complexes. This in turn results in the extracellular release of the polymorph granule contents, particularly when the complex is deposited on a basement membrane and cannot be phagocytosed (so-called "frustrated phagocytosis"). The proteolytic enzymes (including neutral proteinases and collagenase), kinin-forming enzymes, polycationic proteins and reactive oxygen and nitrogen intermediates which are released from the polymorph will damage local tissues and intensify the inflammatory responses. Under appropriate conditions, platelets may be aggregated with two consequences: they provide yet a further source of vasoactive amines and they may also form microthrombi, which can lead to local ischemia. Insoluble complexes taken up by macrophages cannot readily be digested and provide a persistent activating stimulus leading to release of the cytokines IL-1 and TNF, reactive oxygen intermediates (ROIs) and nitric oxide (NO) (figure 14.10) which further damage the tissue.

The outcome of the formation of immune complexes *in vivo* depends not only on the absolute amounts of antigen and antibody, but also on their *relative* proportions which govern the nature of the complexes and hence their distribution within the body. Between **antibody excess** and **mild antigen excess**, the complexes are rapidly precipitated and tend to be localized to the site of introduction of antigen, whereas in **moderate** to **gross antigen excess**, soluble complexes are formed. These small complexes containing C3b bind by immune adherence to CR1 complement receptors on the human erythrocyte and are transported to fixed macrophages in the liver where they are safely inactivated. If there are defects in this system, for example deficiencies in classical complement pathway components or perhaps if the system is overloaded, then the immune complexes are free in the plasma and widespread disease involving deposition in the kidneys, joints and skin may result.

Inflammatory lesions due to locally formed complexes

The Arthus reaction

Maurice Arthus found that injection of soluble antigen intradermally into hyper-immunized rabbits with high levels of antibody produced an erythematous and edematous reaction reaching a peak at 3–8 h and then usually resolving. The lesion was characterized by an intense infiltration with polymorphonuclear leukocytes. The injected antigen precipitates with antibody and binds complement. Using fluorescent reagents, antigen, Ig and complement components can all be demonstrated in this lesion. Anaphylatoxin is soon generated and causes mast cell degranulation,

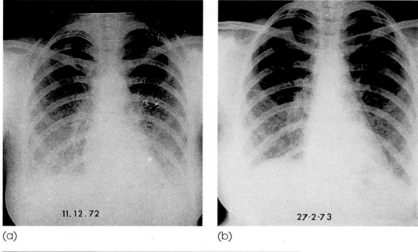

(a)   (b)

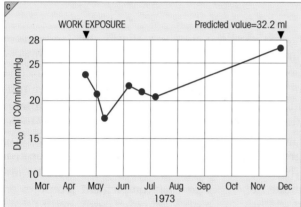

Figure 14.11 Extrinsic allergic alveolitis due to rat serum proteins in a research assistant handling rats (type III hypersensitivity). Typical systemic and pulmonary reactions on inhalation and positive prick tests were elicited by rat serum proteins; precipitins against serum proteins in rat urine were present in the patient's serum. (a) Bilateral micronodular shadowing during acute episodes. (b) Marked clearing within 11 days after cessation of exposure to rats. (c) Temporary fall in pulmonary gas exchange measured by DL_{co} (gas transfer, single breath) following a 3-day exposure to rats at work (arrowed). (From K.B. Carroll, J. Pepys, J.L. Longbottom, D.T.D. Hughes & H.G. Benson (1975) *Clinical Allergy* **5**, 443; figures kindly provided by Professor J. Pepys.)

influx of polymorphs with release of polymorph granules, and local tissue injury. Local intravascular complexes will also cause platelet aggregation and vasoactive amine release resulting in erythema and edema.

Reactions to inhaled antigens

Intrapulmonary Arthus-type reactions to exogenous inhaled antigen appear to be responsible for the condition of hypersensitivity pneumonitis. The severe respiratory difficulties associated with farmer's lung occur within 6–8 h of exposure to the dust from moldy hay. These patients are sensitized to thermophilic actinomycetes which grow in the moldy hay, and extracts of these organisms give precipitin reactions with the subject's serum and Arthus reactions on intradermal injection. Inhalation of bacterial spores present in dust from the hay introduces antigen into the lungs and a complex-mediated hypersensitivity reaction ensues. Similar situations arise in pigeon-fancier's disease, where the antigen is probably serum protein present in the

dust from dried feces and in rat handlers sensitized to rat serum proteins excreted in the urine (figure 14.11). There are many other quaintly named cases of extrinsic allergic alveolitis resulting from continual inhalation of organic particles; for example, cheese washer's disease (*Penicillium casei spores*), furrier's lung (fox fur proteins) and maple bark stripper's disease (spores of *Cryptostroma*). Although the initial damage in the lung is due to localized immune complexes, subsequent infiltration of macrophages and T-cells will result in the release of a variety of proinflammatory cytokines which produce further tissue damage.

Disease resulting from circulating complexes

Serum sickness

Injection of relatively large doses of foreign serum (e.g. horse antidiphtheria) used to be employed for various therapeutic purposes. Horse serum containing specific antibodies is still used therapeutically (such as for the treatment of snake bite) but immune complex disease is nowadays more likely to be seen in patients treated with monoclonal antibodies originating in mice.

Some individuals receiving foreign serum will synthesize antibodies against the foreign protein, giving rise to a condition known as "serum sickness," which appears about 8 days after the injection. It results from the deposition of soluble antigen–antibody complexes, formed in antigen excess, in small vessels throughout the body. The clinical manifestations include a rise in temperature, swollen lymph nodes, a generalized urticarial rash and painful swollen joints associated with low serum complement levels and transient albuminuria. To be pathogenic, the complexes have to be of the right size—too big and they are snapped up smartly by the macrophages of the mononuclear phagocyte system; too small and they fail to induce an inflammatory reaction. Even when they are the right size, it seems that they will only localize in vessel walls if there is a change in vascular permeability. This may come about through release of 5-hydroxytryptamine (5HT; serotonin) from platelets reacting with larger complexes or through an IgE or complement-mediated degranulation of basophils and mast cells to produce histamine, leukotrienes and

PAF. The effect on the capillaries is to cause separation of the endothelial cells and exposure of the basement membrane to which the appropriately sized complexes attach and attract neutrophils that give rise to the vasculitis so typical of immune complex-mediated disease. The skin, joints, kidneys and heart are particularly affected. As antibody synthesis increases, antigen is cleared and the patient normally recovers.

Immune complex glomerulonephritis

Many cases of glomerulonephritis are associated with circulating complexes. These are retained in or on the endothelial side of the glomerular basement membrane (figure 14.12) where they build up as "lumpy" granules staining for antigen, Ig and complement. The inflammatory process damages the basement membrane, causing leakage of serum proteins and consequent proteinuria. Because serum albumin molecules are small they appear in the urine even with just minor degrees of glomerular damage. Figure 14.9b depicts DNA/anti-DNA/complement deposits in the kidney of a patient with systemic lupus erythematosus (SLE). Similar immune complex disease may follow various bacterial infections with certain strains of so-called

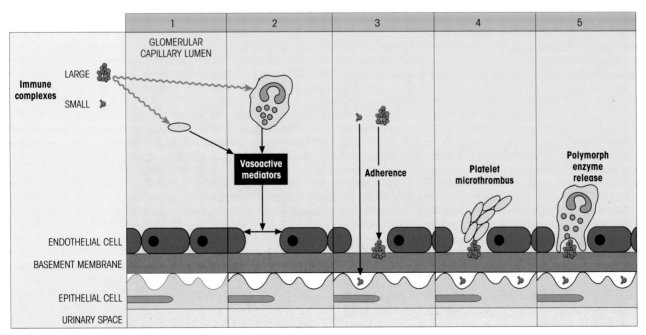

Figure 14.12 Deposition of immune complexes in the kidney glomerulus. (1) Complexes induce release of vasoactive mediators from basophils and platelets which cause (2) separation of endothelial cells, (3) attachment of larger complexes to exposed basement membrane, while smaller complexes pass through to epithelial side; (4) complexes induce platelet aggregation; (5) chemotactically attracted neutrophils release granule contents in "frustrated phagocytosis" to damage basement membrane and cause leakage of serum proteins. Complex deposition is favored in the glomerular capillary because it is a major filtration site and has a high hydrodynamic pressure. Deposition is greatly reduced in animals depleted of platelets or treated with vasoactive amine antagonists.

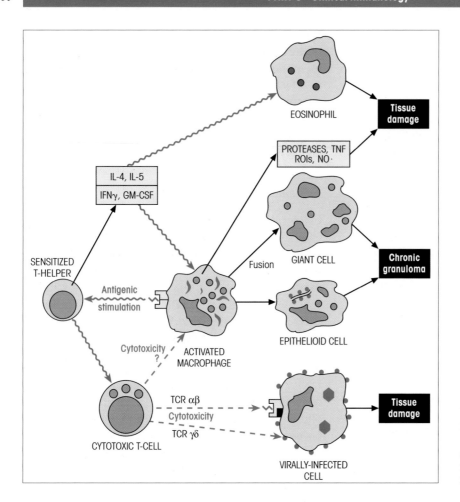

Figure 14.13 The cellular basis of type IV hypersensitivity. GM-CSF, granulocyte-macrophage colony-stimulating factor; IFNγ, interferon γ; IL, interleukin; NO·, nitric oxide; ROIs, reactive oxygen intermediates; TCR, T-cell receptor; TNF, tumor necrosis factor.

"nephritogenic" streptococci, in chronic parasitic infections such as quartan malaria, and in the course of chronic viral infections.

Deposition of immune complexes at other sites

The favored sites for immune complex deposition are the skin, joints and kidney. The vasculitic skin rashes which are a major feature of serum sickness are also characteristic of systemic and discoid lupus erythematosus (figure 14.5c), where biopsies of the lesions reveal amorphous deposits of Ig and C3 at the basement membrane of the dermal–epidermal junction. The necrotizing arteritis produced in rabbits by experimental serum sickness closely resembles the histology of polyarteritis nodosa, where immune complexes containing the hepatitis B surface (HBs) antigen of the hepatitis B virus are present in the lesions (figure 14.5d). In some instances drugs such as penicillin become antigenic after conjugation with body proteins and form complexes that mediate hypersensitivity reactions. The choroid plexus, being a major filtration site, is also favored for immune complex deposition, and this could account for the frequency of central nervous disorders in SLE. Similarly, in subacute sclerosing panencephalitis, deposits containing Ig and measles antigen may be found in neural tissue.

TYPE IV: CELL-MEDIATED (DELAYED-TYPE) HYPERSENSITIVITY

This form of hypersensitivity results from an exaggerated interaction between antigen and the *normal* cell-mediated immune mechanisms. T-cell responses may be autoreactive or directed against microorganisms, transplants or against fixed antigens such as chemicals found on the skin in cases of contact dermatitis. Following earlier priming, memory T-cells recognize the antigen together with class II major histocompatibility complex (MHC) molecules on an antigen-presenting cell, and are stimulated into blast cell transformation and proliferation. The stimulated T-cells release a number of proinflammatory cytokines which function as mediators of the ensuing hypersensitivity response, particularly by attracting and activating macrophages and cytotoxic T-cells (figure 14.13).

Perhaps the best-known example is the **Mantoux reaction** obtained by injection of tuberculin into the skin of an individual in whom previous infection with the mycobacterium has induced a state of cell-mediated immunity (CMI). The reaction is characterized by erythema and induration (figure 14.5e), which appears only after several hours (hence the term "delayed") and reaches a maximum at 24–48 h. Histologically, the earliest phase of the reaction is seen as a perivascular cuffing with mononuclear cells followed by a more extensive exudation of mono and polymorphonuclear cells. The latter soon migrate out of the lesion leaving behind a predominantly mononuclear cell infiltrate consisting of lymphocytes and cells of the monocyte–macrophage series. This contrasts with the essentially "polymorph" character of the Arthus reaction.

Tissue damage produced by type IV reactions

Infections

The development of a state of cell-mediated hypersensitivity against intracellular bacteria is probably responsible for the lesions associated with bacterial allergy such as the cavitation and caseation seen in human tuberculosis, and the granulomatous skin lesions found in patients with the borderline form of leprosy. Chronic infection with these organisms leads to continual release of cytokines from sensitized T-lymphocytes. The macrophage accumulation and activation that follows is responsible for tissue injury due to release of ROIs and NO. Macrophages may differentiate into epithelioid and giant cells, which with the proliferating lymphocytes and fibroblasts form the structure termed a **chronic granuloma**. This represents an attempt by the body to wall off a site of persistent infection (figure 14.13).

The skin rashes in smallpox and measles and the lesions of herpes simplex may be largely attributed to delayed-type allergic reactions with extensive damage to virally infected cells by cytotoxic T-cells. Cell-mediated hypersensitivity has also been demonstra-

ted in pathologic lesions of the fungal diseases candidiasis, dermatomycosis, coccidioidomycosis and histoplasmosis, and in the parasitic disease leishmaniasis.

Contact dermatitis and atopic eczema

Contact hypersensitivity in the skin is often produced by foreign materials capable of binding to body constituents, possibly surface molecules of the Langerhans' cell, to form new antigens. This may occur in people who become sensitized while working with chemicals such as picryl chloride and chromates, or who repeatedly come into contact with the substance urushiol from the poison ivy plant. p-Phenylene diamine in certain hair dyes, neomycin in topically applied ointments, and nickel salts formed from articles such as nickel jewellery clasps (figure 14.5f), can provoke similar reactions. Eczema is not a specific disease but is skin inflammation induced by atopic allergens, irritants or contact allergens which produce T-cell mediated skin damage. The epidermal route of inoculation tends to favor the development of a T-cell response through processing by class II-rich dendritic Langerhans' cells, which migrate to the lymph nodes and present antigen to T-lymphocytes. These then migrate back to the skin where they release interferon γ (IFNγ) that upregulates Fas on keratinocytes. These in turn become susceptible to apoptosis induced by activated T-cells which express FasL (Fas ligand). Thus, these delayed-type reactions are characterized by a mononuclear cell infiltrate peaking at 12–15 h, accompanied by edema of the epidermis with microvesicle formation. As would be expected, effective therapy for contact dermatitis and eczema should be directed at suppressing T-cell function. Topical corticosteroids are the most potent anti-inflammatory drugs but a number of trials have now shown the effectiveness of oral cyclosporin in treating these disorders.

Other examples

Delayed hypersensitivity contributes significantly to the prolonged reactions which result from insect bites. In numerous organ-specific autoimmune diseases, such as type I diabetes, cell-mediated hypersensitivity reactions undoubtedly provide the major engine for tissue destruction. The immunopathogenesis of these disorders will be discussed in Chapter 17.

REVISION

Excessive stimulation of the normal effector mechanisms of the immune system can lead to tissue damage, and we speak of hypersensitivity reactions, of which several types can be distinguished.

Type I: Anaphylactic hypersensitivity

• Anaphylaxis involves contraction of smooth muscle and dilatation of capillaries.

• This depends upon the reaction of antigen with specific immunoglobulin E (IgE) antibody bound through its Fc to the mast cell.

• Cross-linking and clustering of the IgE receptors leads to release from the granules of mediators including histamine, leukotrienes and platelet activating factor (PAF), plus eosinophil and neutrophil chemotactic factors and the cytokines interleukin-3 (IL-3), IL-4, IL-5 and granulocyte-macrophage colony-stimulating factor (GM-CSF).

• Interleukin-4 is involved in the isotype switch to IgE.

Atopic allergy

• Atopy stems from an excessive IgE response to extrinsic antigens (allergens) which leads to local anaphylactic reactions at sites of contact with allergen.

• Hay fever and extrinsic asthma represent the most common atopic allergic disorders resulting from exposure to inhaled allergens.

• Serious prolongation of the response to allergen is caused by T-cells of Th2-type, which recruit tissue-damaging eosinophils through release of IL-5. This Th2 bias is reinforced by nitric oxide (NO·) produced by cytokine-stimulated airway epithelial cells.

• Many food allergies involve type I hypersensitivity.

• Strong genetic factors include the propensity to make the IgE isotype.

• The offending antigen is identified by intradermal prick tests giving immediate wheal and erythema reactions, by provocation testing and also by an ELISA type test.

• Where possible, allergen avoidance is the best treatment.

• Symptomatic treatment involves the use of long-acting β_2-agonists and newly developed leukotriene antagonists. Chromones, such as sodium cromoglycate, block chloride channel activity thereby stabilizing mast cells and inhibiting bronchoconstriction. Theophylline, the single most prescribed drug for asthma, is a phosphodiesterase (PDE) inhibitor which raises intracellular calcium; this causes bronchodilatation and inhibition of IL-5 effects on eosinophils. Chronic asthma is dominated by activated Th2 cells and is treated with topical steroids, supplemented where necessary by long-acting β_2-agonists and theophylline.

• Courses of antigen injection may desensitize by formation of blocking IgG or IgA antibodies or through T-cell regulation.

Type II: Antibody-dependent cytotoxic hypersensitivity

• This involves the death of cells bearing antibody attached to a surface antigen.

• The cells may be taken up by phagocytic cells to which they adhere through their coating of IgG or C3b, or they may be lysed by the operation of the full complement system.

• Cells bearing IgG may also be killed by polymorphs and monocytes or by natural killer (NK) -cells through the extracellular mechanism of antibody-dependent cellular cytotoxicity (ADCC).

• Examples are: transfusion reactions, hemolytic disease of the newborn through rhesus (Rh) incompatibility, antibody-mediated graft destruction, autoimmune reactions directed against the formed elements of the blood and kidney glomerular basement membranes, and hypersensitivity resulting from the coating of erythrocytes or platelets by a drug.

Type III: Immune complex-mediated hypersensitivity

• This results from the effects of antigen–antibody complexes through (i) activation of complement and attraction of polymorphonuclear leukocytes which release tissue-damaging mediators on contact with the complex, and (ii) aggregation of platelets to cause microthrombi and vasoactive amine release.

• Where circulating antibody levels are high, the antigen is precipitated near the site of entry into the body. The reaction in the skin is characterized by polymorph infiltration, edema and erythema maximal at 3–8 h (Arthus reaction).

• Examples are: farmer's lung, pigeon-fancier's disease and pulmonary aspergillosis, where inhaled antigens provoke high antibody levels; reactions to an abrupt increase in antigen caused by microbial cell death during chemotherapy for leprosy or syphilis; and an element of the synovial lesion in rheumatoid arthritis.

• In relative *antigen excess*, soluble complexes are formed which are removed by binding to the CR1 (C3b) receptors on red cells. If this system is overloaded or if the classical complement components are deficient, the complexes circulate in the free state and are deposited under circumstances of increased vascular permeability at certain preferred sites—kidney glomerulus, joints, skin and choroid plexus.

• Examples are: serum sickness following injection of large quantities of foreign protein; glomerulonephritis associated with systemic lupus erythematosus (SLE) or infections with streptococci, malaria and other parasites; neurological disturbances in SLE and subacute sclerosing panencephalitis; polyarteritis nodosa linked to hepatitis B virus; and hemorrhagic shock in dengue viral infection.

Type IV: Cell-mediated or delayed-type hypersensitivity

• This is based upon the interaction of antigen with primed T-cells and represents tissue damage resulting from inappropriate cell-mediated immunity (CMI) reactions.

• A number of soluble cytokines including interferon γ (IFNγ) are released which activate macrophages and account for the events that occur in a typical delayed hypersensitivity response such as the Mantoux reaction to tuberculin; i.e. the delayed appearance of an indurated and erythematous reaction that reaches a maximum at 24–48 h and is characterized histologically by infiltration with mononuclear phagocytes and lymphocytes.

• Continuing provocation of delayed hypersensitivity by persisting antigen leads to formation of chronic granulomas.

• Th2-type cells producing IL-4 and IL-5 can also produce tissue damage through their ability to recruit eosinophils.

• CD8 T-cells are activated by class I major histocompatibility antigens to become directly cytotoxic to target cells bearing the appropriate antigen.

• Examples are: tissue damage occurring in bacterial (tuberculosis, leprosy), viral (smallpox, measles, herpes), fungal (candidiasis, histoplasmosis) and parasitic (leishmaniasis, schistosomiasis) infections; contact dermatitis from exposure to chromates and poison ivy; insect bites; and psoriasis.

> See the accompanying website (**www.roitt.com**) for multiple choice questions

FURTHER READING

Erb, K.J. (1999) Atopic disorders: A default pathway in the absence of infection? *Immunology Today*, **20**, 317–22.

Geha, R.S. (2003) Section on allergy and hypersensitivity. *Current Opinion in Immunology*, **15**, 603–46.

Haeney, M., Chapel, H., Snowden, N. & Misbah, S. (1999) *Essentials of Clinical Immunology*, 4th edn. Blackwell Science, Oxford. [A very broad account of the diseases involving the immune system. Good illustration by case histories and the laboratory tests available: also MCQs.]

Trautmann, A., Akdis, M., Brocker, E.B. *et al.* (2001) New insights into the role of T cells in atopic dermatitis and allergic contact dermatitis. *Trends in Immunology*, **22**, 530–2.

Transplantation

GRAFT REJECTION IS IMMUNOLOGIC

The replacement of diseased organs by a transplant of healthy tissue has long been an objective in medicine but has been frustrated to no mean degree by the uncooperative attempts by the body to reject grafts from other individuals. Before discussing the nature and implications of this rejection phenomenon, it would be helpful to define the terms used for transplants between individuals and species:

Autograft—the tissue is grafted back onto the original donor.

Isograft—graft between syngeneic individuals (i.e. of identical genetic constitution) such as identical twins or mice of the same pure line strain.

Allograft—graft between allogeneic individuals (i.e. members of the same species but different genetic constitution), e.g. human to human and one mouse strain to another.

Xenograft—graft between xenogeneic individuals (i.e. of different species), e.g. pig to human.

It is with the allograft reaction that we are most concerned. The most common allografting procedure is blood transfusion where the unfortunate consequences of mismatching are well known. Considerable attention has been paid to the rejection of solid grafts such as skin, and the sequence of events is worth describing. After suturing the allogeneic skin in place, the graft becomes vascularized within a few days, but between the third and ninth day the circulation gradually diminishes and there is increasing infiltration of the graft bed with lymphocytes and monocytes but very few plasma cells. Necrosis begins to be visible macroscopically and within a day or so the graft is sloughed completely (figure M15.1.1).

First and second set rejection

As would be expected in an immunological reaction, second contact with antigen would produce a more explosive event than the first. Indeed the rejection of a second graft from the same donor is much accelerated (Milestone 15.1). In this second set rejection the initial vascularization is poor and may not occur at all. There is rapid invasion by polymorphonuclear leukocytes and lymphoid cells, including plasma cells, and thrombosis and acute cell destruction can be seen by 3–4 days. Second set rejection is not the fate of all subsequent allografts but only of those derived from the original donor or a related strain (figure M15.1.2). Grafts from new donors are rejected as first set reactions. Rejection therefore has all the hallmarks of an immunological response in that it shows both memory and specificity.

CONSEQUENCES OF MAJOR HISTOCOMPATIBILITY COMPLEX (MHC) INCOMPATIBILITY

Class II MHC differences produce a mixed lymphocyte reaction (MLR)

When lymphocytes from individuals of different class II haplotype are cultured together *in vitro*, blast cell transformation and mitosis occurs, the T-cells of each population of lymphocytes reacting against MHC class II complexes on the surface of the other population (see "allograft recognition" below). This constitutes the MLR. The responding cells belong predominantly to a population of CD4$^+$ T-lymphocytes and are stimulated by the class II molecules present mostly on B-cells, macrophages and, especially, dendritic antigen-presenting cells. For many years the MLR was employed in transplantation laboratories to determine the degree of compatibility between individuals. With the introduction of very accurate molecular human leukocyte antigen (HLA) testing the MLR is no longer routinely performed.

The graft-vs-host (g.v.h.) reaction

When competent T-cells are transferred from an HLA-incompatible donor to an immunosuppressed recipient who is incapable of rejecting them, the grafted cells survive and have time to recognize the host antigens and react immunologically against them. Instead of the normal transplantation reaction of host against

Milestone 15.1—The Immunologic Basis of Graft Rejection

The field of transplantation owes a tremendous debt to Sir Peter Medawar, the outstanding scientist who kick-started and inspired its development. Even at the turn of the century it was an accepted paradigm that grafts between unrelated members of a species would be unceremoniously rejected after a brief initial period of acceptance (figure M15.1.1). That there was an underlying genetic basis for rejection became apparent from Padgett's observations in Kansas City in 1932 that skin allografts between family members tended to survive for longer than those between unrelated individuals, and J.B. Brown's critical demonstration in St Louis in 1937 that monozygotic (i.e. genetically identical) twins accepted skin grafts from each other. However, it was not until Medawar's research in the early part of the Second World War, motivated by the need to treat aircrew with appalling burns, that rejection was laid at immunology's door. He showed that a second graft from a given donor was rejected more rapidly and more vigorously than the first, and further that an unrelated graft was rejected with the kinetics of a first-set reaction (figure M15.1.2). This **second-set rejection** is characterized by **memory** and **specificity** and thereby bears the hallmarks of an immunologic response. This of course was later confirmed by transferring the ability to express a second set reaction with lymphocytes.

The message was clear: to achieve successful transplantation of tissues and organs in the human, it would be necessary to overcome this immunogenetic barrier. Limited success was obtained by Murray, at the Peter Bent Brigham

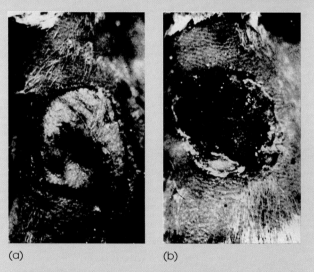

(a)   (b)

Figure M15.1.1 Rejection of CBA skin graft by strain A mouse. (a) Ten days after transplantation; discolored areas caused by destruction of epithelium and drying of the exposed dermis. (b) Thirteen days after transplantation; the scabby surface indicates total destruction of the graft. (Photographs courtesy of Professor L. Brent.)

Hospital in Boston, and Hamburger in Paris, who grafted kidneys between dizygotic twins using sublethal X-irradiation. The key breakthrough came when Schwartz and Damashek's report on the immunosuppressive effects of the antimitotic drug 6-mercaptopurine was applied independently by Calne and Zukowski in 1960 to the prolongation of renal allografts in dogs. This was followed very

(continued)

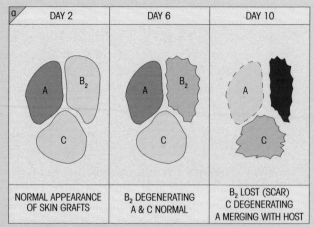
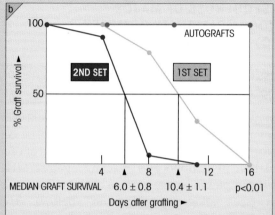

Figure M15.1.2 Memory and specificity in skin allograft rejection in rabbits. (a) Autografts and allografts from two unrelated donors, B and C, are applied to the thoracic wall skin of rabbit A which has already rejected a first graft from B (B₁). While the autograft A remains intact, graft C seen for the first time undergoes first set rejection, whereas a *second* graft from B (B₂) is sloughed off very rapidly. (b) Median survival times of first and second set skin allografts showing faster second set rejection. (From P.B. Medawar (1944) *Journal of Anatomy*, **78**, 176.)

rapidly by Murray's successful grafting in 1962 of an unrelated cadaveric kidney under the immunosuppressive umbrella of azathioprine, the more effective derivative of 6-mercaptopurine devised by Hutchings and Elion.

This story is studded with Nobel Prize winners. Readers interested in the historical aspects will gain further insight into the development of this field and the minds of the scientists who gave medicine this wonderful prize in P.I. Terasaki's (ed.) (1991) *History of Transplantation; Thirty-five Recollections*. UCLA Tissue Typing Laboratory, Los Angeles, CA.

graft, we have the reverse, the so-called graft-vs-host (g.v.h.) reaction. In the human, fever, anemia, weight loss, rash, diarrhea and splenomegaly are observed, with cytokines, especially tumor necrosis factor (TNF), being thought to be the major mediators of pathology. The greater the transplantation antigen difference, the more severe that reaction. Graft-vs-host may therefore be observed in immunologically anergic subjects receiving bone marrow grafts, for example for combined immunodeficiency (see p. 142) or for the reestablishment of bone marrow in subjects whose own marrow has been destroyed by massive doses of chemotherapy used to treat malignant disease (figure 15.1).

MECHANISMS OF GRAFT REJECTION

Allograft recognition

Remember, we defined the MHC by its ability to provoke the most powerful rejection of grafts between members of the same species. It transpires that **normal individuals have a very high frequency of alloreac-**

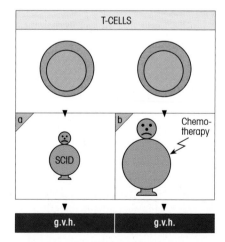

Figure 15.1 Graft-vs-host (g.v.h.) reaction. When competent T-cells are inoculated into a host incapable of reacting against them, the grafted cells are free to react against the antigens on the host's cells which they recognize as foreign. The ensuing reaction may be fatal. Two of many possible situations are illustrated. (a) A patient with severe combined immunodeficiency (SCID) receives a graft from an HLA incompatible donor. (b) A leukemia patient post-chemotherapy receives a bone marrow transplant from an allogeneic donor.

tive cells (i.e. cells that react with allografts), which presumably accounts for the intensity of MHC-mismatched rejection. Whereas merely a fraction of 1% of the normal T-cell population is specific for a given single peptide, upwards of 10% of the T-cells react with alloantigens. The reason for this is that very large numbers of T-cells, each specific for a foreign peptide presented in the groove of self MHC molecules, may cross-react with an allogeneic MHC molecule containing host peptides in its groove. Such a complex mimics self MHC with foreign peptide in its groove and, because the T-cell repertoire is recognizing large numbers of previously unseen foreign antigens, large numbers of recipient T-cells are activated. This is the so-called "direct pathway." In addition, T-cells may recognize some allogeneic peptides presented on self MHC molecules, a process called the "indirect pathway." T-cells recognizing peptides derived from graft proteins are present in low frequency comparable to that observed with any foreign antigen. Nonetheless, a graft, which has been in place for an extended period, will have the time to expand this small population significantly so that later rejection will depend progressively on this pathway.

Lymphocytes mediate acute rejection

A primary role of lymphoid cells in first set rejection would be consistent with the histology of the early reaction showing infiltration by mononuclear cells especially CD8[+] T-cells, with very few polymorphs or plasma cells (figure 15.2). Activated CD8[+] cytotoxic cells proliferate and form specific alloreactive clones which recognize class I alloantigens on the graft. They then mount a cytotoxic reaction against graft parenchymal and endothelial cells by releasing perforin, granzyme and toxic cytokines such as TNFα. CD4[+] cells also play a major role in graft rejection by the secretion of the cytokines which mediate delayed hypersensitivity reactions. These include interferon γ (IFNγ), which activates and recruits macrophages and upregulates MHC antigen expression on the graft, interleukin-2 (IL-2), which promotes T-cell proliferation and CD8[+] cell activation and lymphotoxin, which is directly cytotoxic to allogeneic cells.

There are different forms of graft rejection

Hyperacute rejection is the most dramatic form of graft rejection, occurring within minutes of transplantation. It is due to the presence in the recipient of preformed antibodies directed against donor HLA or ABO antigens. Such antibodies will attach to the

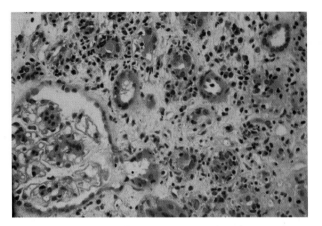

Figure 15.2 Acute rejection of human renal allograft showing dense cellular infiltration of interstitium by mononuclear cells. (Photograph courtesy of Drs M. Thompson and A. Dorling.)

endothelial cells of the donor organ, fix complement and cause endothelial damage. This will initiate blood clotting and produce aggregation of platelets which contributes to the vascular occlusion, seen in renal transplantation as glomerular microthrombi. Fortunately, by ABO matching and by performing cross-matches in which patients are screened for pre-existing antibodies, hyperacute rejection is no longer a major problem in most transplant centers. It is worth pointing out that, because humans have a variety of natural antibodies against animal tissue, hyperacute rejection is the major hurdle to xenogeneic transplants.

Acute early rejection, which occurs up to 10 days after transplantation, is characterized by a dense cellular infiltration (figure 15.2) and rupture of peritubular capillaries. This is a cell-mediated hypersensitivity reaction mainly involving an attack by CD8[+] cells on graft cells whose MHC antigen expression has been upregulated by IFNγ.

Acute late rejection, which occurs from 11 days onwards in patients suppressed with prednisone and azathioprine, is probably caused by the binding of immunoglobulin (presumably antibody) and complement to the arterioles and glomerular capillaries, where they can be visualized by immunofluorescent techniques. These immunoglobulin deposits on the vessel walls induce platelet aggregation in the glomerular capillaries leading to acute renal shutdown (figure 15.3). The possibility of damage to antibody-coated cells through antibody-dependent cell-mediated cytotoxicity must also be considered.

Chronic or late rejection may occur months or years after the initial transplant depending on the success of immunosuppressive therapy. The main pathologic

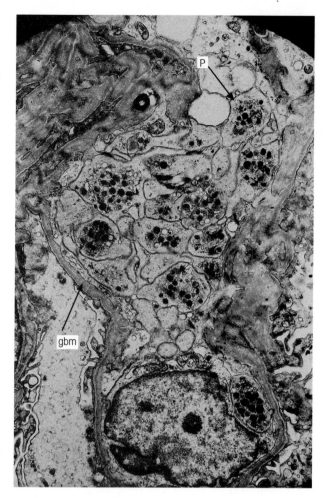

Figure 15.3 Acute late rejection of human renal allograft showing platelet (P) aggregation in a glomerular capillary (gbm) induced by deposition of antibody on the vessel wall (electron micrograph). (Photograph courtesy of Professor K. Porter.)

feature is vascular injury and occlusion of the vessels. This is due to proliferation of smooth muscle cells, and accumulation of T-cells and macrophages in the intima of the vessel wall. The cause of this graft arteriosclerosis is predominantly activation of macrophages in the vessel wall with the release of proinflammatory cytokines and various smooth muscle growth factors. There is also evidence of a humoral component in that deposits of antibody directed against donor tissue, or antigen–antibody complexes have been detected in vascular endothelial cells and may give rise to occlusion of the vessels. It has been noticed that chronic rejection is more prominent in patients who initially showed even mild acute rejection and also in those who have chronic viral infections, especially with cytomegalovirus.

The complexity of the interaction of cellular and humoral factors in graft rejection is presented in figure 15.4.

THE PREVENTION OF GRAFT REJECTION

Matching tissue types on graft donor and recipient

Improvements in operative techniques and the use of drugs have greatly diminished the effects of mismatching HLA specificities on solid graft survival. Nevertheless for the best graft survival a high degree of matching, especially at the MHC class II loci, is indicated (figure 15.5). The consensus is that matching at the DR loci is of greater benefit than the B loci, which in turn are of more relevance to graft survival than the A loci. Bone marrow grafts, however, require a high degree of compatibility, which is now afforded by the greater accuracy of the modern DNA typing methods.

Because of the many thousands of different HLA phenotypes (figure 15.5), it is usual to work with a large pool of potential recipients so that when graft material becomes available the best possible match can be made. The position will be improved when the pool of available organs can be increased through the development of long-term tissue storage banks, but techniques are not good enough for this at present. Bone marrow cells fortunately can be kept viable even after freezing and thawing. With a paired organ such as the kidney, living donors may be used and siblings provide the best chance of a good match (figure 15.5).

Agents producing general immunosuppression

The use of agents that nonspecifically interfere with the induction or expression of the immune response (figure 15.6) can control graft rejection. Because these agents act on various parts of the cellular immune response, patients on immunosuppressive therapy tend to be susceptible to infections and more prone to the development of lymphoreticular cancers, particularly those with a known viral etiology.

Immunosuppressive drugs

Many of the immunosuppressive drugs now employed were first used in cancer chemotherapy because of their toxicity to dividing cells. Aside from the complications of blanket immunosuppression mentioned above, these antimitotic drugs are especially toxic for cells of the bone marrow and small intestine and must therefore be used with great care.

For many years the major drugs used for immuno-

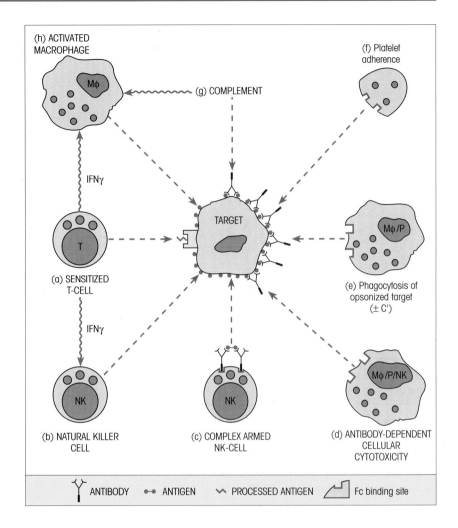

Figure 15.4 Mechanisms of target cell destruction. (a) Direct killing by cytotoxic T-cells (Tc) and indirect tissue damage through release of cytokines from delayed-type hypersensitivity T-cells. (b) Killing by natural killer (NK) cells enhanced by interferon (IFN). (c) Specific killing by immune complex-armed NK cell. (d) Attack by antibody-dependent cellular cytotoxicity. (e) Phagocytosis of target coated with antibody. (f) Sticking of platelets to antibody bound to the surface of graft vascular endothelium leading to formation of microthrombi. (g) Complement-mediated cytotoxicity. (h) Activated macrophages. Mφ, macrophage; P, polymorph.

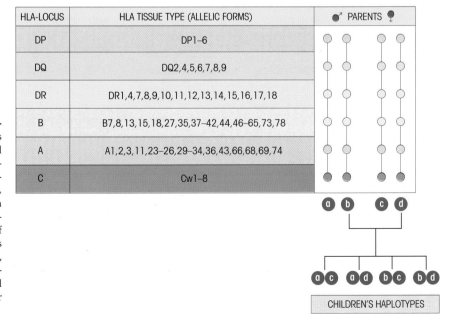

Figure 15.5 Polymorphic HLA specificities and their inheritance. The complex lies on chromosome 6. Since there are several possible alleles at each locus, the probability of a random pair of subjects from the general population having identical HLA specificities is very low. However, there is a 1 : 4 chance that two siblings will be identical in this respect because each group of specificities on a single chromosome forms a haplotype which will be inherited *en bloc*, giving four possible combinations of paternal and maternal chromosomes. Parent and offspring can only be identical if the mother and father have one haplotype in common.

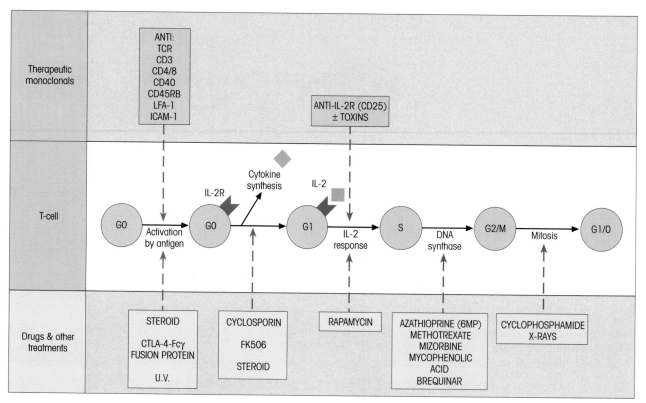

Figure 15.6 Immunosuppressive agents used to control graft rejection. These drugs act at many different points in the immune response. Simultaneous treatment with agents acting at sequential stages in development of the rejection response would be expected to synergize strongly and this is clearly seen with cyclosporin and rapamycin. ICAM-1, intercellular adhesion molecule-1; IL, interleukin; LFA-1, lymphocyte function-associated antigen-1; TCR, T-cell receptor.

suppression were **azathioprine** (Imuran), which inhibits the synthesis of nucleic acid, **cyclophosphamide**, which acts on DNA preventing correct duplication during cell division, and corticosteroids such as prednisolone. The latter intervenes at many points in the immune response, affecting lymphocyte recirculation and the generation of cytotoxic effector cells. In addition, their outstanding anti-inflammatory potency rests on features such as inhibition of neutrophil adherence to vascular endothelium and suppression of monocyte/macrophage functions including release of proinflammatory cytokines. Corticosteroids form complexes with intracellular receptors, which then bind to regulatory genes and block transcription of TNF, IFNγ, IL-1, IL-2, IL-3 and IL-6, i.e. they block expression of cytokines.

Several new agents (figure 15.6) are having a dramatic effect in human transplantation. They include mycophenolic acid, which has a similar but more effective mode of action to azathioprine. The fungal metabolites **cyclosporin** and **FK506** (Tacrolimus) complex with proteins termed immunophilins, and this complex interferes with calcineurin which is crucial for the transcription of IL-2 in activated T-cells. In addition they also block the synthesis of other cytokines and thereby interfere with activated CD4+ helper function. **Rapamycin** (Sirolimus) is a macrolide like FK506, but in contrast acts to block signals induced by combination of cytokines with their receptors such as IL-2R, IL-4R, IL-10R and IL-15R.

These drugs are used not only for prophylaxis and treatment of transplant rejection, but also in a wide range of disorders due to T-cell-mediated hypersensitivity. Indeed, the benefits of cyclosporin in diseases such as idiopathic nephrotic syndrome, type 1 insulin-dependent diabetes, Behçet's syndrome, active Crohn's disease, aplastic anemia, severe corticosteroid-dependent asthma and psoriasis have confirmed the pathogenic role of the cellular immune system.

Targeting lymphoid populations

Anti-CD3 monoclonal antibodies (OKT-3) are in widespread use as anti-T-cell reagents to successfully reverse acute graft rejection. Their benefits were initially constrained by their immunogenicity but this problem has been circumvented by "humanizing" the antibody. The antibody suppresses T-cell-mediated rejection by binding to a subunit of the CD3 molecule, and interfering with CD3–T-cell receptor complex-mediated activation of T-cells. Unfortunately a major side effect is a cytokine release syndrome, which manifests clinically as a variable constellation of symptoms including fever, chills, tremor, nausea and vomiting, diarrhea, rash, and especially pulmonary edema.

The IL-2 receptor, expressed by activated but not resting T-cells, represents another potential target for blocking the immune response. A humanized version of a murine monoclonal anti-IL-2R antibody (Daclizumab or Basiliximab) has, in association with other immunosuppressive drugs, been shown to reduce the frequency of acute kidney rejection. Attention is now turning to the use of anti-adhesion molecule monoclonal antibodies such as an anti-LFA (lymphocyte function-associated antigen), as immunosuppressant therapy for transplanted patients.

IS XENOGRAFTING A PRACTICAL PROPOSITION?

Because the supply of donor human organs for transplantation lags seriously behind the demand, a widespread interest in the feasibility of using animal organs has emerged. Of even greater practical use is the possible transplantation of animal cells and tissues to treat disease. Transplants of animal pancreatic islet cells could cure diabetes, and implants of neuronal cells would be useful in Parkinson's disease and other brain disorders. Pigs are more favored than primates as donors, both on grounds of ethical acceptability and the hazards of zoonoses, although these animals have been shown to harbor endogenous retroviruses that can infect human cells *in vitro*. The first hurdle to be overcome is **hyperacute rejection** due to the presence in all humans of xenoreactive natural antibodies. These activate complement in the absence of regulators of the human complement system such as CD46, CD55 and CD59 (cf. p. 137), which precipitates the hyperacute rejection phenomenon.

The next crisis is acute vascular rejection occurring within 6 days as antibodies are formed to the xenoantigens and attack donor endothelial cells. This results in damage to the vessel walls and intravascular thrombosis.

Even as the immunologic problems are being overcome, the question of whether animal viruses might infect humans and cause man-made pandemics (xenozoonosis), still needs to be considered.

CLINICAL EXPERIENCE IN GRAFTING

Privileged sites

The vast majority of corneal grafts survive without the need for immunosuppression. This is due to unique qualities of the cornea that interfere with the induction and expression of graft rejection. These include the absence of donor-derived antigen-presenting cells in the corneal graft which also has the ability to deflect the systemic immune response from a Th1 to a Th2 pathway. It has also been shown that the corneal allograft expresses FasL (Fas ligand) that attaches to Fas resulting in apoptosis of attacking T-cells.

Kidney grafts

Renal transplantation is now the treatment of choice for end-stage renal failure. With improvement in patient management there is a high rate of survival, and outcomes for transplant recipients continue to improve with a 5-year patient survival of around 80% when the kidney is derived from a deceased donor (figure 15.7) and 90% when it is obtained from a living donor. Matching at the HLA-DR locus has a strong effect on graft survival, but in the long term (5 years or more) the desirability of reasonable HLA-B, and to a lesser extent HLA-A, matching also becomes apparent.

When transplantation is performed because of immune complex-induced glomerulonephritis, the immunosuppressive treatment used may help to prevent

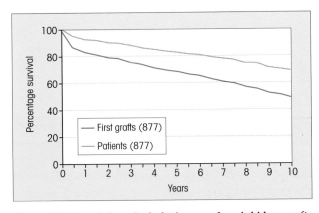

Figure 15.7 Actuarial survival of primary cadaveric kidney grafts in 877 patients treated at the Oxford Transplant Centre with triple therapy of cyclosporin, azathioprine and prednisolone.

a similar lesion developing in the grafted kidney. Patients with glomerular basement membrane antibodies (e.g. Goodpasture's syndrome) are likely to destroy their renal transplants unless first treated with plasmapheresis and immunosuppressive drugs.

The number of requests for **simultaneous kidney–pancreas transplants** continues to rise as patients with type 1 diabetes have noted the benefits of this type of therapy. Regrettably there are inadequate tissues for all the patients requiring them.

Thoracic organ transplantation

The overall 1-year survival figure for heart transplants has moved up to over the 70% mark. More specific modalities of immunosuppression continue to decrease the impact of acute and chronic rejection and immunosuppression related side effects. Full HLA matching is of course not practical, but a single mismatch at the DR locus gave 90% survival at 3 years compared with a figure of 65% for two DR mismatches. Aside from the rejection problem, it is likely that the number of patients who would benefit from cardiac replacement is much greater than the number dying with adequately healthy hearts. More attention will have to be given to the possibility of xenogeneic grafts and mechanical substitutes.

The number of lung transplants also continues to increase. The current indications for single lung transplantation include restrictive lung disease, emphysema, pulmonary hypertension and other nonseptic, end-stage pulmonary disease. Indications for bilateral sequential lung transplantation include cystic fibrosis and patients in whom there is chronic infection with end-stage pulmonary failure including patients with bronchiectasis. There are still several problems, however, that need to be worked out before lung transplantation will offer consistent and long-term relief of symptoms and increased longevity for the vast majority of patients. The problem of chronic rejection, as manifested by obliterative bronchiolitis is a major concern. There is now some progress in the use of single lobes from living related donors for certain groups of patients, most notably, patients with cystic fibrosis. There is also considerable interest in investigating the establishment of chimerism with consequent induction of tolerance where recipients of cadaveric tissues are also given donor bone marrow at the time of their transplant. These individuals seem to develop some degree of chimerism and show a trend toward donor specific nonreactivity and increasing survival.

Liver and intestine transplantation

Survival rates for orthotopic liver grafts continue to improve and this is now the second most common transplant after renal transplantation. An increasing number of these have been grafts of a portion of the liver from living donors. To improve the prognosis of patients with inoperable primary hepatic or bile duct malignancies, transplantation of organ clusters with liver as the central organ may be employed. These include liver and pancreas, or liver, pancreas, stomach and small bowel or even colon. As with other transplants combined immunosuppressive therapy attacking several facets of the rejection process are most effective. Over 700 intestine transplants have been performed with an overall 5-year patient survival of 50%.

Hematopoietic stem cell transplantation

Patients with certain immunodeficiency disorders and aplastic anemia are obvious candidates for treatment with bone marrow stem cells, as are leukemia patients treated radically with marrow ablative chemoradiotherapy to eradicate the neoplastic cells. The source of these stem cells may be bone marrow, umbilical cord blood or peripheral blood following the administration of granulocyte colony-stimulating factor (G-CSF) to increase the number of stem cells. The major problems still restricting the use of this form of therapy are infectious complications, veno-occlusive disease of the liver and g.v.h. disease. To reduce the use of the highly toxic myeloablative regimens thought to be essential for eradication of malignant cells in the marrow, nonmyeloablative conditioning regimens are now being used. The success of this approach depends on a graft-vs-malignancy effect provided by the allogeneic transplant. This allows for safer conditioning of the patient, fewer side effects with equivalent results and fewer leukemic relapses.

Graft-vs-host disease is a major problem in bone marrow grafting

Graft-vs-host disease resulting from recognition of recipient antigens by allogeneic T-cells in the bone marrow inoculum represents a serious, sometimes fatal complication. The incidence of g.v.h. disease is reduced if T-cells in the grafted marrow are first purged with a cytotoxic cocktail of anti-T-cell monoclonals. Two forms of the disease are recognized, an acute form which occurs in the first 2–3 months after transplantation and a chronic form which usually develops after 3 months. The acute form presents with severe dermatitis, hepatitis and enteritis due to production of inflammatory cytokines by activated donor T-cells recognising recipient HLA. Some of these patients can be successfully treated with anti-IL-2 receptor monoclonal antibody and anti-TNF monoclonal antibody. The chronic g.v.h. reaction has a clinical picture similar to that seen in the autoimmune disease scleroderma. There is increased collagen deposition in the skin resulting from stimulation of fibroblast collagen production by cytokines such as IL-1, IL-4 and TNFα.

Successful results with bone marrow transfers require highly compatible donors if g.v.h. reactions are to be avoided. Siblings offer the best chance of finding a matched donor (figure 15.5). Several methods have been used to deplete donor T-cells from the graft and, although this reduces the incidence of g.v.h., there is a higher incidence of leukemia relapse secondary to the decrease in the graft-vs-leukemia effect.

Other organs

It is to be expected that improvement in techniques of control of the rejection process will encourage transplantation in several other areas such as in diabetes, where the number of transplants recorded is rising rapidly with a success rate of around 40%. The 5-year survival rate of 47% for lung transplants is still less than satisfactory and one looks forward to the successful transplantation of skin for lethal burns.

Reports are coming in of experimental forays into the grafting of **neural tissues**. Mutant mice with degenerate cerebellar Purkinje cells which mimic the human condition, cerebellar ataxia, can be restored by engraftment of donor cerebellar cells at the appropriate sites. Clinical trials with transplantation of human embryonic dopamine neurons to reverse the neurological deficit in Parkinson's disease have been severely hampered by the excessive death of the grafted cells.

ASSOCIATION OF HLA TYPE WITH DISEASE

Association with immunologic diseases

There are numerous examples of diseases that are associated with a specific HLA genotype (table 15.1). A significant association between a disease and a given *HLA* specificity does not imply that we have identified the disease susceptibility gene, because there may be even better correlation with another *HLA* gene in linkage disequilibrium with the first. Linkage disequilibrium describes a state where closely linked genes on a chro-

Table 15.1 Association of HLA with disease. (Data mainly from L.P. Ryder, E. Andersen & A. Svejgaard (1979) *Tissue Antigens* (Suppl.) and E. Thorsby (1995) *The Immunologist*, 3, 51.)

DISEASE	HLA ALLELE	RELATIVE RISK
a Class II associated		
Hashimoto's disease	DR11	3.2
Primary myxedema	DR17	5.7
Graves' disease	DR17	3.7
Insulin-dependent diabetes	DQ8	14
	DQ2/8	20
	DQ6	0.2
Addison's disease (adrenal)	DR17	6.3
Goodpasture's syndrome	DR2	13.1
Rheumatoid arthritis	DR4	5.8
Juvenile rheumatoid arthritis	DR8	8.1
Sjögren's syndrome	DR17	9.7
Chronic active hepatitis (autoimmune)	DR17	13.9
Multiple sclerosis	DR2,DQ6	12
Narcolepsy	DQ6	38
Dermatitis herpetiformis	DR17	56.4
Celiac disease	DQ2	3.6
Tuberculoid leprosy	DR2	8.1
b Class I, HLA-B27 associated		
Ankylosing spondylitis	B27	87.4
Reiter's disease	B27	37.0
Post-salmonella arthritis	B27	29.7
Post-shigella arthritis	B27	20.7
Post-yersinia arthritis	B27	17.6
Post-gonococcal arthritis	B27	14.0
Uveitis	B27	14.6
Amyloidosis in rheumatoid arthritis	B27	8.2
c Other class I associations		
Subacute thyroiditis	B35	13.7
Psoriasis vulgaris	Cw6	13.3
Idiopathic hemochromatosis	A3	8.2
Myasthenia gravis	B8	4.4

mosome tend to remain associated rather than being genetically randomized throughout the population.

Many, but not all, of the HLA-linked diseases are autoimmune in nature and the reasons for this are not clear. Most of these diseases are associated with specific class II MHC genes suggesting that they control the type of reaction which will result from the presentation of autoantigens or other causative antigens to T-cells. Alternatively the MHC complex with particular self peptides could positively or negatively select either reactive or suppressive T-cells. Another possibility is that HLA antigens might affect the susceptibility of a cell to viral attachment or infection, thereby influencing the development of autoimmunity to associated surface components.

Insulin-dependent diabetes mellitus is associated with *DQ8* and *DQ2* but the strongest susceptibility is seen in the ***DQ2/8* heterozygote**. The fact that two genes are necessary to determine the strongest susceptibility and the universality of this finding in all populations studied implies that the DQ molecules themselves, not other molecules in linkage disequilibrium, are primarily involved in disease susceptibility. Possession of some subtypes of *DQ6* gives a dominantly protective effect (table 15.1).

DR4 and, to a lesser extent, *DR1* are risk factors for **rheumatoid arthritis** in white Caucasians. Analysis of *DR4* subgroups, and of other ethnic populations where the influence of *DR4* is minimal, has identified a particular linear sequence from residues 67–74 as the disease susceptibility element, and the variations observed are based on sharing of this sequence with other *HLA-DR* specificities. This stretch of amino acids is highly polymorphic and forms particular pockets in the peptide-binding cleft. As in diabetes, the *DR2* allele is under-represented and *DR2*-positive patients have less severe disease, implying that a *DR2*-linked gene might be protective in some way.

There is a very strong association of *HLA-B27* with **ankylosing spondylitis**. Approximately 95% of patients are of B27 phenotype as compared with around 5% in controls. The incidence of *B27* is also markedly raised in other conditions accompanied by sacroiliitis, for example Reiter's disease, acute anterior uveitis, psoriasis and other forms of infective sacroiliitis such as *Yersinia*, gonococcal and *Salmonella* arthritis. One suggestion is that a bacterial peptide may cross-react with a *B27*-derived sequence and provoke an autoreactive T-cell response.

Deficiencies in C4 and C2, which are MHC class III molecules, clearly predispose to the development of immune complex disease. This could be due to abnormal clearance of immune complexes in the absence of a classical complement pathway.

REPRODUCTIVE IMMUNOLOGY

The fetus is a potential allograft

One of the mysteries of immunology is why a fetus that carries paternal MHC is not normally rejected by the mother. In the human hemochorial placenta, maternal blood with immunocompetent lymphocytes does circulate in contact with the fetal trophoblast and maternal responses to fetal antigens do result in the production of antibodies to the father's MHC. These antibodies do not produce damage to the maternal trophoblast because of the presence there of inhibitors of complement proteins. Some of the many speculations to explain how the fetus avoids allograft rejection are summarized in figure 15.8.

A well-documented factor is the lack of both conventional class I and class II MHC antigens on the placen-

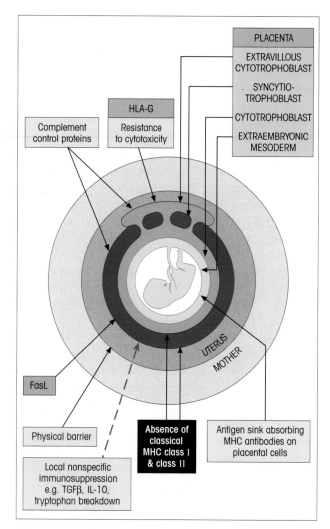

Figure 15.8 Mechanisms postulated to account for the survival of the fetus as an allograft in the mother. FasL, Fas ligand; IL, interleukin; MHC, major histocompatibility complex; TGFβ, transforming growth factor-β.

tal villous trophoblast. This makes the trophoblast resistant to attack by maternal T-cells. There is also the unique expression of the nonclassical HLA-G protein on the extravillous cytotrophoblast. This is a minimally polymorphic class I MHC protein that protects the trophoblast from killing by uterine natural killer (NK) cells, by binding to inhibitory NK cell receptors.

There is now evidence that the placenta itself may produce inhibitory cytokines such as IL-10, transforming growth factor-β (TGFβ) and IL-4 which promote Th2 responses and inhibit Th1 responses. Other factors that may protect the fetus are the presence of FasL at the trophoblast maternal–fetal interface, and the suppression of T-cell activity through tryptophan degradation brought about by the catabolic enzyme indoleamine 2,3-dioxygenase present in trophoblast cells and macrophages.

REVISION

Graft rejection is an immunologic reaction

• It shows specificity, the second set response is brisk, it is mediated by lymphocytes, and antibodies specific for the graft are formed.

Consequences of major histocompatibility complex (MHC) incompatibility

• Class II MHC molecules provoke a mixed lymphocyte reaction (MLR) of proliferation and blast transformation when genetically dissimilar lymphocytes interact.

• Class II differences are largely responsible for the reaction of tolerated grafted lymphocytes against host antigen (graft-vs-host (g.v.h.) reaction).

Mechanisms of graft rejection

• CD8 lymphocytes play a major role in the acute early rejection of first set responses.

• The strength of allograft rejection is due to the surprisingly large number of allospecific precursor cells. These derive mainly from the variety of T-cells which recognize allo-MHC plus self peptides plus a small number which directly recognize the allo-MHC molecule itself; later rejection increasingly involves allogeneic peptides presented by self MHC.

Different forms of graft rejection exist

• Preformed antibodies cause hyperacute rejection within minutes.

• Acute graft rejection is mediated mainly by cytotoxic T-cells.

• Chronic or late rejection is due to release of proinflammatory cytokines by macrophages in the vessel wall. This arteriosclerosis may also be due to antibody directed against the donor or to immune complex deposition.

Prevention of graft rejection

• Rejection can be minimized by cross-matching donor and graft for ABO and MHC tissue types.

• Rejection can be blocked by agents producing general immunosuppression such as antimitotic drugs like azathioprine, or anti-inflammatory steroids. Cyclosporin and FK506 prevent interleukin-2 (IL-2) production, and rapamycin blocks signal transduction triggered by activation of the IL-2 receptor.

• A number of T-cell specific monoclonal antibodies, such as anti-CD3 and anti-IL-2R, are useful in controlling graft rejection.

Xenografting

• The major hurdle to the use of animal organs is hyperacute rejection due to the presence of xenoreactive cross-reacting antibodies in the host.

Clinical experience in grafting

• Cornea and cartilage grafts are avascular and comparatively well tolerated.

• Kidney grafting gives excellent results, although immunosuppression must normally be continuous.

• High success rates are also being achieved with heart, liver and, to a lesser extent, lung transplants.

• Bone marrow grafts for immunodeficiency and aplastic anemia are accepted from matched siblings but it is difficult to avoid g.v.h. disease with allogeneic marrow. Stem cells may be obtained from umbilical cord blood or from peripheral blood, especially after administration of granulocyte colony-stimulating factor (G-CSF).

• There are two forms of g.v.h disease, an acute form with severe skin, liver and bowel involvement and a chronic form which resembles scleroderma.

Association of HLA type with disease

• HLA specificities are often associated with particular diseases, e.g. *HLA-B27* with ankylosing spondylitis, *DR4* with rheumatoid arthritis and *DQ2* and *DQ8* with type 1 insulin-dependent diabetes. The reason for these disease associations is not known.

The fetus as an allograft

• Differences between MHC of mother and fetus may be beneficial to the fetus but as a potential graft it must be protected against transplantation attack by the mother.

• A major defense mechanism is the lack of classical class I and II MHC antigens on syncytiotrophoblast and cytotrophoblast which form the outer layers of the placenta.

• The extravillous cytotrophoblast expresses a nonclassical nonpolymorphic MHC class I protein, HLA-G, which inhibits cytotoxicity by maternal natural killer (NK) cells.

• The placenta produces inhibitory cytokines and other factors that protect against maternal T-cells.

See the accompanying website (**www.roitt.com**) for multiple choice questions

FURTHER READING

Buckley, R.H. (2003) Transplantation immunology: Organ and bone marrow assessment and modulation of the immune response. *Journal of Allergy and Clinical Immunology*, **111**, S733–44.

Daar, A.S. (Chairman) (1999) Animal-to-human organ transplants — a solution or a new problem? *Bulletin of the World Health Organization*, **77**, 54–61. [An in-depth round table discussion.]

Mellor, A.L. & Munn, D.H. (2000) Immunology at the maternal–fetal interface: Lessons for T-cell tolerance and suppression. *Annual Review of Immunology*, **18**, 367–91.

Morris, P.J. (ed.) (2000) *Kidney Transplantation: Principles and Practice*, 5th edn. W.B. Saunders & Company, Philadelphia.

Murphy, W.J. & Blazar, B.R. (1999) New strategies for preventing graft-versus-host disease. *Current Opinion in Immunology*, **11**, 509–15.

Niederkorn, J.Y. (1999) The immune privilege of corneal allografts. *Transplantation*, **67**, 1503–8.

Reisner, Y. & Martelli, M.J. (1999) Stem cell escalation enables HLA-disparate haematopoietic transplants in leukaemia patients. *Immunology Today*, **20**, 343–7.

Tabbara, I.A. (2002) Allogeneic hematopoietic stem cell transplantation: Complications and results. *Archives of Internal Medicine*, **162**, 1558–66.

Thorsby, E. (1995) HLA-associated disease susceptibility. *The Immunologist*, **3**, 51–8.

Waldmann, H. (ed.) (2003) Section on transplantation. *Current Opinion in Immunology*, **15**, 477–511.

Tumor immunology

It has long been suggested that the allograft rejection mechanism represented a means by which the body's cells could be kept under **immunologic surveillance** so that altered cells with a neoplastic potential could be identified and summarily eliminated. For this to operate, cancer cells must display some new discriminating surface structure which can be recognized by the immune system. Indeed tumor antigens can be recognized by raising monoclonal antibodies against them or by specific cytotoxic T-cells (Tc). Identification of tumor antigens recognized by T-cells is crucial for the future production of vaccines which target solid tumors.

CHANGES ON THE SURFACE OF TUMOR CELLS (figure 16.1)

Virally controlled antigens

A substantial minority of tumors arise through infection with **oncogenic DNA viruses** including Epstein–Barr virus (EBV) in lymphomas and human papilloma virus (HPV) in cervical cancers, or RNA viruses such as the human T-cell leukemia virus-1 (HTLV-1). After infection, the viruses express genes homologous with cellular oncogenes which encode factors affecting growth, cell division and apoptosis. Failure to control these genes therefore leads potentially to malignant transformation. Virally derived peptides associated with surface major histocompatibility complex (MHC) on the tumor cell behave as powerful transplantation antigens which generate specific Tc.

Expression of normally silent genes

The dysregulated uncontrolled cell division of the cancer cell creates a milieu in which the products of normally silent genes may be expressed. Sometimes these encode differentiation antigens normally associated with an earlier fetal stage. Thus, tumors may express proteins normally expressed on fetal but not adult tissue. Such **oncofetal antigens** include α-fetoprotein (AFP), found on primary hepatocellular carcinoma cells, and carcinoembryonic antigen (CEA) expressed by gastrointestinal and breast carcinomas. These oncofetal antigens may also be released in various inflammatory conditions but measurement of their levels in the blood may be helpful in the diagnosis of malignant disease and in the monitoring of progression of the disease.

The majority of tumor-specific antigens are either completely abnormal peptides or mutated forms of normal cellular proteins produced by tumor cells and complexed to class I MHC products. These peptides, which are not normally destined to be positioned in the surface plasma membrane, can still signal their presence to T-cells in the outer world by a processed peptide/MHC mechanism. One such group of tumor-specific antigens is encoded by families of genes that

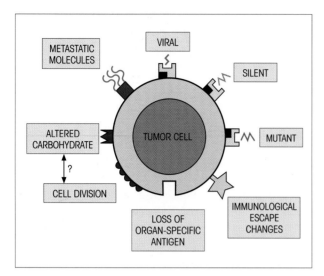

Figure 16.1 Tumor-associated surface changes. Surface carbohydrate changes may occur during cell division. An immunoglobulin idiotype on B-cell leukemia would be a unique antigen.

are normally silent in most normal tissues For example the *MAGE* gene (melanoma antigen gene) which codes for proteins found on the surface of melanomas and other tumors is normally found only on human testis. Patients with these tumors often have circulating cytotoxic T-lymphocytes (CTLs) specific for these peptides, indicating that these antigens can induce immune responses and therefore could be ideal targets for immunotherapy.

Mutant antigens

Other antigens are encoded by genes that are expressed in normal cells but are mutated in tumor cells. Such mutations may change as few as one amino acid. Single point mutations in oncogenes or tumor suppressor genes can account for the large diversity of antigens found on carcinogen-induced tumors. The gene encoding the p53 cell cycle inhibitor is a hotspot for mutation in cancer, while the oncogenic human *ras* genes differ from their normal counterpart by point mutations usually leading to single amino acid substitutions. Such mutations have been recorded in 40% of human colorectal cancers and their preneoplastic lesions, in more than 90% of pancreatic carcinomas, in acute myelogenous leukemia and in preleukemic syndromes. The oncogene *HER-2/neu* encodes a membrane protein that is present on various human tumors, especially ovarian and breast carcinomas, where it could serve as a target for either monoclonal antibodies or Tc.

Tissue-specific differentiation antigens

A tumor arising from a particular tissue may express normal differentiation antigens specific for that tissue. For example, prostatic tumors may carry prostate-specific antigen (PSA), which is also released into the serum and can be measured as a screening test for prostate cancer. Lymphoid cells at almost any stage in their differentiation or maturation may become malignant and proliferate to form a clone of cells which are virtually "frozen" at a particular developmental stage because of defects in maturation. The malignant cells bear the markers one would expect of normal lymphocytes reaching the stage at which maturation had been arrested. Thus, chronic lymphocytic leukemia cells resemble mature B-cells in expressing surface MHC class II and immunoglobulin (Ig), albeit of a single idiotype in a given patient. B-cell lymphomas will express on their surface CD19, CD20 and either κ or λ light chains depending on which light chain the original cell was carrying. Similarly, T-cell malignancies will carry the T-cell receptor (TCR) with CD3 and other T-cell-specific cell surface antigens such as CD4, CD8, CD2, CD7 or the interleukin-2 (IL-2) receptor CD25. Using monoclonal antibodies directed against these specific antigens on T- or B-cells, it has been possible to classify the lymphoid malignancies in terms of the phenotype of the equivalent normal cell (figure 16.2).

Malignant tumors may lack class I MHC molecules

Malignant transformation of cells may be associated with loss or downregulation of class I MHC expression linked in most cases to increased metastatic potential. This presumably reflects their decreased vulnerability to T-cells but not natural killer (NK) cells. In breast cancer, for example, around 60% of metastatic tumors lack MHC class I.

Changes in glycoprotein structure

The chaotic internal control of metabolism within neoplastic cells often leads to the presentation of abnormal surface glycoproteins or glycolipids. Some of these are useful in the diagnosis and follow-up of patients with cancer, such as CA-125 which is found in increased amounts on the cell surface of ovarian or uterine cancers. Similarly CA-19-9 is expressed at high levels in most patients with gastrointestinal or breast carcinoma. Abnormal mucin found in pancreatic and breast tissue can have immunologic consequences and can be recognized by CTL or by antibody.

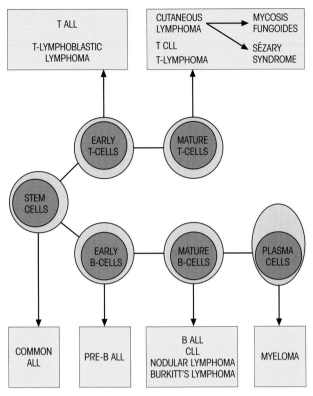

Figure 16.2 Cellular phenotype of human lymphoid malignancies. (After M.F. Greaves & G. Janossy, personal communication.) ALL, acute lymphoblastic leukemia; CLL, chronic lymphocytic leukemia.

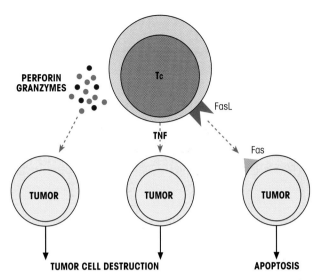

Figure 16.3 Mechanisms involved in cytotoxic T-lymphocyte destruction of tumors by cytotoxic T-cells (Tc). FasL, Fas ligand; TNF, tumor necrosis factor.

IMMUNE RESPONSE TO TUMORS

Immune surveillance against strongly immunogenic tumors

The **immune surveillance theory** would predict that there should be more tumors in individuals whose immune systems are suppressed. This undoubtedly seems to be the case for **strongly immunogenic tumors**. There is a considerable increase in skin cancer in immunosuppressed patients living in high sunshine regions and, in general, transplant patients on immunosuppressive drugs are unduly susceptible to skin cancers, largely associated with papilloma virus, and EBV-positive lymphomas. Likewise, the lymphomas that arise in children with T-cell deficiency linked to Wiskott–Aldrich syndrome or ataxia telangiectasia express EBV genes. On the other hand, there is no clear evidence that nonvirally induced, spontaneously developing tumors, such as the common tumors in humans, have an increased incidence in immunodeficient individuals or athymic (nude) mice.

A role for acquired immune responses?

Various immunologic effector mechanisms against tumors have been described but it is unclear which of these mechanisms are important as protective antitumor responses. Cytotoxic T-lymphocytes are thought to provide surveillance by recognizing and destroying tumor cells. They employ a variety of mechanisms to destroy tumor cells including exocytosis of granules containing the cytotoxic effector molecules perforin and granzyme and secretion of tumor necrosis factor (TNF) which also has tumoricidal activities. Another and perhaps more important mechanism is based on direct effector–target interaction between Fas on target cells and FasL (Fas ligand) expressed on the Tc. FasL activation of the membrane-bound Fas present on target cells leads to apoptosis of the tumor cell (figure 16.3). The role that CTL play in tumor immunity is unclear, but patients with malignant disease have been shown to have both circulating and tumor-infiltrating lymphocytes which show cytotoxicity *in vitro* against the tumor cells. The mechanisms by which tumor cells resist this attack will be dealt with later.

A role for innate immunity?

Perhaps in speaking of immunity to tumors, one too readily thinks only in terms of acquired responses whereas it is now accepted that innate mechanisms are of significance. Macrophages, which often infiltrate a tumor mass, can destroy tumor cells in tissue culture through the copious production of reactive oxygen intermediates (ROIs) and TNF. Similarly, NK cells subserve a function as the earliest cellular effector mechanism against dissemination of blood-borne metastases. Powerful evidence implicating these cells in protection against cancer is provided by beige mice which congenitally lack NK cells. They die with spontaneous tumors earlier than their nondeficient littermates.

Resting NK cells are spontaneously cytolytic for certain, but by no means all, tumor targets; IL-2-activated cells (lymphokine-activated killer cells or LAK cells) display a wider lethality. As was mentioned previously, recognition of class I imparts a **negative inactivating** signal to the NK cell implying conversely that downregulation of MHC class I, which tumors employ as a strategy to escape Tc cells, would make them more **susceptible to NK attack**.

Tumors develop mechanisms to evade the immune response

Most tumors occur in individuals who are not immunosuppressed, indicating that tumors themselves have mechanisms for escaping the innate or acquired immune systems. Several such mechanisms have been suggested (figure 16.4). Most important of these is that tumor cells have an inherent defect in antigen processing or presentation as they lack costimulatory molecules such as the B7 (CD80 and CD86) molecules. T-cell anergy occurs following antigen–MHC complex recognition in the absence of costimulation. Tumor cells also lack other molecules important in activating T-cells, especially MHC class II or adhesion molecules such as ICAM-1 (intercellular adhesion molecule-1) or LFA-3 (lymphocyte function-associated antigen-3). Furthermore, as has been previously indicated, many tumors express reduced or absent levels of class I MHC, which imparts resistance to Tc although presumably increasing susceptibility to NK cells. Other tumors express functional FasL, which confers resistance by inducing apoptosis of autologous infiltrating lymphocytes that express Fas. Tumors themselves may release various immunosuppressive factors such as transforming growth factor-β (TGFβ), which is a potent immunosuppressive cytokine having effects on many mediators of the immune response including a potent inhibitory effect on differentiation of CTL. It is also likely that as tumors grow they tend to favor the selective outgrowth of antigen-negative variants, or they may produce mucins that conceal or mask their antigens so that they are not recognized by the immune response.

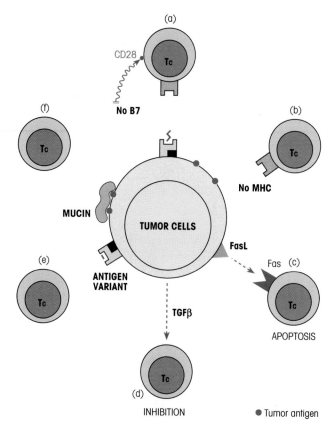

Figure 16.4 Mechanisms by which tumor cells escape destruction by the immune response. Tumor cells may (a) lack costimulatory molecules such as B7; (b) express reduced levels of class I major histocompatibility complex (MHC); (c) express FasL (Fas ligand), which causes apoptosis of attacking cytotoxic T-cells (Tc); (d) produce various cytokines which inhibit the immune response; (e) develop antigen-negative variants; (f) produce mucins which disguise their antigens. TGFβ, transforming growth factor-β.

APPROACHES TO CANCER IMMUNOTHERAPY

Although immune surveillance seems to operate only against strongly immunogenic tumors, the exciting new information on the antigenicity of mutant and previously silent proteins (table 16.1), raises the possibility of developing effective immunotherapeutic approaches against cancer. This will almost certainly only succeed once the tumor load is first reduced by surgery, irradiation or chemotherapy.

Antigen-independent cytokine therapy

Treatment with cytokines

As has been pointed out previously, the cytokine network is extremely complex, and administration of a cytokine designed to stimulate one branch of the

Table 16.1 Potential tumor antigens for immunotherapy. (Reproduced with permission from L. Fong & E.G. Engleman (2000) Dendritic cells in cancer immunotherapy. *Annual Review of Immunology* **18**, 245–73.)

Antigen	Malignancy
Tumor specific	
Immunoglobulin V-region	B-cell non-Hodgkin's lymphoma, multiple myeloma
TCR V-region	T-cell non-Hodgkin's lymphoma
Mutant p21/ras	Pancreatic, colon, lung cancer
Mutant p53	Colorectal, lung, bladder, head and neck cancer
Developmental	
p210/bcr-abl fusion product	Chronic myelogenous leukemia, acute lymphoblastic leukemia
MART-1/Melan A	Melanoma
MAGE-1, MAGE-3	Melanoma, colorectal, lung, gastric cancers
GAGE family	Melanoma
Telomerase	Various
Viral	
Human papilloma virus	Cervical, penile cancer
Epstein–Barr virus	Burkitt's lymphoma, nasopharyngeal carcinoma, post-transplant lymphoproliferative disorders
Tissue specific	
Tyrosinase	Melanoma
gp100	Melanoma
Prostatic acid phosphatase	Prostate cancer
Prostate-specific antigen	Prostate cancer
Prostate-specific membrane antigen	Prostate cancer
Thyroglobulin	Thyroid cancer
α-fetoprotein	Liver cancer
Overexpressed	
HER-2/neu	Breast and lung cancers
Carcinoembryonic antigen	Colorectal, lung, breast cancer
Muc-1	Colorectal, pancreatic, ovarian, lung cancer

get the tumor cells. Administration of autologous LAK cells together with high doses of IL-2 has led, in one study, to a considerable reduction in tumor burden in renal cancer patients.

Tumor necrosis factor has powerful tumor-killing capability and can cause hemorrhagic necrosis and tumor regression. Unfortunately its systemic administration is associated with very severe toxicity due to its activation of the cytokine cascade.

In trials using interferon α (IFNα) and IFNβ, significant responses were seen in patients with various malignancies, including a remarkable response rate of 80–90% among patients with hairy cell leukemia and mycosis fungoides.

With regard to the mechanisms of the antitumor effects, in certain tumors IFNs may serve primarily as antiproliferative agents. In others, activation of NK cells and macrophages may be important, while augmenting the expression of class I MHC molecules may make the tumors more susceptible to control by immune effector mechanisms. In some circumstances the antiviral effect could be contributory.

For diseases like renal cell cancer and hairy cell leukemia, IFNs have induced responses in a significantly higher proportion of patients than conventional therapies. However, in the wider setting, most investigators consider that the role of IFNs will be in combination therapy, for example, with active immunotherapy or with various chemotherapeutic agents.

Exploitation of cell-mediated immune responses

Immunization with viral antigens

Based on the not unreasonable belief that certain forms of cancer (e.g. lymphoma) are caused by oncogenic viruses, attempts are being made to isolate the virus and prepare a suitable vaccine from it. In fact, large-scale protection of chickens against the development of Marek's disease lymphoma has been successfully achieved by vaccination with another herpesvirus native to turkeys. In human Burkitt's lymphoma, work is in progress to develop a vaccine to exploit the ability of Tc cells to target the EBV-related antigens present on the cells of all Burkitt's tumors. Similarly in patients with cervical cancer Tc against the causative HPV can be successfully induced using vaccinia virus expressing HPV genes.

Immunization with whole tumor cells

This has the advantage that we do not necessarily have to know the identity of the antigen concerned. The dis-

immune response may lead to inhibition of another portion of the response. In some cases administration of systemic cytokine has produced serious side effects with life-threatening consequences.

Interleukin-2 has been used in a number of experimental protocols with the idea of expanding Tc and NK cells. A number of these patients had serious side effects due to the production of other cytokines, which produced fever, shock and a vascular leak syndrome. Another approach is to expand peripheral blood lymphocytes with IL-2 to generate large numbers of LAK cells which can be infused back into the patient to tar-

advantage is that the majority of tumors are weakly immunogenic and do not present antigen effectively, and so cannot activate resting T-cells. Remember, the surface MHC–peptide complex on its own is not enough and will result in T-cell anergy, which is a major limitation to the effective development of an immune response. Costimulation with molecules such as B7.1 (CD80) and B7.2 (CD86) and possibly certain cytokines is required to push the resting T-cell into active proliferation and differentiation. Once the T-cells are activated, accessory costimulation is no longer required due to upregulation of accessory binding molecules such as CD2 and LFA-1. In murine studies vaccination with B7-transfected melanoma cells generated CD8$^+$ cytolytic effectors which protected against subsequent tumor challenge; in other words, the introduction of the costimulatory molecule B7 enhances the immunogenicity of the tumor so that the B7-transfected cells can activate resting T-cells to recognize and attack even nontransfected tumor cells (figure 16.5). Another approach is to transfect tumor cells with syngeneic MHC class II genes, to enable the transfected cells to present endogenously encoded tumor peptides to CD4 cells. A less sophisticated but more convenient approach involves the administration of irradiated melanoma cells together with BCG (bacille bilié de Calmette–Guérin) or other adjuvant, which, by generating a plethora of inflammatory cytokines, increases the efficiency of presentation of tumor antigens. It would be exciting to suppose that in the future we might transfect a tumor *in situ* by firing gold particles bearing appropriate gene constructs such as B7, IFNγ (to upregulate MHC class I and II), granulocyte-macrophage colony-stimulating factor (GM-CSF) and IL-2.

Therapy with subunit vaccines

The variety of potential protein targets so far identified (table 16.1) has spawned a considerable investment in clinical therapeutic trials using peptides as vaccines. Because of the pioneering work in characterizing melanoma-specific antigens, this tumor has been the focus of numerous studies. Encouraging results in terms of clinical benefit, linked to the generation of CTLs, have been obtained following vaccination with peptides with or without adjuvants. The inclusion of accessory factors, such as IL-2 or GM-CSF, and blockade of CTLA-4 (cytotoxic T-lymphocyte antigen-4) can be crucial for success.

The unique **idiotype** on monoclonal B-cell tumors with surface Ig offers a potentially feasible target for immunotherapy. This form of therapy, however, requires the preparation of a different vaccine for each patient. Other tumor-specific antigens and mutant peptide sequences are all possible candidates for immunotherapy such as the human melanoma-specific MAGE antigenic peptides. Various forms of immunization are possible, including the injection of peptide alone or with adjuvant and the use of recombinant defective viruses carrying the sequence encoding the protein.

VACCINATION WITH DENDRITIC CELLS (DCs)

The sheer power of the dendritic antigen-presenting cell for the initiation of T-cell responses has been the focus of an ever-burgeoning series of immunotherapeutic strategies. These have elicited tumor-specific protective immune responses after injection of isolated DCs loaded with tumor lysates, tumor antigens, or peptides derived from them. Administration of DCs transfected with tumor cell derived RNA has been shown to induce the expansion of tumor-specific T-cells in cancer patients and considerable success has been achieved in animal models and increasingly with human patients (figure 16.6). The copious numbers of DCs needed for each patient's individual therapy are obtained by expansion of CD34$^+$ precursors in bone marrow by culture with cytokines including GM-CSF, IL-4 and TNF. Alternatively CD14$^+$ monocytes from peripheral blood generate DC in the presence of GM-CSF plus IL-4. It is unclear why the administration of small numbers of antigen-pulsed DCs induces specific T-cell responses and tumor regression in patients in whom both the antigen and DCs are already plentiful. The suggestion has been made that DCs in or near malignant tissues may be ineffective, perhaps due to IL-10 secretion by the tumor.

Therapy with monoclonal antibodies

The strategies

Immunologists have for a long time been bemused by the idea of eliminating tumor cells with specific antibody or antibody linked to a killer molecule. Such immunotoxins represent a class of magic bullet in which the toxin of plant or bacterial origin is attached to an antibody or growth factor. After binding to the cell surface, the toxin is internalized and

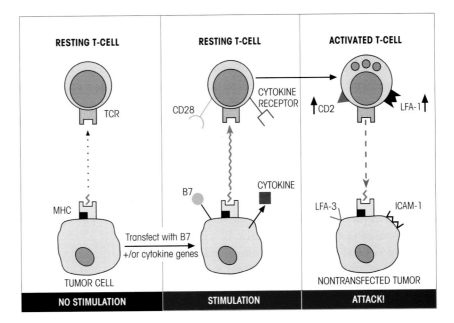

Figure 16.5 Immunotherapy by transfection with costimulatory molecules. The tumor can only stimulate the resting T-cell with the costimulatory help of B7 and/or cytokines such as granulocyte-macrophage colony-stimulating factor (GM-CSF), interferon γ (IFNγ) and interleukin-2 (IL-2), IL-4 and IL-7. Once activated, the T-cell with upregulated accessory molecules can now attack the original tumor lacking costimulators. ICAM-1, intercellular adhesion molecule-1; LFA, lymphocyte function-associated antigen; MHC, major histocompatibility complex; TCR, T-cell receptor.

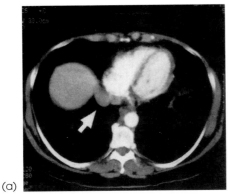

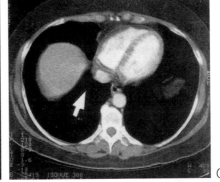

(a)   (b)

Figure 16.6 Clinical response to autologous vaccine utilizing dendritic cells pulsed with idiotype from a B-cell lymphoma. Computed tomography scan through patient's chest (a) prevaccine and (b) 10 months after completion of three vaccine treatments. The arrow in (a) points to a paracardiac mass. All sites of disease had resolved and the patient remained in remission 24 months after beginning treatment. (Photography kindly supplied by Professor R. Levy from the article by F.J. Hsu, C. Benike, F. Fagnoni *et al.* (1996) *Nature Medicine* **2**, 52; reproduced by kind permission of Nature America Inc.)

kills the cell by catalytic inhibition of protein synthesis. One such immunotoxin consists of anti-idiotype antibody conjugated with ricin, a toxin of such devastating potency that one molecule entering the cell is lethal. Such immunotoxins need to have a reasonable half-life in the circulation, to be able to penetrate into tumors and not bind significantly to nontumor cells. Other practical problems include difficulties in moving the antibodies through the tortuous vessels found in tumors, and the development in the tumor of mutant cells that fail to express the target antigens. Along the same lines, internalizing a photo-sensitizer renders the cells vulnerable to photodynamic therapy.

Radioimmunoconjugates that carry a radiation source to the tumor site for therapy or imaging are being intensively developed and have two advantages over toxins: they are nonimmunogenic and they can destroy adjacent tumor cells which have lost antigen. Radioimmunotherapy, using isotopes such as yttrium-90 (^{90}Y), indium-111 (^{111}In) or iodine-131 (^{131}I) linked to antibody, delivers doses of radiation to tumor tissue which would be impossibly toxic with external beam sources. Results are even better when used in synergy with chemotherapy. A potent antilymphoma drug (Zevalin or Bexaar) employs a monoclonal antibody to the B-cell surface antigen CD20, to which is attached radioactive ^{90}Y or ^{131}I. These **radiolabeled monoclonal antibodies** destroy B-cell lymphomas by antibody-dependent cellular cytotoxicity (ADCC) and by signaling-induced apoptosis, acting in synergy with DNA damage due to gamma-radiation. Therapy with this agent has been spectacularly successful. Likewise, radionuclide conjugates of a humanized anti-CD33 (Mylotarg) are very useful in patients with myeloid leukemia and can destroy even large tumor burdens.

Another strategy is to target **growth factor receptors** present on the surface of tumor cells. Blocking of such receptors should deprive the cells of crucial growth signals. Herceptin is a monoclonal antibody that recognizes and binds to the HER-2/neu protein found on 30% of breast cancer cells. Because the protein is not present on normal cells, the antibody selectively attacks the tumor causing its shrinkage in a substantial proportion of cases. In a similar manner, a humanized anti-CD52 (Campath-1H or alemtuzumab) has shown benefit in a range of hematological tumors, and antibodies to the epidermal growth factor receptor (EGFR) enhanced the effects of conventional chemotherapy and radiation therapy. Another new approach is to target the tumor blood supply. Tumors generally cannot grow beyond the size of 1 mm in diameter without the support of blood vessels and, because the tumor is new tissue, its blood vessels will also have to be new. These vessels form through the process known as angiogenesis, the sprouting of new blood vessels from existing ones, but they are biochemically and structurally different from normal resting blood vessels and so provide differential targets for therapeutic monoclonal antibodies.

Genetic technology has now allowed the development of **chimeric antibodies** that have the variable antigen-binding region of a mouse monoclonal antibody but with a human constant region. Taking this one stage further, the mouse variable region framework regions can be replaced with human frameworks, creating the "humanized" antibodies mentioned above (cf. figure 3.11). Both chimeric and humanized antibodies retain the specificity of the monoclonal but are much less immunogenic. Other options for immunologic attack using monoclonal antibodies are possible. For example, a mixture of two **bispecific heteroconjugates** of antitumor/anti-CD3 and antitumor/anti-CD28 should act synergistically to induce contact between a T-cell and the tumor to activate direct cytotoxicity (figure 16.7).

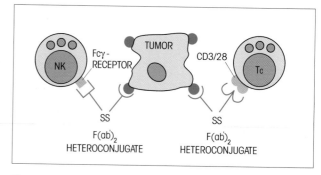

Figure 16.7 Focusing effector cells by heteroconjugates. Coupling F(ab')$_2$ fragments of monoclonal antibodies specific for the tumor and an appropriate molecule on the surface of natural killer (NK) or cytotoxic T-cells (Tc), provides the specificity to bring the effectors into intimate contact with the target cell.

Another use of monoclonal antibodies is to **purge bone marrow grafts** of unwanted cells *in vitro* in the presence of complement from a foreign species. Thus, differentiation antigens present on leukemic cells but absent from bone marrow stem cells can be used to prepare tumor-free autologous stem cells to restore function in patients treated with chemotherapy or X-irradiation (figure 16.8).

Immunologic diagnosis of lymphoid neoplasias

With the availability of a range of monoclonal antibodies and improvements in immuno-enzymic and flow cytometric technology, great strides have been made in exploiting, for diagnostic purposes, the fact that malignant lymphoid cells, especially leukemias and lymphomas, display the markers of the normal lymphocytes which are their counterparts. Thus in the diagnosis of non-Hodgkin's lymphomas, the majority of which are of B-cell origin, the feature that is diagnostic is the synthesis of monotypic Ig, i.e. of one light chain only (figure 16.9a). In contrast, the population of cells at a site of reactive B-cell hyperplasia will stain for both κ and λ chains (figure 16.9b).

Plasma cell dyscrasias

Multiple myeloma

This is defined as a malignant proliferation of a clone of plasma cells secreting a monoclonal Ig. The myeloma or "M" component in serum is recognized as a tight band on gel electrophoresis (figure 16.10) as all molecules in the clone are, of course, identical and have the same mobility. Since Ig-secreting cells produce an ex-

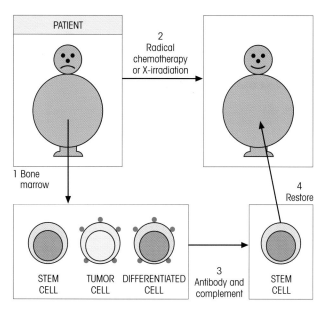

Figure 16.8 Treatment of leukemias by autologous bone marrow rescue. By using cytotoxic antibodies to a differentiation antigen present on leukemic cells and even on other normal differentiated cells, but absent from stem cells, it is possible to obtain a tumor-free population of the latter which can be used to restore hematopoietic function in patients subsequently treated radically to destroy the leukemic cells.

cess of light chains, free light chains are present in the plasma of multiple myeloma patients, and can be recognized in the urine as Bence-Jones protein.

Waldenström's macroglobulinemia

This disorder is produced by the unregulated proliferation of cells of an intermediate appearance called lymphoplasmacytoid cells which secrete a monoclonal IgM, the Waldenström macroglobulin. Since the IgM is secreted in large amounts and is confined to the intravascular compartment, there is a marked rise in serum viscosity, the consequences of which can be temporarily mitigated by vigorous plasmapheresis. The disease runs a fairly benign course and the prognosis is quite good, although the appearance of lymphoplasmacytoid tumor cells in the blood is an ominous sign.

Heavy chain disease

Heavy chain disease is a rare condition in which quantities of abnormal heavy chains are excreted in the urine. The amino acid sequences of the N-terminal regions of these heavy chains are normal, but they have a deletion extending from part of the variable domain through most of the C_H1 region so that they lack the

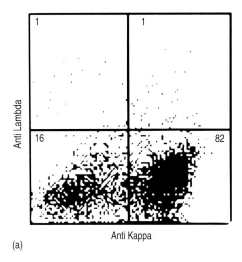

(a)

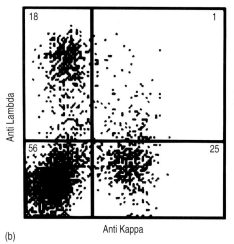

(b)

Figure 16.9 Use of flow cytometry to diagnose malignant lymphoma. Cells are dispersed and stained with fluorescein-labeled antibodies against κ (kappa) and λ (lambda) light chains. Lymphoma cells are monotypic and in this case stain with anti-κ (a) while normal lymphocytes are polytypic and stain with both anti-κ and anti-λ (b).

cysteine required to form the disulphide bond to the light chains.

Immunodeficiency secondary to lymphoproliferative disorders

Immunodeficiency is a common feature in patients with lymphoid malignancies. The reasons for this are still obscure, but it appears that the malignant cells interfere with the development of the corresponding normal cells. Thus, in multiple myeloma the levels of normal B-cells and of non-myeloma Ig may be grossly depressed and the patients susceptible to infection with pyogenic bacteria.

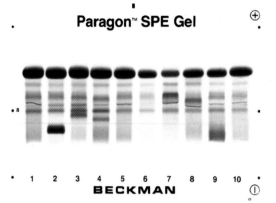

Figure 16.10 Myeloma paraprotein demonstrated by gel electrophoresis of serum. Lane 1, normal; lane 2, γ-paraprotein; lane 3, near β-paraprotein; lane 4, fibrinogen band in the γ-region of a *plasma* sample; lane 5, normal serum; lane 6, immunoglobulin (Ig) deficiency (low γ); lane 7, nephrotic syndrome (raised α_2-macroglobulin, low albumin and Igs); lane 8, hemolysed sample (raised hemoglobin/haptoglobin in α_2 region); lane 9, polyclonal increase in Igs (e.g. infection, autoimmune disease); lane 10, normal serum. (Gel kindly provided by Mr A. Heys.)

REVISION

Changes on the surface of tumor cells

• Processed peptides derived from oncogenic viruses are powerful major histocompatibility complex (MHC)—associated transplantation antigens.

• Some tumors express genes that are silent in normal tissues; sometimes they have been expressed previously in embryonic life (oncofetal antigens).

• Many tumors express weak antigens associated with point mutations in oncogenes such as *ras* and *HER-2/neu.*

• Many tumors express normal differentiation antigens specific for that tissue.

• Tumors may lack class I MHC molecules.

• Dysregulation of tumor cells frequently causes structural abnormalities in surface glycoprotein or glycolipid structures.

Immune response to tumors

• T-cells generally mount effective surveillance against tumors associated with oncogenic viruses or ultraviolet induction which are strongly immunogenic.

• More weakly immunogenic tumors are not controlled by T-cell surveillance, although sometimes low-grade responses are evoked.

• Cytotoxic T-cells (Tc) may provide surveillance and cause tumor cell destruction or apoptosis.

• Natural killer (NK) cells probably play a role in containing tumor growth and metastases. They can attack MHC class I negative tumor cells because the class I molecule normally imparts a negative inactivation signal to NK cells.

Tumor cells have a variety of mechanisms to evade the immune response

• Tumor cells lack costimulatory molecules for antigen presentation and this may result in T-cell anergy.

• Tumors express reduced levels of MHC class I or class II.

• Some tumors express FasL (Fas ligand) which causes apotosis of attacking lymphocytes with Fas on their surface.

• Tumors may release inhibitory cytokines such as transforming growth factor-β (TGFβ).

• Tumors may produce mucins that mask their tumor specific antigens.

Approaches to cancer immunotherapy

• Systemic cytokine therapy may be used to stimulate specific effector cells but is associated with severe side effects.

• Interleukin-2 (IL-2)-stimulated NK cells (LAK) are active against renal carcinoma. Interferon γ (IFNγ) and IFNβ are very effective in the T-cell disorders, hairy cell leukemia and mycosis fungoides.

• Cancer vaccines based on oncogenic viral proteins can be expected.

• Immunization with tumor-specific peptides may be useful, but a different vaccine may be required for each patient. Effective melanoma-specific antigens have been identified. Immunogenic potency of a tumor antigen is greatly enhanced by dendritic cells (DCs) pulsed with the antigen.

• Weakly immunogenic tumors provoke effective anti-cancer responses if transfected with costimulatory molecules such as B7 or with MHC class II genes.

• Vaccination with DCs loaded with tumor antigens or tumor-derived RNA yields tumor-specific immune responses.

• Monoclonal antibodies conjugated to toxins or radionuclides can target tumor cells or antigens associated with malignancy.

• Monoclonal antibodies targeting growth factor receptors on tumor cells or the blood supply to the tumor are useful in treatment.

• Bifunctional antibodies can bring effectors such as NK and Tc close to the tumor target.

• Monoclonal antibodies attached to an isotope may be used to image tumors.

Lymphoid malignancies

• The surface phenotype aids in the diagnosis and classification of lymphomas and leukemias.

• Multiple myeloma represents a malignant proliferation of a single clone of plasma cells producing a single "M" band on electrophoresis.

• Bence-Jones protein consists of free light chains found in the urine of patients with multiple myeloma.

• Waldenström's macroglobulinemia is associated with large amounts of serum IgM causing hyperviscosity.

• Malignant lymphoid cells produce secondary immunodeficiency by suppressing differentiation of the corresponding normal lineage.

See the accompanying website (**www.roitt.com**) for multiple choice questions

FURTHER READING

Begent, R.H.J., Verhaar, M.J., Chester, K.A. *et al.* (1996) Clinical evidence of efficient tumor targeting based on single-chain Fv antibody selected from a combinatorial library. *Nature Medicine*, **2**, 979–84.

Chattopadhyay, U. (1999) Tumour immunotherapy: Developments and strategies. *Immunology Today*, **20**, 480–2.

Dunn, G.P., Old, L.J. & Schreiber, R.D. (2004) The three Es of cancer. *Annual Review of Immunology*, **22**, 329–60.

Finn, O.J. (2003) Cancer vaccines: Between the idea and the reality. *Nature Reviews. Immunology*, **3**, 630–41.

Finn, O.J. (ed.) (2004) Section on tumor immunology. *Current Opinion in Immunology*, **16**, 127–62.

Autoimmune diseases

THE SCOPE OF AUTOIMMUNE DISEASES

The monumental repertoire of the adaptive immune system has evolved to allow it to recognize and ensnare microbial molecules of virtually any shape. In so doing it has been unable to avoid the generation of lymphocytes which react with the body's own constituents. The term "**autoimmune disease**" applies to conditions where the **autoimmune process contributes to the pathogenesis of the disease**. This is different to situations where apparently harmless autoantibodies are formed following tissue damage, for example heart antibodies appearing after a myocardial infarction. Autoimmune diseases count amongst the major medical problems of today's societies. There are, for example, over 6.5 million cases of rheumatoid arthritis (RA) in the USA, and type 1 diabetes is the leading cause of end-stage renal disease.

The spectrum of autoimmune diseases

These disorders may be looked upon as forming a spectrum. At one end we have "**organ-specific diseases**" with organ-specific autoantibodies. **Hashimoto's disease** of the thyroid is an example: there is a specific lesion in the thyroid involving infiltration by mononuclear cells (lymphocytes, macrophages and plasma cells), destruction of follicular cells and germinal center formation accompanied by the production of circulating antibodies with absolute specificity for certain thyroid constituents (Milestone 17.1).

Moving towards the center of the spectrum are those disorders where the lesion tends to be localized to a single organ but the antibodies are nonorgan-specific. A typical example would be **primary biliary cirrhosis** where the small bile ductule is the main target of inflammatory cell infiltration but the serum antibodies present—mainly mitochondrial—are not liver-specific.

At the other end of the spectrum are the "**nonorgan-specific**" or "**systemic autoimmune diseases**" broadly belonging to the class of rheumatologic disorders, exemplified by **systemic lupus erythematosus (SLE)**, where neither lesions nor autoantibodies are confined to any one organ. Pathologic changes are widespread and are primarily lesions of connective tissue with fibrinoid necrosis. They are seen in the skin (the "lupus" butterfly rash on the face is characteristic), kidney glomeruli, joints, serous membranes and blood vessels. In addition, the formed elements of the blood are often affected. A bizarre collection of autoantibodies is found some of which react with the DNA and other nuclear constituents found in all cells of the body.

An attempt to fit the major diseases considered to be associated with autoimmunity into this spectrum is shown in table 17.1.

Overlap of autoimmune disorders

There is a tendency for more than one autoimmune disorder to occur in the same individual; for example,

Milestone 17.1—The Discovery of Thyroid Autoimmunity

In an attempt to confirm Paul Ehrlich's concept of "horror autotoxicus"—the body's dread of making antibodies to self, Rose and Witebsky immunized rabbits with rabbit thyroid extract in complete Freund's adjuvant. This procedure, which could also be carried out in other species such as the rat, resulted in the production of thyroid autoantibodies and chronic inflammatory destruction of the thyroid gland architecture (figure M17.1.1a and b).

Having noted the fall in serum gammaglobulin which followed removal of the goiter in Hashimoto's thyroiditis and the similarity of the histology (figure M17.1.1c) to that of Rose and Witebsky's rabbits, Roitt, Doniach and Campbell tested the hypothesis that the plasma cells in the gland might be making an autoantibody to a thyroid component, so causing the tissue damage and chronic inflammatory response. Sure enough, the sera of the first patients tested had precipitating antibodies to an autoantigen in normal thyroid extracts, which was soon identified as thyroglobulin (figure M17.1.2).

Adams and Purves, in seeking a circulating factor that

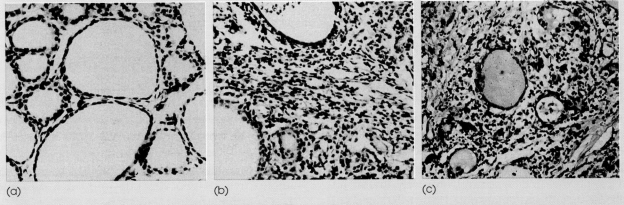

(a)   (b)   (c)

Figure M17.1.1 Experimental autoimmune thyroiditis. (a) Control rat thyroid showing normal follicular architecture. (b) Thyroiditis produced by immunization with rat thyroid extract in complete Freund's adjuvant; the invading chronic inflammatory cells have destroyed the follicular structure. (Based on the experiments of N.R. Rose & E. Witebsky (1956) *Journal of Immunology*, **76**, 417.) (c) Similarity of lesions in spontaneous human autoimmune disease to those induced in the experimental model. Other features of Hashimoto's disease such as the eosinophilic metaplasia of acinar cells (Askenazy cells) and local lymphoid follicles are not seen in this experiment model, although the latter occur in the spontaneous thyroiditis of Obese strain chickens.

(continued)

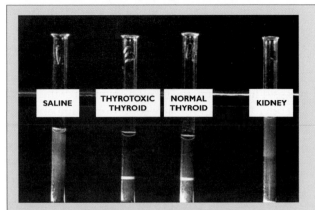

Figure M17.1.2 Thyroid autoantibodies in the serum of a patient with Hashimoto's disease demonstrated by precipitation in agar. Test serum is incorporated in agar in the bottom of the tube; the middle layer contains agar only while the autoantigen is present in the top layer. As serum antibody and thyroid autoantigen diffuse towards each other, they form a zone of opaque precipitate in the middle layer. Saline and kidney extract controls are negative (Based on I.M. Roitt, D. Doniach, P.N. Campbell & R.V. Hudson (1956) *Lancet*, **ii**, 820.)

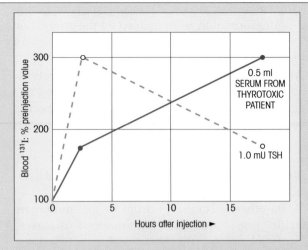

Figure M17.1.3 The long-acting thyroid stimulator in Graves' disease. Injection of thyroid-stimulating hormone (TSH) causes a rapid release of iodine-131 (^{131}I) from the pre-labeled animal thyroid in contrast to the prolonged release which follows injection of serum from a thyrotoxic patient. (Based on D.D. Adams & H.D. Purves (1956) *Proceedings of the University of Otago Medical School*, **34**, 11.)

might be responsible for the hyperthyroidism of Graves' thyrotoxicosis, injected patient's serum into guinea-pigs whose thyroids had been prelabeled with iodine-131 (^{131}I), and followed the release of radiolabeled material from the gland with time. Whereas the natural thyroid-stimulating hormone (TSH) produced a peak in serum radioactivity some 4 h after injection of the test animal, serum from thyrotoxic patients had a prolonged stimulatory effect (figure M17.1.3). The so-called *long-acting thyroid stimulator* (LATS) was ultimately shown to be an immunoglobulin G (IgG) mimicking TSH thorough its reaction with the TSH receptor but differing in its time-course of action, largely due to its longer half-life in the circulation.

patients with autoimmune thyroiditis (Hashimoto's disease or primary myxedema) have a much higher incidence of pernicious anemia than would be expected in a random population matched for age and sex (10.0% as against 0.2%). Conversely, both thyroiditis and thyrotoxicosis are diagnosed in pernicious anemia patients with an unexpectedly high frequency.

There is an even greater overlap in serological findings (table 17.2). Thirty percent of patients with autoimmune thyroid disease have concomitant parietal cell antibodies in their serum. Conversely, thyroid antibodies have been demonstrated in up to 50% of pernicious anemia patients. It should be stressed that these are not cross-reacting antibodies. The thyroid-specific antibodies will not react with stomach and vice versa. When a serum reacts with both organs it means that two populations of antibodies are present, one with specificity for thyroid and the other for stomach.

NATURE AND NURTURE

Autoimmune disorders are multifactorial

The breakdown of mechanisms required for maintaining self tolerance has a multifactorial etiology. Superimposed upon a genetically complex susceptibility, we have the influence of sex hormones and various environmental factors. Particularly important are microbial agents, which could promote the movement of autoreactive lymphocytes into infected tissues and there contribute to their activation.

Genetic factors in autoimmune disease

Autoimmune phenomena tend to aggregate in certain families. For example, the first-degree relatives (siblings, parents and children) of patients with

Table 17.1 Spectrum of autoimmune diseases.

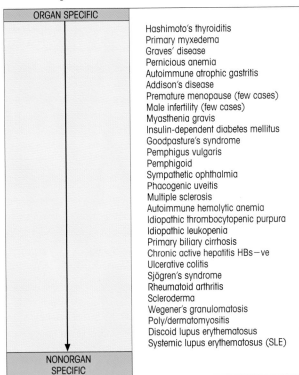

ORGAN SPECIFIC

Hashimoto's thyroiditis
Primary myxedema
Graves' disease
Pernicious anemia
Autoimmune atrophic gastritis
Addison's disease
Premature menopause (few cases)
Male infertility (few cases)
Myasthenia gravis
Insulin-dependent diabetes mellitus
Goodpasture's syndrome
Pemphigus vulgaris
Pemphigoid
Sympathetic ophthalmia
Phacogenic uveitis
Multiple sclerosis
Autoimmune hemolytic anemia
Idiopathic thrombocytopenic purpura
Idiopathic leukopenia
Primary biliary cirrhosis
Chronic active hepatitis HBs−ve
Ulcerative colitis
Sjögren's syndrome
Rheumatoid arthritis
Scleroderma
Wegener's granulomatosis
Poly/dermatomyositis
Discoid lupus erythematosus
Systemic lupus erythematosus (SLE)

NONORGAN SPECIFIC

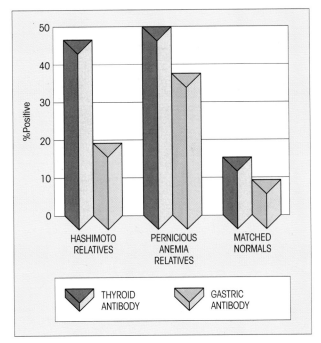

Figure 17.1 The high incidence of thyroid and gastric autoantibodies in the first-degree relatives of patients with Hashimoto's disease or pernicious anemia. Note the overlap of gastric and thyroid autoimmunity and the higher incidence of gastric autoantibodies in pernicious anemia relatives. In general, titers were much higher in patients than in controls. (Data from D. Doniach & I.M. Roitt (1964) *Seminars in Haematology*, **1**, 313.)

Table 17.2 Organ-specific and nonorgan-specific serological interrelationships in human disease.

DISEASE	% POSITIVE REACTIONS FOR ANTIBODIES TO:			
	THYROID*	STOMACH*	NUCLEI*	IgG†
Hashimoto's thyroiditis	99.9	32	8	2
Pernicious anemia	55	89	11	
Sjögren's syndrome	45	14	56	75
Rheumatoid arthritis	11	16	50	75
SLE	2	2	99	35
Controls‡	0–15	0–16	0–19	2–5

*Immunofluorescence test
†Rheumatoid factor classical tests
‡Incidence increases with age and females > males
IgG, immunoglobulin G; SLE, systemic lupus erythematosus.

Hashimoto's disease show a high incidence of thyroid autoantibodies (figure 17.1) and of overt and subclinical thyroiditis. Parallel studies have disclosed similar relationships in the families of pernicious anemia patients, in that gastric parietal cell antibodies are prevalent in relatives. There is now powerful evidence that multiple genetic components must be involved. The data on **twins** are unequivocal. When thyrotoxicosis or type I diabetes (insulin-dependent diabetes mellitus, IDDM) occurs in twins there is a far greater concordance rate (ie. both twins affected) in identical than in nonidentical twins. Furthermore, lines of animals have been bred which spontaneously develop autoimmune disease. In other words, **the autoimmunity is genetically programmed**.

Most autoimmune diseases are multigenic with patients inheriting multiple genetic polymorphisms which may vary among different ethnic populations. Dominant amongst the genetic associations with autoimmune diseases is linkage to the major histocom-

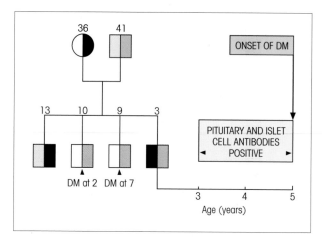

Figure 17.2 HLA-haplotype linkage and onset of insulin-dependent diabetes (DM). Haplotypes: (□) A3, B14, DR6; (■) A3, B7, DR4; (▨) A28, B51, DR4; and (▨) A2, B62, C3, DR4. Disease is linked to possession of the A2, B62, C3, DR4 haplotype. The 3-year-old brother had complement-fixing antibodies to the islet cell surface for 2 years before developing frank diabetes. (From A.N. Gorsuch, K.M. Spencer, J. Lister *et al.* (1981) *Lancet*, **ii**, 1363.)

patibility complex (MHC). Numerous examples have been described, including the association between B27 and ankylosing spondylitis, the increased risk of IDDM for DQ8 individuals, the higher incidence of DR3 in Addison's disease and of DR4 in RA (see table 15.1). Some HLA molecules are associated with protection against autoimmune disease. In IDDM some molecules are associated with susceptibility, others with protection, whereas others appear neutral. Figure 17.2 shows a multiplex family with IDDM in which the disease is closely linked to a particular HLA-haplotype.

It is not clear how particular structural variants of MHC molecules participate in autoimmunization. In fact the association may not be with the identified allele but with closely related polymorphic genes such as that encoding tumor necrosis factor (TNF) or other cytokines. For example, the gene for familial hemochromatosis, a disorder that causes severe iron overload, is tightly linked to HLA-A3 and is said to be in linkage disequilibrium with it. Similarly the association of IDDM with DR3 and DR4 is almost certainly related to the linkage disequilibrium between these DR alleles and the susceptibility genes at the DQ locus. It is possible that the MHC glycoprotein may influence the outcome of positive and negative selection within the thymus and allow immature T-cells which are reactive with particular self antigens, to escape negative selection. It is most likely, however, that a particular allelic form of the MHC molecule may have an exceptional capacity to present disease-inciting peptides to cytotoxic or helper T-cells.

Several other gene families, which encode molecules important in the immune response, may show polymorphisms that increase susceptibility to autoimmune disease. Of particular interest are allelic variants of CTLA-4 (cytotoxic T-lymphocyte antigen-4), which is normally an important inhibitor of T-cell activation. Polymorphisms have been shown in Graves' disease, RA, Addison's disease, multiple sclerosis (MS), SLE and many other autoimmune diseases. There is now interest in the association between SLE and polymorphism of the Fcγ receptor and the CD19 receptor normally present on human B-cells. There are also indications that genetic polymorphisms of cytokines, chemokines and their respective receptors could be linked to autoimmune disease; for example, chemokine or chemokine receptor gene polymorphisms might be related to susceptibility or the severity of MS. These polymorphisms may control the pattern of cytokine secretion or influence the balance of Th1/Th2 subsets, which could enhance susceptibility to autoimmune diseases. We should remember too, that congenital deficiencies of the early classical complement components predispose to vasculitis and a SLE-like syndrome.

Hormonal influences in autoimmunity

There is a general trend for autoimmune disease to occur far more frequently in women than in men (figure 17.3), probably due to differences in hormonal patterns. Although the reason for the higher incidence of autoimmune disease in females is not clear, it is known that sex hormones can affect immune responses by modifying patterns of gene expression. Females generally produce higher levels of antibodies after immune responses which are often more likely to be proinflammatory Th1 responses. Similarly, administration of male hormones to mice with SLE reduces the severity of disease. Pregnancy is often associated with amelioration of disease severity, particularly in RA, and there is sometimes a striking relapse after giving birth.

Does the environment contribute?

Twin studies

Although the 50% concordance rate for the development of the autoimmune disease IDDM in identical twins is considerably higher than that in dizygotic twins, and suggests a strong genetic element, there is still 50% unaccounted for. In nonorgan-specific diseases such as SLE there is an even lower genetic contri-

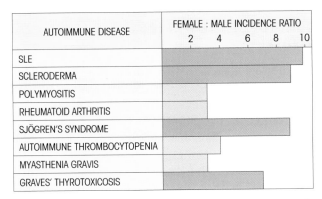

Figure 17.3 Increased incidence of autoimmune disease in females.

Table 17.3 Molecular mimicry: homologies between microbes and body components as potential cross-reacting T-cell epitopes.

Microbial molecule	Body component
Bacteria:	
Arthritogenic *Shigella flexneri*	HLA-B27
Klebsiella nitrogenase	HLA-B27
Proteus mirabilis urease	HLA-DR4
Mycobact. tuberculosis 65 kDa hsp	Joint (adjuvant arthritis)
Viruses:	
Coxsackie B	Myocardium
Coxsackie B	Glutamic acid decarboxylase
EBV gp110 }	RA shared Dw4 T-cell epitope
(*E.coli* DNAJ hsp) }	
HBV octamer	Myelin basic protein
HSV glycoprotein	Acetylcholine receptor
Measles hemagglutinin	T-cell subset
Retroviral gag p32	U-1 RNA

bution with a concordance rate of only 23% in same-sex monozygotic twins. This compares with 9% in same-sex dizygotic twins. There are also many examples where clinically unaffected relatives of patients with SLE have a higher incidence of nuclear autoantibodies if they are household contacts than if they live apart from the proband. Summing up, in some disorders the major factors are genetic, whereas in others, environmental influences seem to dominate.

Microbes

A number of autoimmune diseases following infectious episodes have been described, usually in genetically predisposed individuals. The reasons for this predisposition are not clear but a number of mechanisms have been proposed:

1 Molecular mimicry in which immune responses directed against viruses or bacteria may cross-react with self antigens (c.f. figure 17.6b(2)). Many organisms have been shown to possess antigenic determinants that are repeated in normal human tissue. For example, two envelope proteins of *Yersinia enterocolitica* share epitopes with the extracellular domain of the human thyroid-stimulating hormone (TSH) receptor. In rheumatic fever, antibodies produced to the *Streptococcus* also react with heart tissue and in the Guillain–Barré syndrome, antibodies against human gangliosides cross-react with the endotoxin of *Campylobacter jejuni*. Colon antibodies present in ulcerative colitis have been found to cross-react with *Escherichia coli* 014. There is also some evidence for the view that antigens present on *Trypanosoma cruzi* may cross-react with cardiac muscle and peripheral nervous system antigens and provoke some of the immunopathologic lesions seen in Chagas' disease.

A large number of microbial peptide sequences having varying degrees of homology with human proteins have been identified (table 17.3) but the mere existence of a homology is no certainty that infection with that organism will necessarily lead to autoimmunity.

2 Microbes may act as adjuvants. Incorporation of many autologous proteins into adjuvants frequently endows them with the power to induce autoimmune disease in laboratory animals. This indicates that autoreactive T-cells are normally present and that they can be activated when presented with suitably altered autoantigens. Microbes often display adjuvant properties through their ability to impart "danger signals" which activate dendritic antigen-presenting cells.

3 Microbes may activate lymphocytes polyclonally. For example, bacterial endotoxins can act by providing a nonspecific inductive signal for B-cell stimulation. The variety of autoantibodies detected in cases of infectious mononucleosis must surely be attributable to the polyclonal activation of B-cells by the Epstein–Barr virus (EBV) again bypassing the need for specific T-cell help. However, unlike the usual situation in human autoimmune disease, these autoantibodies tend to be immunoglobulin M (IgM) and, normally, do not persist when the microbial components are cleared from the body. In some instances microbes can act as superantigens that link CD4+ T-cells to antigen-presenting cells (APCs) through the outer surfaces of the Vβ chain and the class II MHC glycoprotein. These may bring about the polyclonal stimulation of certain T-cell receptor (TCR) Vβ families.

AUTOREACTIVITY COMES NATURALLY

It used to be thought that self–nonself discrimination was a simple matter of deleting autoreactive cells in the

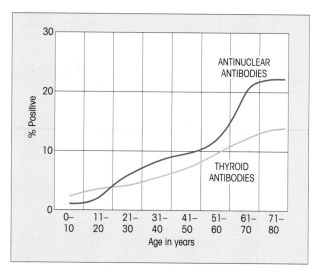

Figure 17.4 Incidence of autoantibodies in the general population. A serum was considered positive for thyroid antibodies if it reacted at a dilution of 1/10 in the tanned red cell test or neat in the immunofluorescent test, and positive for antinuclear antibodies if it reacted at a dilution of 1/4 by immunofluorescence.

thymus, but it is now clear that this mechanism does not destroy all self-reactive lymphocytes. Immune cells that recognize self proteins do exist in normal people and in the vast majority of cases produce no harm. Thus autoreactive T-cells specific for self antigens will survive in the repertoire but are not normally activated. There is also a subpopulation of B-cells that make low-affinity IgM autoantibodies. These antibodies, which do not normally cause tissue damage, are demonstrable in comparatively low titer in the general population and their incidence increases steadily with age (figure 17.4).

Is autoantigen available to the lymphocytes?

Our earliest view, with respect to organ-specific antibodies at least, was that the antigens were sequestered within the organ and, through lack of contact with the immune system, failed to establish immunologic tolerance. Any mishap that caused a release of the antigen would then provide an opportunity for autoantibody formation. For a few body constituents this holds true. In the case of sperm, lens and heart, for example, release of certain components directly into the circulation can provoke autoantibodies. In general, the experience has been that injection of *unmodified* extracts of those tissues concerned in the organ-specific autoimmune disorders does not readily elicit antibody formation.

CONTROL OF THE T-HELPER CELL IS PIVOTAL

The message then is that we are all sitting on a mine-field of self-reactive cells, with potential access to their respective autoantigens, but since autoimmune disease is more the exception than the rule, the body has homeostatic mechanisms, such as regulatory T-cells, that prevent them being triggered under normal circumstances. Accepting its limitations, figure 17.5 provides a framework for us to examine ways in which these mechanisms may be circumvented to allow autoimmunity to develop. It is assumed that the key to the system is control of the autoreactive T-helper cell since the evidence heavily favors the T-dependence of virtually all autoimmune responses; thus, interaction between the T-cell and MHC-associated peptide becomes the core consideration. We start with the assumption that these cells are unresponsive because of clonal deletion, clonal anergy, T-suppression or inadequate autoantigen presentation.

AUTOIMMUNITY CAN ARISE THROUGH BYPASS OF T-HELPERS

Provision of new carrier determinant

If autoreactive T-cells are tolerized and thereby unable to collaborate with B-cells to generate autoantibodies (figure 17.6a), provision of new carrier determinants to which no self tolerance had been established would bypass this mechanism and lead to autoantibody production (figure 17.6b). Modification can be achieved through combination with a drug (figure 17.6b(3)); for example, the autoimmune hemolytic anemia associated with administration of α-methyldopa might be attributable to modification of the red-cell surface in such a way as to provide a carrier for stimulating B-cells which recognize the rhesus antigen. Similarly, a new helper determinant may arise through the insertion of viral antigen into the membrane of an infected cell (figure 17.6b(4)).

Polyclonal activation

As indicated above, microbes such as EBV can activate B-cells in a polyclonal manner, and this has been suggested as an important mechanism for the induction of autoimmunity. It is, however, difficult to see how a pan-specific polyclonal activation could give rise to the patterns of autoantibodies characteristic of the different autoimmune disorders without the operation of some antigen-directing factor.

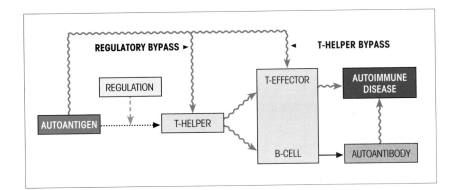

Figure 17.5 Autoimmunity arises through bypass of the control of autoreactivity. The constraints on the stimulation of self-reactive helper T-cells by autoantigen can be circumvented either through bypassing the helper cell or by disturbance of the regulatory mechanisms.

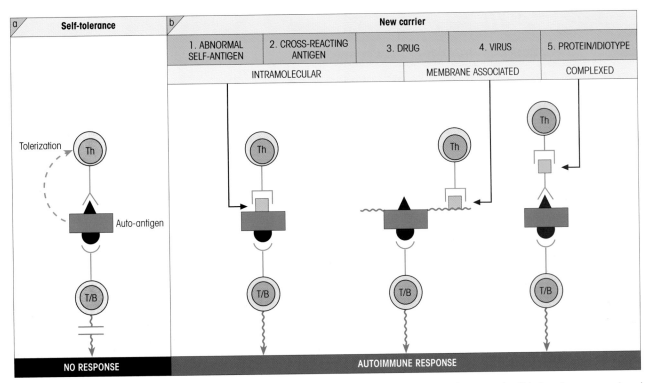

Figure 17.6 T-helper bypass through new carrier epitope (▢) generates autoimmunity. For simplicity, processing for major histocompatibility complex (MHC) association has been omitted from the diagram. (a) The pivotal autoreactive T-helper is unresponsive either through tolerance or inability to see a cryptic epitope. (b) Different mechanisms providing a new carrier epitope. Th, T-helper cell.

BYPASS OF REGULATORY MECHANISMS RESULTS IN AUTOIMMUNE DISEASE

Failure of Fas–FasL (Fas ligand) interaction

The Fas pathway normally mediates apoptosis which is a key mechanism in the down-regulation of immune responses. Failure of this interaction, resulting from either absence of Fas or of FasL, has been shown to be associated with autoimmune disease due to persistence and survival of normally deleted helper T-cells specific for self antigens. This is seen in **autoimmune lympho-**

proliferative syndrome, a human genetic disorder due to a defect in the Fas protein or the Fas receptor. Interleukin-2 (IL-2) also has an important role in the apoptosis of T-cells, and animals defective in IL-2 production or which lack the IL-2 receptor fail to undergo Fas mediated apoptosis resulting in autoimmunity.

Polymorphism of CTLA-4

We have previously indicated that CTLA-4 is important in regulating T-cell activity, and animals with knockout of the *CTLA-4* gene develop severe autoimmune disease. There is some evidence in humans that polymorphism of the *CTLA-4* gene may lead to IDDM and other autoimmune problems.

Upregulation of T-cell interaction molecules

The majority of organ-specific autoantigens normally appear on the surface of the cells of the target organ in the context of class I but not class II MHC molecules. As such they cannot communicate with T-helpers and are therefore immunologically silent. When class II genes are expressed, they endow the surface molecules with potential autoantigenicity (figure 17.7). For example, human thyroid cells in tissue culture express surface HLA-DR (class II) molecules after stimulation with interferon γ (IFNγ), and the glands of patients with Graves' disease (thyrotoxicosis) stain strongly with anti-HLA-DR reagents, indicating active synthesis of class II polypeptide chains. Inappropriate class II expression has also been reported on the bile ductules in primary biliary cirrhosis and on endothelial cells and some β-cells in the type I diabetic pancreas.

Th1–Th2 imbalance with resulting overproduction of cytokines may induce autoimmunity

Th1 responses appear to be involved in the pathogenesis of a number of organ-specific autoimmune diseases by producing large quantities of inflammatory cytokines. Under normal circumstances this overproduction can be controlled by Th2-derived cytokines, especially IL-10, which antagonizes IL-12, a cytokine crucial for the development of Th1 cells. If an imbalance exists, unregulated IL-2 and IFNγ production can initiate autoimmunity. This may occur by increasing the concentration of processed intracellular autoantigens available to professional APCs and increasing their avidity for naive T-cells by upregulating adhesion molecules, or even by making previously anergic cells responsive to antigen (figure 17.7).

Autoimmunity results from inadequate regulatory cell activity

Populations of regulatory cells must hold normally present self-reactive T-cells in check. This function is performed by CD4+CD25+ T-cells derived from the thymus, which suppress the proliferation of other T-cells. The importance of this subpopulation of T-cells is shown in animals depleted of this population, which

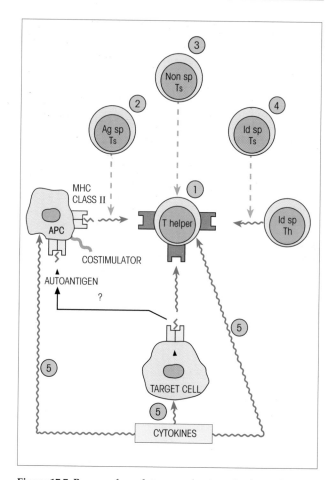

Figure 17.7 Bypass of regulatory mechanisms leads to triggering of autoreactive T-helper cells through defects in (1) tolerizability or ability to respond to or induce T-regulatory cells, or (2) expression of antigen-specific, (3) nonspecific or (4) idiotype-specific T-regulators, or through (5) imbalance of the cytokine network producing derepression of class II genes with inappropriate cellular expression of class II and presentation of antigen on target cell, stimulation of antigen-presenting cell (APC), and possible activation of anergic T-helper. Ag sp, antigen specific; Id sp, idiotype specific; MHC, major histocompatibility complex; Non sp, nonspecific; Th, T-helper cell; Ts, T-suppressor.

die of autoimmune disease. Furthermore in animal models of type I diabetes and inflammatory bowel disease, transfer of normal CD4+CD25+ cells can control the disease.

TISSUE MAY BE DAMAGED BOTH BY AUTOANTIBODIES AND BY AUTOREACTIVE T-CELLS

The tissue damage in many autoimmune diseases is produced both by humoral and cell mediated mechanisms. Autoantibodies, by activating the complement cascade may cause cytotoxicity of target tissue or they

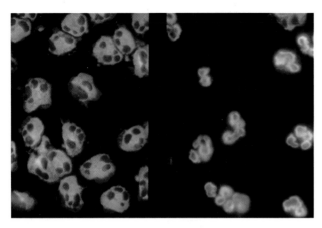

Figure 17.8 Antineutrophil cytoplasmic antibodies (ANCAs). *Left:* cytoplasmic ANCA (cANCA) diffuse staining specific for proteinase III in Wegener's granulomatosis. *Right:* perinuclear ANCA (p-ANCA) staining by myeloperoxidase antibodies in periarteritis nodosa. Fixed neutrophils are treated first with patient's serum then fluorescein-conjugated antihuman immunoglobulin. (Kindly provided by Dr G. Cambridge.)

may promote phagocytosis of target cells or antibody-dependent cellular cytotoxicity (ADCC). Some antibodies initiate damage by forming immune complexes and others interfere with the physiology of the target cell either by blocking or stimulating receptors. Autoreactive CD8+ T-cells can produce cytolysis of tissue by perforin and granzyme-B activity, and CD4+ cells amplify attack on the target by recruitment of inflammatory cells and by stimulating release of their mediators.

PATHOGENIC EFFECTS OF HUMORAL AUTOANTIBODY

Blood

Erythrocyte antibodies play a dominant role in the destruction of red cells in **autoimmune hemolytic anemia**. Normal red cells coated with autoantibody have a shortened half-life essentially as a result of their adherence to Fcγ receptors on phagocytic cells in the spleen. Lymphopenia occurring in patients with SLE and RA may also be a direct result of antibody, since nonagglutinating antibodies coating these white cells have been reported in such cases.

In **Wegener's granulomatosis** antibodies to the usually intracellular proteinase III, the so-called antineutrophil cytoplasmic antibodies (ANCAs) (figure 17.8) may react with the antigen on the surface of the cell, causing activation and resulting degranulation and generation of reactive oxygen intermediates (ROIs).

Endothelial cell injury would then be a consequence of the release of superoxide anion and other ROI.

Platelet antibodies are responsible for **idiopathic thrombocytopenic purpura (ITP)** as IgG from a patient's serum when given to a normal individual causes a decrease in the platelet count. The transient neonatal thrombocytopenia, which may be seen in infants of mothers with ITP, is explicable in terms of transplacental passage of IgG antibodies to the child.

The primary **antiphospholipid syndrome** is characterized by recurrent venous and arterial thromboembolic phenomena, recurrent fetal loss, thrombocytopenia and the presence of cardiolipin antibodies. Passive transfer of such antibodies into mice is fairly devastating, resulting in lower fecundity rates and recurrent fetal loss. The effect seems to be mediated through reaction of the autoantibodies with a complex of cardiolipin and β_2-glycoprotein 1, which inhibits triggering of the coagulation cascade, but may also activate the endothelial cells to increase prostacyclin metabolism, produce proinflammatory cytokines such as IL-6, and upregulate adhesion molecules.

Thyroid

Under certain circumstances antibodies to the surface of a cell may stimulate rather than destroy. This is the case in **Graves' disease**, which is due to the presence of antibodies to thyroid-stimulating hormone receptors (TSH-R) which act in the same manner as TSH. Both stimulate the production of thyroid hormones by activating the adenylate cyclase system after binding to the TSH-R. When thyroid-stimulating immunoglobulins (TSIs) from a mother with Graves' disease cross the placenta they cause the production of neonatal hyperthyroidism (figure 17.9), which resolves after a few weeks as the maternal IgG is catabolized.

Thyroid-stimulating immunoglobulins act independently of the pituitary–thyroid axis and patients with this form of hyperthyroidism will have very low serum TSH levels. Graves' disease is often associated with exophthalmos, which might be due to a cross-reaction of antibodies to a 64kDa membrane protein present on both thyroid and eye muscle.

Muscle

Myasthenia gravis is due to an autoantibody directed against the acetylcholine receptors (ACh-R) on the motor end-plates of muscle cells. These antibodies deplete these receptors by a combination of complement-dependent lysis of the post-synaptic membrane and by

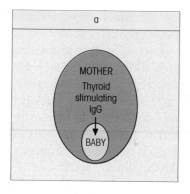
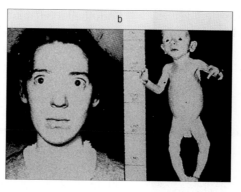

Figure 17.9 Neonatal thyrotoxicosis. (a) The autoantibodies that stimulate the thyroid through the thyroid-stimulating hormone receptors are immunoglobulins G (IgG) that cross the placenta. (b) The thyrotoxic mother therefore gives birth to a baby with thyroid hyperactivity, which spontaneously resolves as the mother's IgG is catabolized. (Photograph courtesy of Professor A. MacGregor.)

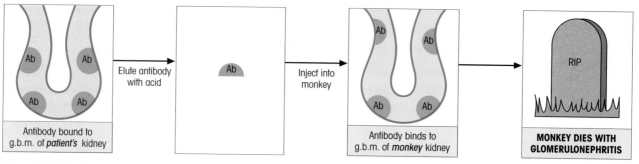

Figure 17.10 Passive transfer of glomerulonephritis to a squirrel monkey by injection of antiglomerular basement membrane (anti-g.b.m.) antibodies isolated by acid elution from the kidney of a patient with Goodpasture's syndrome. (After R.A. Lerner, R.J. Glascock & F.J. Dixon (1967) *Journal of Experimental Medicine*, **126**, 989.) Ab, antibody.

blocking ACh-R function. This results in inhibition of acetylcholine binding and muscular weakness. The transient muscle weakness seen in a proportion of babies born to mothers with myasthenia gravis is compatible with the transplacental passage of an IgG capable of inhibiting neuromuscular transmission. In addition, myasthenic symptoms can be induced in animals by injection of monoclonal antibodies to ACh-R or by active immunization with the purified receptors themselves.

Glomerular basement membrane (g.b.m.)

Goodpasture's syndrome is an autoimmune disease characterized by progressive glomerulonephritis and pulmonary hemorrhage. As with many other autoimmune disorders it is restricted by the MHC. Susceptibility is increased by HLA-DRβ1*1501 and DRβ1*1502. It is due to antibodies directed against the α3.α4.α5(IV) component of type IV collagen, the major component of basement membrane in the lungs and the glomeruli. These antibodies can be detected by immunofluorescent staining of kidney biopsies that show *linear* deposition of IgG and C3 along the basement membrane of

the glomerular capillaries (see figure 14.9a; p. 156). If the antibody is eluted from a diseased kidney and injected into a squirrel monkey it rapidly fixes to type IV collagen on the g.b.m. of the recipient animal and produces a fatal nephritis (figure 17.10).

Heart

Neonatal lupus erythematosus is the most common cause of permanent **congenital complete heart block**. Almost all cases have been associated with high maternal titers of anti-Ro/SS-A antibodies. The key observation is that anti-Ro binds to neonatal rather than adult cardiac tissue and alters the transmembrane action potential by inhibiting repolarization. Immunoglobulin G anti-Ro reaches the fetal circulation by transplacental passage but although maternal and fetal hearts are exposed to the autoantibody, only the latter is affected.

The ability of β-hemolytic streptococci to elicit cross-reactive autoantibodies which damage heart muscle underlies the pathogenesis of acute rheumatic fever. Although antibodies to the streptolysin O exotoxin (ASO) are found in low titer in many patients following streptococcal infection, high and increasing titers are strongly suggestive of acute rheumatic fever. Although molecular mimicry initiates the production of cross-reacting antibodies, CD4 lymphocytes, cytokines and adhesion molecules also play a crucial role in the pathogenesis of this disease.

Stomach

Pernicious anemia, which manifests as a deficiency of vitamin B12, is an autoimmune disease of the stomach commonly due to autoantibodies directed against gastric parietal cells (parietal cell antibodies). The relevant antigen on these cells is the gastric adenosine triphosphatase (ATPase), which is the major protein of the membrane lining the secretory canaliculi of parietal cells. Patients develop an atrophic gastritis in which a chronic inflammatory mononuclear invasion is associated with degeneration of secretory glands and failure to produce gastric acid. In many patients additional abnormal antibodies may be directed against the B12-binding site of intrinsic factor or to the intrinsic factor-B12 complex so blocking the uptake of B12 into the body.

Other tissues

Many other organ-specific autoimmune diseases are associated with specific antibodies directed to those organs. Patients with idiopathic Addison's disease have circulating antibodies to adrenal antigens and the serum of patients with idiopathic hypoparathyroidism contains antibodies to cytoplasmic antigens of parathyroid cells. Women with premature ovarian failure may show antibodies to the cytoplasm of cells of the ovary and in some **infertile males**, agglutinating antibodies cause aggregation of the spermatozoa and interfere with their penetration into the cervical mucus. An antibody pathogenesis for **pemphigus vulgaris** is favored by the recognition of an autoantigen on stratified squamous epithelial cells. Antibodies to this keratinocyte transmembrane adhesion molecule are easily seen on direct immunofluorescent microscopy of affected skin.

PATHOGENIC EFFECTS OF COMPLEXES WITH AUTOANTIGENS

Systemic lupus erythematosus (SLE)

Systemic lupus erythematosus is a relapsing and remitting multisystem disease where autoantibodies are formed against soluble components to which they have continual access. The complexes that are gener-

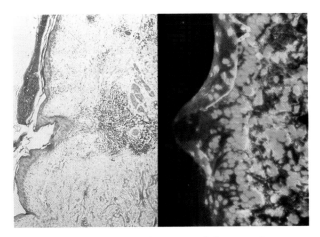

Figure 17.11 The "lupus band" in systemic lupus erythematosus. *Left*: section of skin showing slight thickening of the dermo-epidermal junction with underlying scattered inflammatory cells and a major inflammatory focus in the deeper layers. Low power H & E. *Right*: green fluorescent staining of a skin biopsy at higher power showing deposition of complexes containing immunoglobulin G (anti-C3 gives the same picture) on the basement membrane at the dermo-epidermal junction. (Kindly provided by Professor D. Isenberg.)

ated give rise to lesions similar to those occurring in serum sickness. A variety of different autoantigens are present in lupus, many of them within the nucleus, with the most pathognomonic being **double-stranded DNA (dsDNA)**. The detection of antinuclear antibodies (ANAs) and particularly the measurement of anti-DNA antibodies are valuable tests for the diagnosis of SLE. Deposition of complexes is widespread, as the name implies, and lesions are often present in the kidney, skin, joints, muscle, lung and brain (figure 17.11). About 40% of patients eventually develop kidney involvement and eluates of renal tissue from patients with lupus nephritis will show anti-dsDNA. Immunofluorescent staining of kidney biopsies from patients with evidence of renal dysfunction will show the presence of antigen-antibody complexes and complement. The staining pattern with a fluorescent anti-IgG or anti-C3 is punctate or "lumpy-bumpy" (see figure 14.9b; p. 156), in marked contrast with the linear pattern caused by the g.b.m. antibodies in Goodpasture's syndrome (figure 14.9a; p. 156). Patients with SLE produce antibodies to a variety of tissue antigens including those on red cells, platelets, lymphocytes and various clotting factors. During the active phase of the disease, serum complement levels fall as components are binding to immune aggregates in the kidney and circulation.

It is worth recalling that normal clearance of immune complexes requires an intact classical complement cascade and that absence of an early complement protein predisposes to immune complex disease. Thus, although homozygous complement deficiency is a rare cause of SLE—the archetypal immune complex disorder—it represents the most powerful disease susceptibility genotype so far identified as more than 80% of cases with homozygous C1q and C4 deficiency develop an SLE-like disease.

T-CELL-MEDIATED HYPERSENSITIVITY AS A PATHOGENIC FACTOR IN AUTOIMMUNE DISEASE

Insulin-dependent diabetes mellitus (IDDM)

Insulin-dependent diabetes mellitus (type I diabetes) is a multifactorial autoimmune disease the major feature of which is a T-cell infiltration of the islets of Langerhans and progressive **T-cell-mediated destruction** of insulin-producing β-cells. Auto-reactive T-cells specific for β-cell antigens such as glutamic acid decarboxylase (GAD) and insulin can be identified in the blood of newly diagnosed diabetic patients. Autoantibodies specific for the same antigens can also be detected in the serum of patients and can be used as a sensitive marker to predict the risk of developing the disease (see figure 17.2; p. 192). It is not clear if these antibodies are the result of T-cell-mediated injury or if they play some role in the causation of the disease. Delay in onset of disease can be achieved by early treatment with cyclosporin, since this drug targets T-cell cytokine synthesis so specifically. The disease has a strong genetic basis and is associated with genes within the MHC, particularly the *DR3.DQ2* and the *DR4.DQ8* haplotypes, and with polymorphisms within the insulin gene region on chromosome 11p15.5.

Multiple sclerosis (MS)

Multiple sclerosis is an autoimmune disorder of the central nervous system mediated by T-cells directed at central nervous system myelin components occurring in individuals with certain class II MHC alleles. The T-cells recognize and attack components of the axonal myelin sheath resulting in destruction of myelin and the underlying axon. The idea that MS could be an autoimmune disease has for long been predicated on the morphological resemblance to experimental allergic encephalomyelitis (EAE). This is a demyelinating disease leading to motor paralysis, which can be produced by immunizing experimental animals with MBP (myelin basic protein) in complete Freund's adjuvant or by transferring Th1-cells from an affected to a naive animal. In human MS damage to the myelin is produced by Th1-cytokines such as TNF and IFNγ and by activated macrophages, which phagocytose myelin constituents. In addition cytotoxic T-cells may directly damage myelin and antibodies directed against myelin constituents can cause demyelination by ADCC, myelin opsonization or complement activation. Antibodies against MBP and MOG (myelin oligodendrocyte glycoprotein) are found in these patients and are associated with more frequent relapses and a worse prognosis. Another feature of MS is the presence of oligoclonal Igs in the cerebrospinal fluid (CSF) of patients: their specificity and significance in the pathogenesis of the disease remains unknown. Although the etiology of MS is unknown, molecular mimicry may play a role. It is of interest that a T-cell clone derived from a patient with the disease, reacted against both MBP and an antigen found in EBV.

Rheumatoid arthritis (RA)

Immunopathogenesis

Rheumatoid arthritis is a common destructive arthropathy of unknown etiology, strongly linked to the MHC class II proteins HLA-DRB1*0404 and *0401. The joint changes are produced by the hyperplasia of the synovial cells associated with increased vascularity and infiltration of inflammatory cells forming a pannus overlaying and destroying cartilage and bone (figure 17.12). The infiltrating cells are primarily CD4+ T-cells, which stimulate monocytes, macrophages and mast cells to secrete IL-1, IL-6, TNF and a variety of chemokines, which recruit neutrophils into the joints. The IL-1 and TNF in the synovium stimulate fibroblasts and chondrocytes to release tissue-destroying proteolytic enzymes which lead to joint damage, and bone destruction follows the stimulation of osteoclasts by these cytokines. As the malign pannus (cover) grows over the cartilage, tissue breakdown can be seen at the margin (figure 17.12c), almost certainly as a result of the release of enzymes, ROIs and especially of IL-1, IL-6 and TNF. B-cells are also activated and plasma cells are frequently observed. Secondary lymphoid follicles with germinal centers may be present in the synovium. Immune complexes of rheumatoid factor and IgG may initiate an Arthus reaction in the joint space leading to an influx of polymorphs. By releasing elastase, collagenase and proteases these cells add to the joint destruction by degrading proteoglycan in the superficial layer of cartilage (figure 17.13).

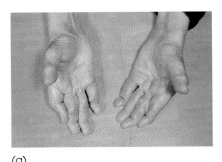

(a)

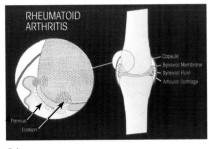

(b)

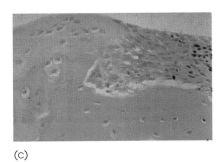

(c)

Figure 17.12 Rheumatoid arthritis (RA). (a) Hands of a patient with chronic RA showing classical swan-neck deformities. (b) Diagrammatic representation of a diarthrodial joint showing bone and cartilaginous erosions beneath the synovial membrane-derived pannus.

(c) Histology of pannus showing clear erosion of bone and cartilage at the cellular margin. ((a) Kindly given by Professor D. Isenberg; (c) by Dr L.E. Glynn.)

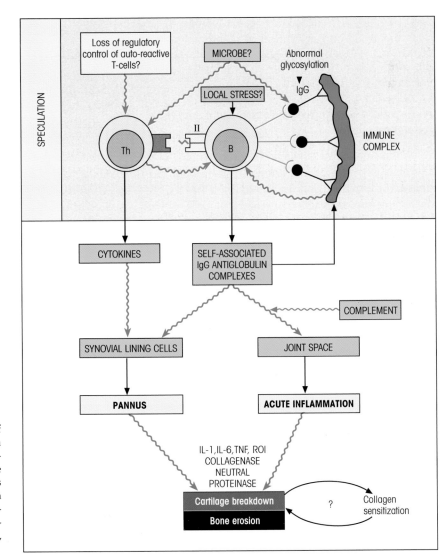

Figure 17.13 Immune pathogenesis of rheumatoid arthritis and speculation on the induction of autoimmunity. The identity of the peptide(s) associated with the class II molecule is unknown. Green arrows indicate stimulation. Black arrows mean "becomes" or "leads to." IgG, immunoglobulin G; IL, interleukin; Th, T-helper cell; TNF, tumor necrosis factor; ROI, reactive oxygen intermediate.

Rheumatoid arthritis can be successfully treated with anticytokine therapy or by blocking T-cell activation

Now that the central role of cytokines in RA is appreciated, a number of anticytokine therapies have been developed. These include a soluble TNF receptor-IgG1 fusion protein (Etanercept) which neutralizes free TNF, and a chimeric monoclonal antibody against TNF itself (Infliximab). By blocking TNF activity, its ability to activate the cytokine cascade of IL-1, IL-6, IL-8 and other inflammatory cytokines is impeded, making this a valuable adjunct to the treatment of RA. Another approach is to block the activation of CD28 on T-cells using a fusion protein made up of CTLA-4 and IgG1. This competes with CD28 for binding to B7.1 (CD80) and B7.2 (CD86) and prevents T-cell activation. By acting so early in the inflammatory cascade CTLA4Ig inhibits the secondary activation of macrophages and B-cells and shows considerable promise in treating patients with RA.

Immunoglobulin G autosensitization and immune complex formation

Autoantibodies to the IgG Fc region, which is abnormally glycosylated, are known as antiglobulins or **rheumatoid factors**, and are the hallmark of the disease, being demonstrable in virtually all patients with RA. The majority are IgM antiglobulins, the detection of which provides a very useful clinical test for RA.

Immunoglobulin G aggregates, presumably products of the infiltrating plasma cells which synthesize self-associating IgG antiglobulins, can be regularly detected in the synovial tissues and in the joint fluid where they give rise to typical acute inflammatory reactions with fluid exudates.

Crohn's disease

Crohn's disease is a chronic granulomatous inflammatory bowel disease which is a complex disorder with immunologic, environmental and genetic components. The etiology is not known but it has been suggested that it is an autoimmune disease; patients produce antibodies to a variety of organisms, and 70% have antibodies to the yeast *Saccharomyces cerevisiae*. The detection of antibodies forms a useful test in the diagnosis of Crohn's disease. The lesions in the bowel are characterized by infiltration of mononuclear cells with increased production of inflammatory cytokines including TNF, IL-1, IL-6 and IL-12. A gene on chromosome 16, called *NOD2*, confers susceptibility to the

disease and a polymorphism of this gene is an important genetic risk factor. It has been suggested that the NOD2 protein has a role in apoptosis which normally regulates the lymphocyte populations and terminates immune responses. Defective apoptosis is one of the features of lamina propria T-cells in patients with Crohn's disease. This results in uncontrolled activation of Th1 cells, with release of IL-12, IFNγ and IL-2, and subsequent activation of monocytes, which respond by releasing TNF and other mediators of inflammation. Indeed neutralization of TNF with the TNF neutralizing antibody, Infliximab, is associated with dramatic clinical responses. This human–mouse chimeric antibody not only has an antiinflammatory effect but may increase apoptosis of lamina propria T-cells.

Celiac disease

The normally acquired tolerance to dietary proteins seems to break down in celiac disease. This is a condition due to an inappropriate T-cell response to the gliadin fraction of ingested gluten. The disease is associated with DQ2 in over 90% of cases and with DQ8 in the rest of the cases. Ingestion of gliadin leads to infiltration of the intestinal mucosa by both CD4+ and CD8+ cells. Patients develop immune responses to gliadin and to a component of the endomysium identified as tissue transglutaminase (TTG). The presence of antibodies, both IgA and IgG, against TTG are both specific and diagnostic for celiac disease.

Chronic autoimmune (Hashimoto's) thyroiditis

T-cells play a crucial role in the development of Hashimoto's thyroiditis, interacting with thyroid follicular cells and extracellular matrix. T-cells may become activated either by molecular mimicry against an infectious agent or by interacting with class II MHC molecules aberrantly present on thyroid cells from these patients. Direct killing of thyroid cells by CD8+ cells is responsible for the hypothyroidism but cytokine secretion may also play a role. Patients also develop serum antibodies to thyroid peroxidase and thyroglobulin but a role for these autoantibodies in the causation or the perpetuation of the disease has not been defined. Titers of these antibodies are closely associated with disease activity but it is not clear whether immune responses to these autoantigens initiate thyroiditis or are secondary to T-cell mediated tissue damage.

We see now that there is considerable diversity in the autoimmune response to the thyroid. This may lead to

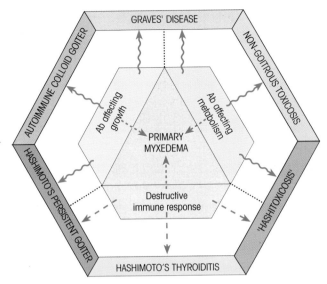

Figure 17.14 Relationship of different autoimmune responses to the circular spectrum of autoimmune thyroid disease. Hashitoxicosis refers to a thyroid which shows Hashimoto's thyroiditis and thyrotoxicosis simultaneously. (Courtesy of Professors D. Doniach and G.F. Bottazzo.) Ab, antibody.

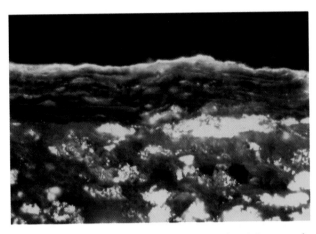

Figure 17.15 Expression of heat-shock protein 60 in an early human arteriosclerotic lesion. Frozen, unfixed, 4 µm thick section of a fatty streak (= early lesion) of a human carotid artery stained in indirect immunofluorescence with a monoclonal antibody to heat-shock protein 60 and a fluorescein-labeled second antibody. A strong reaction with endothelial cells as well as cells infiltrating the intima, including foam cells, is evident. (Original magnification ×400.) (Photograph kindly provided by Professor G. Wick.)

tissue destruction, metabolic stimulation, growth promotion or mitotic inhibition, which in different combinations account for the variety of forms in which autoimmune thyroid disease presents (figure 17.14).

Atherosclerosis

Cells of the immune system and the numerous inflammatory mediators that they produce are important in the initiation, growth and even rupture of atherosclerotic plaques. The targets of the postulated autoimmune attack are epitopes produced by oxidation of low-density lipoproteins (LDLs) which have accumulated in the intima of the vessel. The modified LDLs stimulate endothelial cells to develop adhesion molecules for lymphocytes and monocytes and also activate the intimal smooth muscle to produce cytokines including IL-1, TNF, IL-6, IL-18, IFNγ and macrophage colony-stimulating factor (M-CSF). Endothelial cells release chemokines, which attract leukocytes to the area, and as a result monocytes and T-cells infiltrate the vessel wall. The monocytes become activated by cytokines such as M-CSF and actively ingest the modified LDL particles becoming so-called foam cells. There is also some evidence that heat shock proteins (HSP) and especially the 60 kDa family could be the culprit autoantigens in the development of early atherosclerosis (figure 17.15). These proteins are found both on endothelial cells and on a number of microorganisms such as *Chlamydia* and *Escherichia coli* and may

facilitate immunological cross-reactions between pathogen and self HSP60. The ultimate result is the continued recruitment of T-cells and macrophages, which together form the fatty streaks which are the earliest manifestations of atherosclerosis. Further cytokine production causes proliferation and migration of smooth muscle cells and atherosclerotic plaques, which can interfere with blood flow or can rupture causing an acute coronary obstruction.

Psoriasis

Psoriasis is primarily a T-cell-mediated inflammatory disease where **keratinocyte hyperproliferation** is driven by proinflammatory Th1 cytokines produced locally by infiltrating T-cells. Activated T-cells within psoriatic lesions elaborate many cytokines, including IFNγ, TNF, IL-1, and IL-2, but only low levels of Th2 cytokines such as IL-4 and IL-10 are present. The nature and location of the initiating antigen is unknown. The crucial role of T-cells is proven by the variety of anti-T-cell biologic agents, which are effective in treating these patients. These include use of CTLA-4Ig, a recombinant fusion protein of CTLA-4 and IgG, which blocks T-cell activation or the use of antibodies against CD4 or against the IL-2 receptor (Daclizumab). Improvement in clinical psoriasis has also been shown using Etanercept, which targets TNF, and Efalizumab, which targets the adhesion molecule LFA-1. Even more exciting is the use of recombinant human IL-4 to

Table 17.4 Autoimmunity tests and diagnosis.

DISEASE	ANTIBODY	COMMENT
Hashimoto's thyroiditis	Thyroid	Distinction from colloid goiter, thyroid cancer and subacute thyroiditis Thyroidectomy usually unnecessary in Hashimoto goiter
Primary myxedema	Thyroid	Tests +ve in 99% of cases.
Thyrotoxicosis	Thyroid	High titers of cytoplasmic Ab indicate active thyroiditis and tendency to post-operative myxedema: anti-thyroid drugs are the treatment of choice although HLA-B8 patients have high chance of relapse
Pernicious anemia	Stomach	Help in diagnosis of latent PA, in differential diagnosis of non-autoimmune megaloblastic anemia and in suspected subacute combined degeneration of the cord
Insulin-dependent diabetes mellitus (IDDM)	Pancreas	Insulin Ab early in disease. GAD Ab standard test for IDDM. Two or more autoAb seen in 80% of new onset children or prediabetic relatives but not in controls
Idiopathic adrenal atrophy	Adrenal	Distinction from tuberculous form
Myasthenia gravis	Muscle ACh receptor	When positive suggests associated thymoma (more likely if HLA-B12), positive in >80%
Pemphigus vulgaris and pemphigoid	Skin	Different fluorescent patterns in the two diseases
Autoimmune hemolytic anemia	Erythrocyte (Coombs' test)	Distinction from other forms of anemia
Sjögren's syndrome	Salivary duct cells, SS-A, SS-B	
Primary biliary cirrhosis	Mitochondrial	Distinction from other forms of obstructive jaundice where test rarely +ve Recognize subgroup within cryptogenic cirrhosis related to PBC with +ve mitochondrial Ab
Active chronic hepatitis	Smooth muscle anti-nuclear and 20% mitochondrial	Smooth muscle Ab distinguish from SLE Type 1 classical in women with Ab to nuclei, smooth muscle, actin and asialoglycoprotein receptor. Type 2 in girls and young women with anti-LKM-1 (cyt P450)
Rheumatoid arthritis	Antiglobulin, e.g. SCAT and latex fixation Antiglobulin + raised agalacto-Ig	High titer indicative of bad prognosis Prognosis of rheumatoid arthritis
SLE	High titer antinuclear, DNA Phospholipid	DNA antibodies present in active phase. Ab to double-stranded DNA characteristic; high affinity complement-fixing Ab give kidney damage, low affinity CNS lesions Thrombosis, recurrent fetal loss and thrombocytopenia
Scleroderma	Nucleolar	Characterization of the disease
Wegener's granulomatosis	Neutrophil cytoplasm	Antiserine protease closely associated with disease; treatment urgent

Ab, antibody; CNS, central nervous sytem; GAD, glutamic acid decarboxylase; Ig, immunoglobulin; PA, pernicious anemia; SLE, systemic lupus erythematosus.

convert the Th1 to a Th2 response resulting in significant clinical improvement.

DIAGNOSTIC VALUE OF AUTOANTIBODY TESTS

Serum autoantibodies frequently provide valuable diagnostic markers, and the salient information is summarized in table 17.4. These tests may prove of value in screening for people at risk, for example relatives of patients with autoimmune diseases such as diabetes, thyroiditis patients for gastric autoimmunity and vice versa, and ultimately the general population if the sociological consequences are fully understood and acceptable.

TREATMENT OF AUTOIMMUNE DISORDERS

Control at the target organ level

The major approach to treatment, not unnaturally, involves manipulation of immunologic responses (fig-

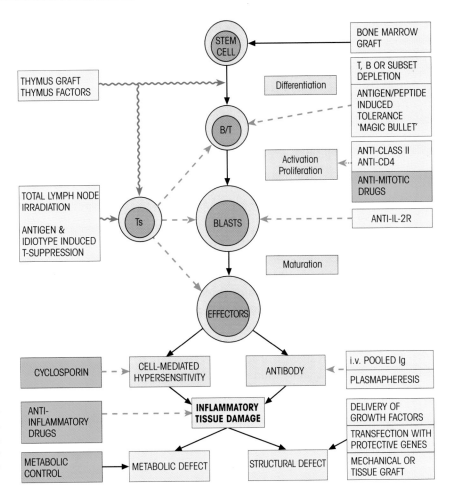

Figure 17.16 The treatment of autoimmune disease. Current conventional treatments are in dark orange; some feasible approaches are given in lighter orange boxes. (In the case of a live graft, bottom right, the immunosuppressive therapy used may protect the tissue from the autoimmune damage which affected the organ being replaced.) Ig, immunoglobulin; IL, interleukin; i.v., intravenous; Ts, T-suppressor.

ure 17.16). However, in many organ-specific diseases, metabolic control is usually sufficient, for example thyroxine replacement in primary myxedema, insulin in juvenile diabetes, vitamin B12 in pernicious anemia and anti-thyroid drugs for Graves' disease. Xenografts of genetically engineered fetal or neonatal pig tissue such as islet cells are under study, and stem cells are being differentiated in culture to produce a variety of tissues that could be used to replace destroyed tissues.

Anti-inflammatory drugs

Corticosteroids have long been used to treat autoimmune diseases as they not only suppress various aspects of the immune response but also control the inflammatory lesions and particularly the influx of neutrophils and other phagocytic cells. Patients with severe myasthenic symptoms respond well to high doses of steroids, and the same is true for serious cases of other autoimmune disorders such as SLE and immune complex nephritis. In RA, steroids are very effective and accelerate the induction of remission.

Selectins, leukocyte integrins and adhesion molecules on endothelial cells appear to be downregulated as a result of treatment and this seriously impedes the influx of inflammatory cells into the joint.

Immunosuppressive drugs

Because it blocks cytokine secretion by T-cells, cyclosporin is an anti-inflammatory drug and, since cytokines like IL-2 are also obligatory for lymphocyte proliferation, cyclosporin is also an antimitotic drug. It is of proven efficacy in a variety of autoimmune diseases, as are the conventional nonspecific antimitotic agents such as azathioprine, cyclophosphamide and methotrexate, usually given in combination with steroids. The general immunosuppressive effect of these agents, however, places the patients at much greater risk from infections.

Plasmapheresis

Successful results have been obtained in a number of

autoimmune diseases, especially when the treatment has been applied in combination with antimitotic drugs. However, plasma exchange to remove the abnormal antibodies and lower the rate of immune complex deposition in SLE provides only temporary benefit.

T-cell control strategies

A range of options is presented in figure 17.17.

Idiotype control with antibody

The powerful immunosuppressive action of anti-idiotype antibodies suggests that it may be useful in controlling autoantibody production. In a number of autoimmune diseases **intravenous injection of Ig pooled from many normal donors** is of benefit and in some conditions is the treatment of choice. The pooled Ig is not only a source of antiidiotype antibodies, which can interact with the idiotype of autoantibodies, but it contains antibodies against numerous cytokines and also has significant anti-inflammatory effects. The effects of intravenous Ig reflect the numerous functions of natural antibodies in maintaining immune homeostasis in healthy individuals.

T-cell vaccination

If we regard autoreactive T-cells as tissue-destroying pathogens, it becomes clear that these T-cells if rendered inactive may be employed as vaccines to prevent and perhaps treat the disease. Administration of such autologous T-cells may induce the regulatory network to specifically control destructive T-cells, and such an approach has been successfully employed to control EAE in experimental animals. Trials in MS using a TCR peptide vaccine embodying the Vβ5.2 sequence expressed on T-cells specific for MBP show promise (figure 17.17(5)).

Manipulation of regulatory mediators

In most solid organ-specific autoimmune diseases it is the Th1 cells that are pathogenic, and attempts to switch the phenotype to Th2 should be beneficial (figure 17.17(1)). Administration of IL-4, which deviates the immune response from Th1 to Th2, has been shown in EAE to downregulate or inhibit the destructive T-cell process. Interferon β inhibits the synthesis of IFNγ and has a number of suppressive effects on T-cell-mediated inflammation. These regulatory activities provide the basis for the therapeutic use of IFNβ in MS,

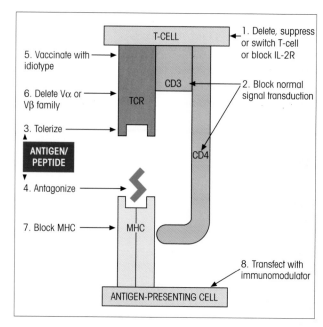

Figure 17.17 Strategic options for therapy based on T-cell targeting. IL, interleukin; MHC, major histocompatibility complex; TCR, T-cell receptor.

where it significantly reduces both the frequency and the severity of the clinical exacerbations and is considered the first drug proven to improve the natural course of the disease.

Manipulation by antigen

The object is to present the offending antigen in sufficient concentration and in a form that will occupy the antigen-binding cleft on MHC molecules to prevent binding by the autoantigen. One strategy is to design high-affinity peptide analogs differing by only one amino acid, which bind to the appropriate MHC molecule and antagonize the response to autoantigen (figure 17.17(4)). Since we express several different MHC molecules, this should not impair microbial defenses unduly.

We have already noted that, because the mucosal surface of the gut is exposed to a horde of powerfully immunogenic microorganisms, it has been important for the immune defenses of the gut to evolve mechanisms which deter Th1-type responses. This objective is attained by the stimulation of cells which release immunosuppressive cytokines. Thus, feeding antigens should tolerize Th1 cells and this has proved to be a successful strategy for blocking EAE and other experimental autoimmune diseases. Regrettably, attempts to induce oral tolerance in humans have not met with success.

The tolerogen can also be delivered by inhalation of peptide aerosols and this could be a very attractive way of generating antigen-specific T-cell suppression. Intranasal peptides have been used successfully to block various experimental autoimmune diseases, and treatment can be effective even after induction of disease.

Other biological agents that inhibit the immune response

A variety of monoclonal antibodies have been produced which, based upon the "magic bullet" concept, selectively home onto lymphocytes bearing specific surface receptors. A number of these antibodies and other forms of biological inhibitors are being tested for the treatment of autoimmune diseases. Their mechanisms of action include:
• Blockade of TNF with a specific monoclonal antibody (Infliximab) or a TNF receptor-IgG1 fusion protein (Etanercept).
• Blockade of IL-1 receptors with a recombinant IL-1-receptor antagonist.
• Blockade of leukocyte recruitment to tissues using chemokine receptor or chemokine antagonists. This form of therapy could target inflammation in an organ specific manner. For example CTACK (CCL27) and its receptor CCR10 are important for the homing of T-cells into the skin but not into other organs. Blocking of this response could be useful in psoriasis and should spare the rest of the immune system.
• CTLA-4Ig, a recombinant fusion protein consisting of CTLA-4 linked to the constant region of IgG, which blocks T-cell activation and turns down primary and secondary antibody responses.
• Blockade of CD4 with a fully human anti-CD4 monoclonal antibody.
• Blockade of the IL-2 receptor CD25 (Daclizumab). Such an antibody targets only activated T-cells and does not affect the overall immune responsiveness of the recipient.
• Blockade of adhesion molecules such as LFA-1, annexin-1 and VAP-1 (vascular adhesion protein-1).
• Antibodies against the CD40 ligand.
• Inhibitors of cell signaling pathways.
• Stem cell transplantation, with a view to restoring homeostasis and regulatory cells.

REVISION

The immune system balances precariously between effective responses to environmental antigens and regulatory control of potentially suicidal attack against self molecules.

The scope of autoimmune diseases
• Autoimmunity is associated with certain diseases which form a spectrum. At one pole, exemplified by Hashimoto's thyroiditis, the autoantibodies and the lesions are organ-specific with the organ acting as the target for autoimmune attack; at the other pole are the nonorgan-specific or systemic autoimmune diseases such as SLE, where the autoantibodies have widespread reactivity and the lesions resemble those of serum sickness relating to deposition of circulating immune complexes.
• There is a tendency for organ-specific disorders such as thyroiditis and pernicious anemia to overlap in given individuals, while overlap of rheumatologic disorders is greater than expected by chance.

Genetic and environmental influences
• Multifactorial genetic factors increase the likelihood of developing autoimmune disease: these include HLA tissue type, predisposition to aggressive autoimmunity and the selection of potential autoantigens.
• Females have a far higher incidence of autoimmunity than males, perhaps due to hormonal influences.
• Twin studies indicate a strong environmental influence in many disorders; both microbial and nonmicrobial factors have been suspected.
• Microbes may initiate autoimmune disease by a number of mechanisms, including molecular mimicry, or by acting as adjuvants or superantigens, or as polyclonal activators of the immune response.

Autoreactivity comes naturally
• Autoantigens are, for the most part, accessible to circulating lymphocytes which normally include autoreactive T- and B-cells. These autoreactive cells are controlled by regulatory CD4$^+$CD25$^+$ T-cells and absence of this population results in autoimmunity.

The T-helper is pivotal for control
• It is assumed that the key to the system is control of autoreactive T-helper cells which are normally unrespon-

(continued)

Table 17.5 Direct pathogenic effects of humoral antibodies.

DISEASE	AUTOANTIGEN	LESION
Autoimmune hemolytic anemia	Red cell	Erythrocyte destruction
Lymphopenia (some cases)	Lymphocyte	Lymphocyte destruction
Idiopathic thrombocytopenic purpura	Platelet	Platelet destruction
Wegener's granulomatosis	PMN proteinase III	PMN induced endothelial injury
Anti-phospholipid syndrome	Cardiolipin/$\beta2$–glycoprotein 1 complex	Recurrent thromboembolic phenomena
Male infertility (some cases)	Sperm	Agglutination of spermatozoa
Pernicious anemia	H^+/K^+-ATPase, gastrin receptor Intrinsic factor	Block acid production Block vitamin B12 uptake
Hashimoto's disease	Thyroid peroxidase surface antigen	Cytotoxic effect on thyroid cells in culture
Primary myxedema	TSH receptor	Blocking of thyroid cell
Graves' disease	TSH receptor	Stimulation of thyroid cell
Goodpasture's syndrome	Glomerular basement membrane	Complement-mediated damage to basement membrane
Myasthenia gravis	Acetylcholine receptor	Blocking and destruction of receptors
Lambert–Eton syndrome	Presynaptic Ca channel	Neuromuscular defect
Acanthosis nigricans (type B) and ataxia telangiectasia with insulin resistance	Insulin receptor	Blocking of receptors
Atopic allergy (some cases)	β-Adrenergic receptors	Blocking of receptors
Congenital heart block	Ro/SS-A	Distort fetal cardiac membrane action potential
Celiac disease	Endomysium	Small intestinal inflammation

ATPase, adenosine triphosphatase; PMN, polymorphonuclear neutrophil; TSH, thyroid-stimulating hormone.

sive because of clonal deletion, clonal anergy, T-suppression or inadequate autoantigen processing.

Autoimmunity can arise through bypass of T-helpers
• Abnormal modification of the autoantigen through synthesis or breakdown, combination with a drug or cross-reaction with exogenous antigens, can provide new carrier determinants, which can activate T-cells.
• B-cells and T-cells can be stimulated directly by polyclonal activators such as EBV or superantigens.
• Failure of the Fas–FasL (Fas ligand) interaction can result in survival of normally deleted T-cells. Interleukin-2 (IL-2) besides its important activation function is also crucial for apoptosis, and absence of IL-2 or its receptor may lead to autoimmunity.

Autoimmunity can arise through bypass of regulatory mechanisms
• The derepression of class II genes could give rise to inappropriate cellular expression of class II so breaking the "silence" between cellular autoantigen and autoreactive T-inducer.

• Th1–Th2 imbalance may result in overproduction of inflammatory cytokines.

Pathogenic effects of humoral autoantibody
• Direct pathogenic effects of human autoantibodies to blood, surface receptors and several other tissues are listed in table 17.5.
• Passive transfer of disease is seen in "experiments of nature" in which transplacental passage of maternal immunoglobulin G (IgG) autoantibody produces a comparable but transient disorder in the fetus.

Pathogenic effects of complexes with autoantigens
• Immune complexes, usually with bound complement, appear in the kidneys, skin and joints of patients with systemic lupus erythematosus (SLE), associated with lesions in the corresponding organs.

T-cell-mediated hypersensitivity as a pathogenic factor
• Type 1 diabetes mellitus (IDDM) has a strong genetic basis linked to MHC class II genes. T-cell destruction of insulin-producing cells is the basis of the disease but

Table 17.6 Comparison of organ-specific and nonorgan-specific diseases.

ORGAN-SPECIFIC (e.g. THYROIDITIS, GASTRITIS, ADRENALITIS)	NONORGAN-SPECIFIC (e.g. SYSTEMIC LUPUS ERYTHEMATOSUS)
DIFFERENCES	
Antigens only available to lymphoid system in low concentration	Antigens accessible at higher concentrations
Antibodies and lesions organ-specific	Antibodies and lesions nonorgan-specific
Clinical and serologic overlap – thyroiditis, gastritis and adrenalitis	Overlap SLE, rheumatoid arthritis, and other connective tissue disorders
Familial tendency to organ-specific autoimmunity	Familial connective tissue disease
Lymphoid invasion, parenchymal destruction by cell-mediated hypersensitivity and/or antibodies	Lesions due to deposition of antigen–antibody complexes
Therapy aimed at controlling metabolic deficit or tolerizing T-cells	Therapy aimed at inhibiting inflammation and antibody synthesis
Tendency to cancer in organ	Tendency to lymphoreticular neoplasia
Antigens evoke organ-specific antibodies in normal animals with complete Freund's adjuvant	No antibodies produced in animals with comparable stimulation
Experimental lesions produced with antigen in Freund's adjuvant	Diseases and autoantibodies arise spontaneously in certain animals (e.g. NZB mice and hybrids)
SIMILARITIES	

Circulating autoantibodies react with normal body constituents
Patients often have increased immunoglobulins in serum
Antibodies may appear in each of the main immunoglobulin classes particularly IgG and are usually high affinity and mutated
Greater incidence in women
Disease process not always progressive; exacerbations and remissions
Association with HLA
Spontaneous diseases in animals genetically programmed
Autoantibody tests of diagnostic value

IgG, immunoglobulin G; SLE, systemic lupus erythematosus.

various autoantibodies are also present.
• Multiple sclerosis (MS) is due to demyelination produced by cytokines and activated macrophages and T-cells. Similarity to experimental autoimmune encephalomyelitis, a demyelinating disease induced by immunization with myelin in complete Freund's adjuvant, suggests that autoimmunity forms the basis of the disease.
• Activated T-cells and macrophages are abundant in the rheumatoid synovium where they give rise to inflammation in the joint space through the release of IL-1, IL-6, tumor necrosis factor (TNF), prostaglandin E_2 (PGE_2), collagenase, neutral proteinase and reactive oxygen intermediates (ROIs).
• Synovial lining cells grow as a malign pannus which produces erosions in the underlying cartilage and bone.
• Rheumatoid arthritis (RA) can be successfully treated with anti-TNF therapy or by competing with CD28 activation of T-cells using CTLA-4Ig. The presence of autoantibodies to IgG, known as rheumatoid factor, are useful in making a diagnosis of RA.

• The lesions of Crohn's disease are characterized by infiltrating mononuclear cells and the presence of cytokines, suggesting a T-cell basis for the disorder. Neutralization of TNF results in clinical improvement.
• Celiac disease is due to T-cell activation against the gliadin fraction of gluten found in wheat products. Anti-tissue transglutaminase antibodies are diagnostic of celiac disease.
• Hashimoto's thyroiditis is produced by cytotoxic T-cells and cytokines. The role of antibodies to thyroid components is unclear but these antibodies are useful in the diagnosis of chronic autoimmune thyroiditis.
• Atherosclerosis is initiated by the movement of mononuclear cells into the vessel wall. The target antigen may be modified low-density lipoproteins or heat shock proteins. Cytokines produced by mononuclear cells and endothelial cells cause proliferation of smooth muscle cells and atherosclerotic plaques.
• Psoriasis results from keratinocyte hyperproliferation induced by Th1 cytokines. Anti-T-cell biologic agents are useful in the treatment.

(continued)

Diagnostic value of autoantibody tests

- A wide range of serum autoantibodies now provide valuable diagnostic markers.

Treatment of autoimmune disorders

- Therapy conventionally involves metabolic control and the use of anti-inflammatory and immunosuppressive drugs.
- Plasma exchange may be of value especially in combination with antimitotic drugs.
- Intravenous Ig is of benefit in a number of autoimmune disorders. This may be due to the presence of anti-idiotype antibodies or anti-cytokine activity.
- A whole variety of potential immunologic control therapies are under intensive investigation. These include T-cell vaccinations, switching the immune response from Th1 to Th2, idiotype manipulations and attempts to induce antigen-specific unresponsiveness particularly for T-cells using peptides.
- Numerous biologic agents that inhibit the immune response are being investigated. These include blockade of cytokines, or adhesion molecules or receptors such as the IL-2 receptor or CD40L (CD40 ligand).
- Blockade of TNF is highly effective therapy for RA and other autoimmune diseases.
- The accompanying comparison of organ-specific and nonorgan-specific autoimmune disorders (table 17.6) gives an overall view of many of the points raised in this chapter.

See the accompanying website (**www.roitt.com**) for multiple choice questions

---

FURTHER READING

Appelmelk, B.J., Faller, G., Claeys, D., Kirchner, T. & Vandenbroucke-Grauls, C.M.J.E. (1998) Bugs on trial: The case of *Helicobacter pylori* and autoimmunity. *Immunology Today*, **19**, 296–9.

Choy, E.H.S & Panayi, G.S. (2001) Cytokine pathways and joint inflammation in rheumatoid arthritis. *New England Journal of Medicine*, **345**, 907–16.

Davidson, A. & Diamond, B. (2001) Advances in immunology. Autoimmune diseases. *New England Journal of Medicine*, **345**, 340–50.

Greaves, D.R. & Channon, K.M. (2002) Inflammation and immune responses in atherosclerosis. *Trends in Immunology*, **23**, 535–41.

Kazatchkine, M.D. & Kaveri, S.V. (2001) Immunomodulation of autoimmune and inflammatory diseases with intravenous immune globulin. *New England Journal of Medicine*, **345**, 747–55.

Kelly, M.A., Rayner, M.L., Mijovic, C.H. & Barnett, A.H. (2003) Molecular aspects of type 1 diabetes. *Molecular Pathology*, **56**, 1–10.

Sarvetnick, N. & Ohashi, P.S. (eds) (2003) Section on autoimmunity. *Current Opinion in Immunology*, **15**, 647–730.

Tian, J., Olcott, A., Hanssen, L., Zekzer, D. & Kaufman, D.L. (1999) Antigen-based immunotherapy for autoimmune disease: From animal models to humans? *Immunology Today*, **20**, 190–5.

Vandenbark, A.A., Chou, Y.K., Whitham, R. *et al*. (1996) Treatment of multiple sclerosis with T-cell receptor peptides. *Nature Medicine*, **2**, 1109–15.

Van Den Brande, J.M.H., Peppelenbosch, M.P. & Van Deventer, S.J.H. (2002) Treating Crohn's disease by inducing T lymphocyte apoptosis. *Annals of the New York Academy of Science*, **973**, 166–80.

Walker, L.S.K. & Abbas, A.K. (2002) The enemy within: Keeping self-reactive T cells at bay in the periphery. *Nature Reviews Immunology*, **2**, 11–19.

Wicker, L. & Wekerle, H. (eds) (1995) Autoimmunity. *Current Opinion in Immunology*, **6**, 783–852. [Several critical essays in each annual volume.]

Glossary

acute phase proteins: Serum proteins, mostly produced in the liver, which rapidly change in concentration (some increase, some decrease) during the initiation of an inflammatory response.

adjuvant: Any substance which nonspecifically enhances the immune response to antigen.

affinity (intrinsic affinity): The strength of binding (affinity constant) between a receptor (e.g. one antigen-binding site on an antibody) and a ligand (e.g. epitope on an antigen).

agglutination: The aggregation of particles such as red cells or bacteria by antibodies.

allele: Variants of a polymorphic gene at a given genetic locus.

allelic exclusion: The phenomenon whereby, following successful rearrangement of one allele of an antigen receptor gene, rearrangement of the other parental allele is suppressed, thereby ensuring each lymphocyte expresses only a single specificity of antigen receptor (although this does not occur for α chains in T-cells).

allotype: An allelic variant of an antigen which, because it is not present in all individuals, may be immunogenic in members of the same species which have a different version of the allele.

anaphylatoxin: A complement breakdown product (e.g. C3a, C4a or C5a) capable of directly triggering mast cell degranulation.

anaphylaxis: An often fatal hypersensitivity reaction, triggered by IgE or anaphylatoxin-mediated mast cell degranulation, leading to anaphylactic shock due to vasodilatation and smooth muscle contraction.

anergy: Potentially reversible specific immunological tolerance in which the lymphocyte becomes functionally nonresponsive.

antibody-dependent cellular cytotoxicity (ADCC): A cytotoxic reaction in which an antibody-coated target cell is directly killed by an Fc receptor-bearing leukocyte, e.g. NK cell, macrophage or neutrophil.

apoptosis: A form of programmed cell death, characterized by endonuclease digestion of DNA.

atopic allergy: IgE-mediated hypersensitivity, i.e. asthma, eczema, hayfever and food allergy.

avidity (functional affinity): The binding strength between two molecules (e.g. antibody and antigen) taking into account the valency of the interaction. Thus the avidity will always be equal to or greater than the intrinsic affinity (*see* affinity).

chemokines: A family of structurally-related cytokines which selectively induce chemotaxis and activation of leukocytes. They also play important roles in lymphoid organ development, cell compartmentalization within lymphoid tissues, Th1/Th2 development, angiogenesis and wound healing.

chemotaxis: The directional migration of cells towards an attractant.

complementarity determining regions (CDR): The hypervariable amino acid sequences within antibody and T-cell receptor variable regions which interact with complementary amino acids on the antigen or peptide–MHC complex.

C-reactive protein: An acute phase protein which is able to bind to the surface of microorganisms where it functions as a stimulator of the classical pathway of complement activation, and as an opsonin for phagocytosis.

cytokines: Low molecular weight proteins that stimulate or inhibit the differentiation, proliferation or function of immune cells.

delayed-type hypersensitivity (DTH): A hypersensitivity reaction occurring within 48–72 h and mediated by cytokine release from sensitized T-cells.

diversity (D) gene segments: Found in the immunoglobulin heavy chain gene and T-cell receptor β and δ gene loci between the *V* and *J* gene segments. Encode part of the third hypervariable region in these antigen receptor chains.

endotoxin: Pathogenic cell wall-associated lipopolysaccharides of Gram-negative bacteria.

epitope: That part of an antigen recognized by an antigen receptor.

Fab: Monovalent antigen-binding fragment obtained following papain digestion of immunoglobulin. Consists of an intact light chain and the N-terminal V_H and C_H1 domains of the heavy chain.

F(ab')$_2$: Bivalent antigen-binding fragment obtained following pepsin digestion of immunoglobulin. Consists of both light chains and the N-terminal part of both heavy chains linked by disulfide bonds.

Fas: A member of the TNF receptor gene family. Engagement of Fas (CD95) on the surface of the cell by the Fas ligand (CD178) present on cytotoxic cells, can trigger apoptosis in the Fas-bearing target cell.

Fc: Crystallizable, non-antigen binding fragment of an immunoglobulin molecule obtained following papain digestion. Consists of the C-terminal portion of both heavy chains which is responsible for binding to Fc receptors and C1q.

fluorescent antibody: An antibody conjugated to a fluorescent dye such as FITC.

framework regions: The relatively conserved amino acid sequences which flank the hypervariable regions in immunoglobulin and T-cell receptor variable regions and maintain a common overall structure for all V-region domains.

gammaglobulin: The serum proteins, mostly immunoglobulins, which have the greatest mobility towards the cathode during electrophoresis.

germ line: The arrangement of the genetic material as transmitted through the gametes.

germinal center: Discrete areas within lymph node and spleen where B-cell maturation and memory development occur.

graft vs host (g.v.h.) reaction: Reaction occurring when T lymphocytes present in a graft recognize and attack host cells.

granuloma: A tissue nodule containing proliferating lymphocytes, fibroblasts, and giant cells and epithelioid cells (both derived from activated macrophages), which forms due to inflammation in response to chronic infection or persistence of antigen in the tissues.

granzymes: Serine esterases present in the granules of cytotoxic T lymphocytes and NK cells. They induce apoptosis in the target cell which they enter through perforin channels inserted into the target cell membrane by the cytotoxic lymphocyte.

haplotype: The set of allelic variants present at a given genetic region.

hapten: A low molecular weight molecule that is recognized by preformed antibody but is not itself immunogenic unless conjugated to a "carrier" molecule which provides epitopes recognized by helper T-cells.

hematopoiesis: The production of erythrocytes and leukocytes.

high endothelial venule (HEV): Capillary venule composed of specialized endothelial cells allowing migration of lymphocytes into lymphoid organs.

HLA (*h*uman *l*eukocyte *a*ntigen): The human major histocompatibility complex (MHC).

humanized antibody: A genetically engineered monoclonal antibody of non-human origin in which all but the antigen-binding CDR sequences have been replaced with sequences derived from human antibodies. This procedure is carried out to minimize the immunogenicity of therapeutic monoclonal antibodies.

humoral: Pertaining to extracellular fluid such as plasma and lymph. The term humoral immunity is used to denote antibody-mediated immune responses.

hybridoma: Hybrid cell line obtained by fusing a lymphoid tumor cell with a lymphocyte which then has both the immortality of the tumor cell and the effector function (e.g. monoclonal antibody secretion) of the lymphocyte.

hypervariable regions: Those amino acid sequences within the immunoglobulin and T-cell receptor variable regions which show the greatest variability and contribute most to the antigen or peptide–MHC binding site.

idiotype: The complete set of idiotopes in the variable region of an antibody or T-cell receptor which react with an anti-idiotypic serum.

idiotype network: A regulatory network based on interactions of idiotypes and anti-idiotypes present on antibodies and T-cell receptors.

immune complex: Complex of antibody bound to antigen which may also contain complement components.

immunofluorescence: Technique for detection of cell or tissue-associated antigens by the use of a fluorescently-tagged ligand (e.g. an anti-immunoglobulin conjugated to fluorescein isothiocyanate).

immunogen: Any substance which elicits an immune response. Whilst all immunogens are antigens, not all antigens are immunogens (*see* hapten).

immunoglobulin superfamily: Large family of proteins characterized by possession of "immunoglobulin-type" domains of approximately 110 amino acids folded into two β-pleated sheets. Members include immunoglobulins, T-cell receptors and MHC molecules.

immunotoxin: A cytotoxic agent produced by chemically coupling a toxic agent to a specific monoclonal antibody.

internal image: An epitope on an anti-idiotype which binds in a way that structurally and functionally mimics the antigen.

isotype: An antibody constant region structure present in all normal individuals, i.e. antibody class or subclass.

ITAM: *Immunoreceptor Tyrosine-based Activation Motifs* are consensus sequences for src-family tyrosine kinases. These motifs are found in the cytoplasmic domains of several signaling molecules including the signal transduction units of lymphocyte antigen receptors and of Fc receptors.

J chain: A molecule which forms part of the structure of pentameric IgM and dimeric IgA.

joining (J) gene segments: Found in the immunoglobulin and T-cell receptor gene loci and, upon gene rearrangement, encode part of the third hypervariable region of the antigen receptors.

lectins: A family of proteins, mostly of plant origin, which bind specific sugars on glycoproteins and glycolipids. Some lectins are mitogenic (e.g. PHA, ConA).

linkage disequilibrium: The occurrence of two alleles being inherited together at a greater frequency than that expected from the product of their individual frequencies.

lipopolysaccharide (LPS): Endotoxin derived from Gram-negative bacterial cell walls which has inflammatory and mitogenic actions.

mannose binding lectin: A member of the collectin family of calcium-dependent lectins, and an acute phase protein. It activates the complement system by binding to mannose residues on the surface of microorganisms.

marginal zone: The outer area of the splenic periarteriolar lymphoid sheath (PALS) which is rich in B cells, particularly those responding to thymus-independent antigens.

margination: Leukocyte adhesion to the endothelium of blood vessels in the early phase of an acute inflammatory reaction.

membrane attack complex (MAC): Complex of complement components C5b–C9 which inserts as a pore into the membrane of target cells leading to cell lysis.

memory cells: Clonally expanded T- and B-cells produced during a primary immune response and which are "primed" to mediate a secondary immune response to the original antigen.

MHC (*major histocompatibility complex*): A genetic region encoding molecules involved in antigen presentation to T-cells. Class I MHC molecules are present on virtually all nucleated cells and are encoded by HLA-A, B, and C in man, whilst class II MHC molecules are expressed on antigen-presenting cells (primarily macrophages, B-cells and interdigitating dendritic cells) and are encoded by HLA-DR, DQ, and DP in man. Allelic differences can be associated with the most intense graft rejection within a species.

MHC restriction: The necessity that T-cells recognize processed antigen only when presented by MHC molecules of the original haplotype associated with T-cell priming.

mitogen: A substance which non-specifically induces lymphocyte proliferation.

monoclonal antibody: Homogeneous antibody derived from a single B-cell clone and therefore all bearing identical antigen-binding sites and isotype.

mucosal-associated lymphoid tissue (MALT): A system of lymphoid tissue found in the gastrointestinal and respiratory tracts.

murine: Pertaining to mice.

myeloma protein: Monoclonal antibody secreted by myeloma cells.

negative selection: Deletion by apoptosis in the thymus of T-cells which recognize self peptides presented by self MHC molecules, thus preventing the development of autoimmune T-cells. Negative selection of developing B-cells is also thought to occur if they encounter high levels of self antigen in the bone marrow.

nude mouse: Mouse which is T-cell deficient due to a homozygous gene defect (*nu/nu*) resulting in the absence of a thymus (and also lack of body hair).

oncofetal antigen: Antigen whose expression is normally restricted to the fetus but which may be expressed during malignancy in adults.

opsonin: Substance, e.g. antibody or C3b, which enhances phagocytosis by promoting adhesion of the antigen to the phagocyte.

opsonization: Coating of antigen with opsonin to enhance phagocytosis.

pathogen-associated molecular pattern (PAMP): Molecules such as lipopolysaccharide, peptidoglycan, lipoteichoic acids and mannans, which are widely expressed by microbial pathogens as repetitive motifs but are not present on host tissues. They are therefore utilized by the pattern recognition receptors (PRRs) of the immune system to distinguish pathogens from self antigens.

pattern recognition receptor (PRR): Receptors on professional antigen-presenting cells and phagocytes which enable them to recognize pathogen-associated molecular patterns (PAMPs). Amongst the large number of different PRRs are the mannose receptor and the macrophage scavenger receptor.

perforin: Molecule produced by cytotoxic T-cells and NK cells which, like complement component C9, polymerizes to form a pore in the membrane of the target cell leading to cell death.

PHA (phytohemagglutinin): A plant lectin which acts as a T-cell mitogen.

phagolysosome: Intracellular vacuole where killing and digestion of phagocytosed material occurs following the fusion of a phagosome with a lysosome.

phagosome: Intracellular vacuole produced following invagination of the cell membrane around phagocytosed material.

positive selection: The selection of those developing T-cells in the thymus which are able to recognize self MHC molecules. This occurs by preventing apoptosis in these cells.

proteasome: Cytoplasmic proteolytic enzyme complex involved in antigen processing for association with MHC.

recombination signal sequence (RSS): Conserved heptamer (7-nucleotide)-nonamer (9-nucleotide) sequences, separated by a 12 or 23 base spacer, which occur 3' of variable gene segments, 5' and 3' of diversity gene segments, and 5' of joining gene segments, in both immunoglobulin and T cell receptor genes. They function as recognition sequences for the recombinase enzymes that mediate the gene rearrangement process involved in the generation of lymphocyte antigen receptor diversity.

respiratory burst: The increased oxidative metabolism which occurs in phagocytic cells following activation.

rheumatoid factor: IgM, IgG and IgA autoantibodies to IgG, particularly the Fc region. These antibodies are usually found in the blood of patients with rheumatoid arthritis.

secretory component: Proteolytic cleavage product of the poly-Ig receptor which remains associated with dimeric IgA in sero-mucus secretions.

somatic hypermutation: The enhanced rate of point mutation in the immunoglobulin variable region genes which occurs following antigenic stimulation and acts as a mechanism for increasing antibody diversity and affinity.

superantigen: An antigen which reacts with all the T-cells belonging to a particular T-cell receptor V region family, and which therefore stimulates (or deletes) a much larger number of cells than does conventional antigen.

TAP: The *Transporters associated with Antigen Processing* (TAP-1 and TAP-2) are molecules which carry antigenic peptides from the cytoplasm into the lumen of the endoplasmic reticulum for incorporation into MHC class I molecules.

T-dependent antigen: An antigen which requires helper T-cells in order to elicit an antibody response.

thymocyte: Developing T-cell in the thymus.

T-independent antigen: An antigen which is able to elicit an antibody response in the absence of T-cells.

titer: Measure of the relative "strength" (a combination of amount and avidity) of an antibody or antiserum, usually given as the highest dilution which is still operationally detectable in, for example, an ELISA.

Toll-like receptors: A family of pattern-recognition receptors that recognize different molecules on bacterial surfaces. Activation of these receptors usually results in cytokine production and upregulation of the adaptive immune response.

variable (V) gene segments: Genes that rearrange together with *D* (diversity) and *J* (joining) gene segments in order to encode the variable region amino acid sequences of immunoglobulins and T-cell receptors.

Index